AF393341

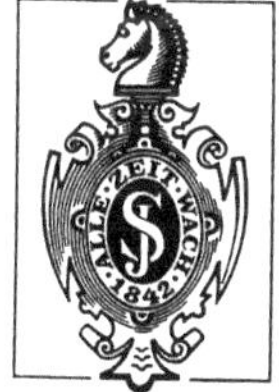

Marton Lanyi

Diagnosis and Differential Diagnosis of Breast Calcifications

With 200 Figures in 383 Separate Illustrations
and 11 Tables

Springer-Verlag
Berlin Heidelberg New York
London Paris Tokyo

Dr. med. MARTON LANYI

Röntgeninstitut
Kaiserstraße 21–27
5270 Gummersbach
FRG

Translated from the German edition by

TERRY C. TELGER

6112 Waco Way
Fort Worth, TX 76133
USA

German edition
Diagnostik und Differentialdiagnostik der Mammaverkalkungen
© Springer-Verlag Berlin Heidelberg 1986

ISBN-13: 978-3-642-71495-5   e-ISBN-13: 978-3-642-71493-1
DOI: 10.1007/978-3-642-71493-1

Library of Congress Cataloging in Publication Data. Lanyi, M. (Marton). Diagnosis and differential diagnosis of breast calcifications.
Translation of: Diagnostik und Differentialdiagnostik der Mammaverkalkungen. Bibliography: p. Includes index. 1. Breast – Calcification – Diagnosis. 2. Diagnosis, Differential. 3. Breast – Radiography. I. Title. [DNLM: 1. Breast Diseases – diagnosis. 2. Calcinosis – radiography. 3. Mammography. WP 840 L296d]   RG496.C34L3613 1987   618.1'907'5   86-31358
ISBN-13: 978-3-642-71495-5 (U.S.)

© Springer-Verlag Berlin Heidelberg 1988
Softcover reprint of the hardcover 1st edition   1988

2121/3130-543210

Preface

*Very thorough knowledge of breast pathology is a
sine qua non for interpretation of breast films . . .
progress in X-ray diagnosis could only be made by
careful comparison of the film with the actual specimen.*

H. INGLEBY

*Multiplication of the same erroneous diagnosis does
not make that diagnosis correct.*

J. G. AZZOPARDI

Paradoxically enough, our specialty considers the radiologist who mistakes a skin fibroma or the calcifications in a sponge kidney for a kidney stone to lack basic knowledge, while the radiologist who immediately calls for the surgeon because of a few white spots on a mammogram is thought to be acting according to the rules of medical practice.

Misunderstandings and confusion with regard to breast pathology as well as the comfortable philosophy that superfluous biopsies are the price we have to pay for the early detection of carcinomas have in many places led to a loss of confidence in mammography. Yet this is a method with which carcinomas can be detected earlier than with any other imaging technique.

A quarter of a century ago, during a population screening for breast cancer in Budapest, I first detected a clinically occult breast carcinoma on grounds of a cluster of microcalcifications. The possibility of being able to make a histological diagnosis of a carcinoma based on tiny, white spots on the X-ray was fascinating. My disappointment was all the greater when the pathologist later found benign processes for apparently similar phenomena. It became clear to me, after reading the book by INGLEBY and GERSHON-COHEN (1960), that it would only be possible to solve the problems of a differential diagnosis of this X-ray phenomena by means of detailed, systematic, and comparative mammographic and histologic analyses. Yet three prerequisites for such an analysis were missing at that time, namely, good mammography technology, sufficient material, and the possibility to collate the image of a microcalcification to its pathological manifestation.

Just 13 years ago I was able to initiate the systematic work. The technological prerequisites were available, I had collected sufficient material about microcalcifications, and I had found someone, my friend and pathologist Professor P. CITOLER, who was ready to determine the spatial relationship between microcalcifications and histological transformations. It took me 7 years to develop the differential diagnosis system described in this book, and another 2 years to test its practical viability. I examined mammograms without prior knowledge of the histology from almost 1000 cases operated on because of microcalcifications (from the Universities of Cologne, Nijmegen, and San Francisco, the Institute Curie in Paris, the Radiological Institute in Cologne, and the Knappschaftskrankenhaus in Dortmund). The results steadily improved. By analyzing the incorrect diagnoses, I was able to further refine the system and determine its limitations.

Now, one year after the publication of the book in German, the English edition is ready and will make the differential diagnostic system accessible throughout the world. It may thus reach radiologists who in their darkened rooms are using a magnifying glass to try to make a definite diagnosis on the basis of a few white spots on a mammogram. I hope that this book may help them.

I would not have been able to write this book without the help of numerous colleagues and friends from Europe and America. They have sent me interesting cases, prepared histophotograms, made material available to me in order to test my system of differential diagnosis, and were the first readers whose probing questions uncovered the weak spots in my manuscript and who drove me to express myself more clearly. I would like to express my gratitude first to them: Dr. E. ALBRING, Gelsenkirchen, Prof. V. BARTH, Esslingen, Prof. K. BREZINA, Vienna, Dr. P.D. C. BROKS, Utrecht, Prof. P. CITOLER, Cologne, Prof. O. FISCHEDICK, Dortmund, Prof. M. FRIEDRICH, Berlin, Dr. J.H.C.L. HENDRIKS, Nijmegen, Prof. W. HOEFFKEN, Cologne, Dr. R. HOLLAND, Nijmegen, Prof. H. KIEFER, Wiesbaden, Dr. M. LEGAL, Paris, Dr. K. LENDVAI, Porz, Prof. K.J. LENNARTZ, Düsseldorf, Prof. H. LENZ, Eschweiler, Dr. R. MÜLLER, Siegburg, Dr. K. NEUFANG, Cologne, Dr. Z. PÉNTEK, Szekszárd, Hungary, Dr. M. RADO, Bergheim, Dr. E. ROSS, Vallendar, Dr. E. SICKLES, San Francisco, Prof. K.H. VAN DE WEYER, Trier, Prof. H.H. ZIPPEL, Marburg.

The illustrations and photographs were prepared by E. STORCH at the Radiological Institute of Cologne, E. WITTE at the Catholic University of Nijmegen, and H. LAMBACH, a graphic artist. The statistics were compiled and checked by Professor P. SCHWANENBERG of the Technical University of Gummersbach.

The translation of a specialized text about radiology and pathology requires linguistic as well as medical knowledge. If, as I hope, the translation of this book is well done, credit is due to TERRY TELGER, the translator, and MICHAEL WILSON, head of copy editing at Springer-Verlag. I am also grateful to the radiologist Dr. J.G. BLICKMAN for reviewing the manuscript. WILLI BISCHOFF is responsible for the good optical presentation of the book.

My special thanks go to BERNHARD LEWERICH, who recognized the importance of the subject at an early stage and who urged and supported the preparation of the English edition.

M. LANYI

Contents

1 Historical Review, Critical Analysis of the Literature, Statement of Problem and Goals

As early as 1913 SALOMON, while taking X-ray films of amputated breasts, noticed "small black spots" at the center of a carcinoma, which he interpreted as "intraductal cancerous masses undergoing cystic degeneration." These spots, barely visible on the X-ray print, were the first microcalcifications of the breast to be visualized radiographically. From then until 1951 nothing of significance occurred in the area of microcalcifications, aside from a case described by FINSTERBUSCH and GROSS (1934) which showed unusual intramammary calcifications suggestive of plasma cell mastitis (Fig. 1.1). At that time the technical quality of the radiographs was relatively poor, and microcalcifications were generally thought to represent artifacts.

In 1951 LEBORGNE published his discovery that microcalcifications were demonstrable in 30% of breast cancers, describing them as "innumerable, punctate, or slightly elongated, resembling grains of salt, and arranged in clusters" (Fig. 1.2 a, b). He noted that the microcalcifications could occur "inside or outside the tumor shadow, or in the absence of a tumor shadow." According to Leborgne, "With sufficient experience, differential diagnosis between calcifications of malignant processes which we have described and calcifications in benign processes is generally easy." Thirteen years later EGAN (1964) likeweise stated that the typical microcalcifications are so pathognomonic that a negative histologic diagnosis would imply either that the surgeon had failed to remove the proper area of the breast, or that the pathologist had erred. Sixteen years later, however, EGAN et al. (1980) expressed a completely different view: "The radiographic signs are so nonspecific that all punctate microcalcifications require histologic evaluation." Thus, the 30-year period from 1951 to 1980 is the history of an ever-dwindling hope of finding a simple way to diagnose breast cancer.

Indeed, it appears that excisional biopsies performed on the basis of breast microcalcifications lead to a positive diagnosis of carcinoma in only a small percentage of cases. At the Cologne University Women's Clinic, for example, 90% of operations performed for breast microcalcifications proved to be unnecessary (CITOLER 1978). RUMMEL et al. (1976) draw a similar conclusion with their 16% yield of breast carcinoma. We must ask ourselves whether this low diagnostic yield is simply a fact of life, or whether it relates to a basic inadequacy in the definitions of "benign" and "malignant" calcifications that have been used by so many authors for more than 30 years. A radiographic finding that is so important yet so difficult to evaluate requires careful, thorough analysis. To draw valid conclusions, we need a volume of case material that is large enough for statistical evaluation.

To establish the radiographic features of microcalcifications of different etiologies, it is not enough to speak of "benign" versus "malignant" calcifications; we must demand a specific histologic classification. In this regard we must not only differentiate between *benign intracystic* and *benign intraductal* calcified secretions or

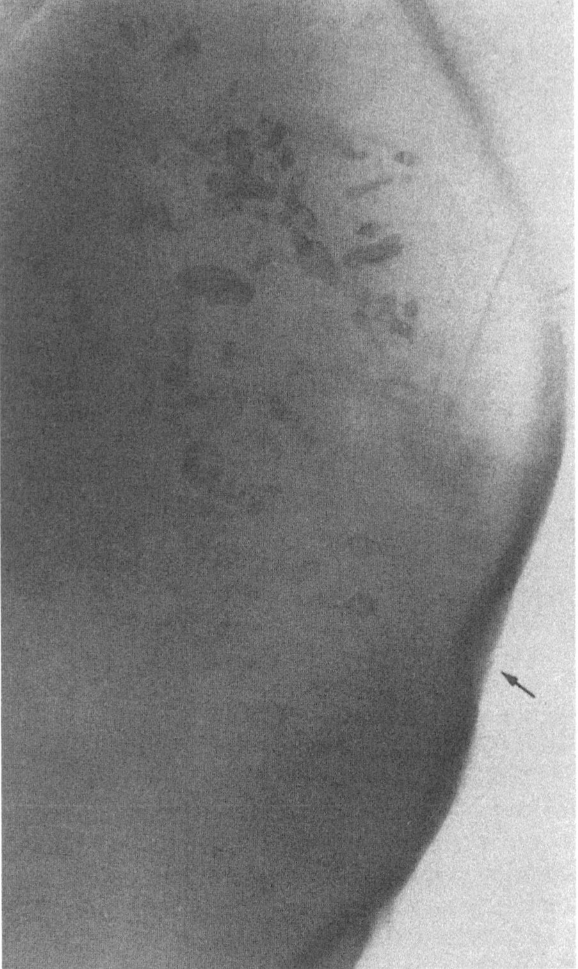

Fig. 1.1. This was the first case of intramammary calcifications associated with carcinoma to be reported in the German literature. Because the calcifications were bilateral, while the carcinoma was unilateral *(arrow),* FINSTERBUSCH and GROSS (1934) correctly surmised that these "calcium deposits in the mammary ducts" were unrelated to the carcinoma. Today we would relate these calcifications to plasma cell mastitis

between *malignant papillary cribriform calcifications* and *comedo calcifications,* but we must also be able to exclude lobular neoplasias (lobular carcinomas in situ, LCIS; see the discussion of these terms in Sect. 4.2). This is important when we consider that lobular neoplasias detected on the basis of microcalcifications may incidentally coexist with benign cystic calcifications (see Table 4.5). We cannot expect these decidedly benign calcifications to help us in our search for the features that characterize malignant patterns of calcification.

It is also important that the pathologist demonstrate the radiographically visible microcalcifications histologically and establish their exact localization. It would

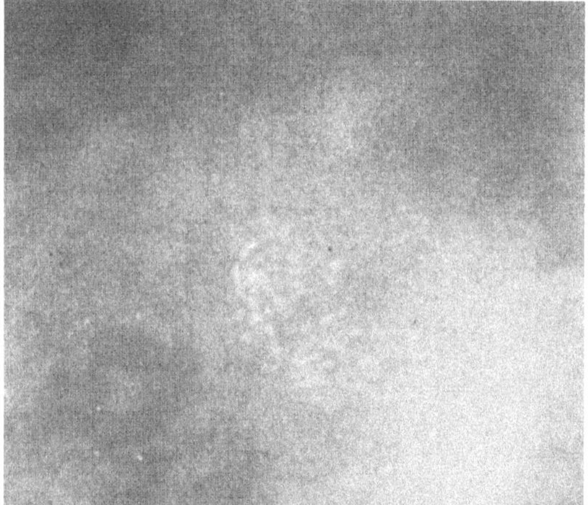

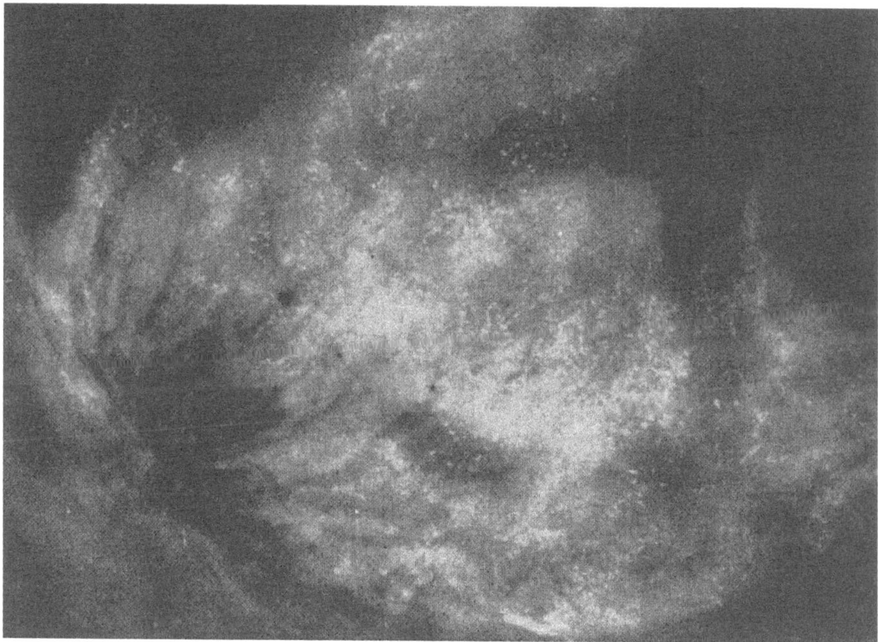

Fig. 1.2a, b. Radiographs of historical importance: microcalcification cluster in a carcinoma (LEBORGNE 1951). **a** Because of technical constraints existing at that time, the calcifications appear faint, but their polymorphism is apparent. **b** Specimen radiograph from the same publication

only result in confusion to attempt to determine the appearance of "malignant" microcalcifications on the basis of the shape of cystic or liponecrotic microcalcifications in the immediate proximity of a clinically and radiographically occult (tubular) carcinoma (see Figs. 4.37, 6.9).

Another important requirement is sufficient magnification of the radiographic image (at least 4 ×) due to the extremely small size of the lesions. Also, a precise and reproducible analysis of all important parameters (size, number, shape, etc.) is necessary for the various benign and malignant processes in order to establish differential diagnostic features. Descriptions such as "dense," "faint," and "flaky," or "very fine" are subjective and not reproducible.

With this in mind, we analyzed 25 studies on breast microcalcifications published between 1951 and 1984 (Table 1.1) to determine the following:

1. Was the number of carcinoma cases in the study large enough for valid conclusions to be drawn?
2. Was a reproducible method used to analyze the benign and malignant microcalcifications, and was sufficient magnification employed? Were subjective terms used (e. g., "resembling grains of sand"), or was the appearance of the microcalcifications described in detail?
3. Were the malignant and benign lesions given a specific histologic classification (e. g., cribriform carcinoma, fibroadenoma), or were microcalcifications classified only in general terms as "benign" or "malignant"? Were the microcalcifications of lobular neoplasia evaluated together with other carcinomas, or were they evaluated separately?

Number of Cases. The number of cases examined was specified in only 13 of the 25 publications reviewed. The number of cases was between 45 and 100 in eight studies, and between 100 and 200 in two studies. There were two other studies in which more than 200 cases were evaluated (LeGal et al. 1984; Sigfusson et al. 1983). The largest number of breasts with microcalcifications (468) were examined by Egan et al. (1980). A total of 666 carcinomas were analyzed – the smallest number (13) by Menges et al. (1973) and the largest (115, including 13 LCIS!) by Egan et al. (1980). Except for LeGal et al. (1984) who analyzed 101 cancers (including 6 LCIS), all the authors evaluated fewer than 100.

It is apparent, then, that of the 25 publications reviewed, only 3 (Egan et al. 1980; LeGal et al. 1984; Sigfusson et al. 1983) had sufficient material and a sufficient number of carcinomas from which to draw meaningful conclusions. Conclusions based on the analysis of 15 carcinomas and 40 benign lesions – such as the conclusion of Colbassini et al. (1982) that "careful study of the microcalcification clusters ... did not show significant differences between the malignant and benign groups that could be helpful to the clinician, in predicting the nature of the lesion" – cannot be taken seriously.

Magnification and Reproducibility. Only six studies met the criterion of adequate magnification and reproducibility. For example, Egan et al. (1980) used a magnifying lens, enlargement by projection onto a screen, and photographic enlargement. Colbassini et al. (1982) worked with an instrument with a resolution to 0.1 mm and magnifications of 9 and 14. A new method was introduced by Galkin et al. (1983), who examined the calcifications on mammograms using a 180 × optical dissecting microscope.

Interestingly, all the studies investigated multiple features of the microcalcifications. In 1973 Menges et al. studied only the number of benign and malignant calcifications and postulated a direct correlation between number and malignancy (i. e., the greater the number of microcalcifications, the more confident the diagnosis of carcinoma – an assumption that has proved false). In 1976 MILLIS et al. evaluated both the size and the spatial distribution of the microcalcifications, and in 1980 EGAN et al. studied the lesions for number, size, spatial arrangement, shape, contour, and density. All but five of the publications used subjective terms to describe malignant-appearing microcalcifications: resembling a grain of salt or sand, crystalline, flaky, needlelike, resembling a broken needle point, bizarre, irregular, teardrop-shaped, pointed, cometlike, trunklike, tadpolelike.

Several authors – LEGAL et al. (1976, 1984), MOSKOWITZ (1979), and SIGFUSSON et al. (1983) – addressed the question of which shapes of clustered microcalcifications were associated with a high risk of carcinoma, and which were not. The authors made the following determinations (Table 1.2):

1. The more irregular, linear, or vermiform the calcifications, the higher the risk of carcinoma.
2. Microcalcifications arranged in a linear or branched pattern signify a high risk.
3. Rounded or ringlike calcifications with evidence of sedimentation ("teacup" sign, see p. 51) are not suggestive of malignancy

However, because the statistical risk is meaningless for the individual case, the range of intermediate risks remains an area of complete uncertainty. From a diagnostic standpoint, it is immaterial whether the radiologist knows that a carcinoma is diagnosable with 17%–22% confidence in the minimal risk group and with 37.9%–40% confidence in the moderate risk group. All but the zero risk group would have to undergo biopsy, as Moskowitz points out. But this means that some 80% of biopsies in the minimal risk group, and more than 50% in the moderate risk group, would be unrewarding. What, then, is the benefit of assessing cancer risk?

Except for the author's description of the "triangular principle" for intraductal cancers (LANYI 1977), no one has yet tried to accurately define the shapes of the microcalcification clusters associated with benign and malignant conditions!

Specification of the Histological Diagnosis. None of the 25 publications that were reviewed attempted to classify lesions in terms more specific than "malignant" or "benign." The ductal carcinomas were not differentiated according to histologic type (papillary, cribriform, comedo). All the authors counted lobular neoplasia among the true carcinomas, which invalidates their results from the outset (lobular neoplasia accounted for 15% of carcinomas in SIGFUSSON et al. 1983, 10% in EGAN et al. 1980, and 6% in LEGAL et al. 1984). In nine publications the benign microcalcifications were specified to a greater or lesser degree, but none of the studies characterized the lesions by their localization, even though, as we shall see, the microcalcifications associated with a *benign lobular* process have a very different presentation from those associated with a *benign ductal* process. This error likewise has been a source of general confusion.

The diagnosis and differential diagnosis of breast calcifications and especially microcalcifications is a problem of major importance in everyday practice. In a series of 1044 consecutive mammograms taken at the Gummersbach Radiology Institute from 2 January to 31 March 1983, 300 (26.7%) different breast calcifications were demonstrated (Table 1.3). The series included 81 (7.7%) clustered calcifications but only 6 ductal carcinomas (0.5% of all cases examined and 7.4% of all

Table 1.1. Survey of the literature on breast microcalcifications

Author	Number			Magnification	Histologic localization of microcalcifications	Finer specification of diagnosis	Number of lobular neoplasias (LCIS) included among carcinomas	Signs pathognomonic for carcinoma
	Mal.	Ben.	Total					
BARTH (1977)	Not stated			Not stated	Not stated	Not stated	Not stated	Needlelike; finely clumped, stippled; arranged along the milk ducts
BARTH and PRECHTEL (1982)	Not stated			Not stated	Not stated	Not stated	Not stated	Needlelike; arranged in fine clumps along the milk ducts
BJURSTAM (1978)	86[a]	52	148	Micrometer eye piece of "Kellner type"	Yes	Only in benign lesions	1	Irregular, bizarre, branched; cluster shape and arrangement were not analyzed
COLBASSINI et al. (1982)	15[b]	40[b]	55[b]	Emoscop S 9 with 0.1 mm resolution ($14\times$)	Yes	Not stated	Not stated	Polymorphism; variability of shape is not typical of carcinoma. Number of microcalcifications per cluster and per cm^2 and their density is somewhat greater with carcinoma. No significant difference between malignant and benign cluster shapes. Cluster shape and arrangement were not analyzed
EGAN (1964)	Not stated			Not stated	Not stated	Not stated	Not stated	Like grains of sand, bizarre or heterogeneous; coarse; smooth; like needle points; wavy; faint; rounded. Cluster shape and arrangement were not analyzed
EGAN (1969)	Not stated			Not stated	Not stated	Not stated	Not stated	Fine; innumerable; confined to measurable area in two planes, not diffuse throughout the breast; no distinct geometric pattern can be detected. When number is 5–10: ⅓ carcinomas, ⅓ borderline, ⅓ hyperplasia, papillomatosis, sclerosing adenosis

EGAN et al. (1980)	115	353	468	Hand magnifying lens and dental (10X)X-ray enlarger; enlarging (60X) by projection onto a screen and photographic enlargement	Not stated	Not stated	13	Clustered microcalcifications of increasing number, variability from very fine to rather coarse, variable density from almost imperceptible to fairly dense, and increasing number in the specimen radiograph provide clues to the presence of carcinoma. There is such a wide overlapping of the calcifications in fibrocystic disease and carcinoma that a mammographer cannot confidently exclude carcinoma
FRISCHBIER and LOHBECK (1977)	Not stated			Not stated	Not stated	Not stated	Not stated	The more numerous the microcalcifications, the higher the risk of malignancy. Calcifications vary from fine/barely perceptible to grossly visible. The more pronounced the size variation, the higher the index of suspicion. Polymorphism; the more bizarre and irregular the shape, the higher the likelihood of malignancy. Irregular configuration is suspicious
GALKIN et al. (1983)	42	58	100^c	Unitron ZST zoom stereo Trinocular optical dissecting microscope	Not stated	Not stated	Not stated	Certain calcification shapes are specific for malignant and benign processes. Malignant types tend to be bizarre, angular, linear, irregular, nonuniform; benign types are rounded, regular, and uniform. While most benign microcalcifications are distinguishable from malignant, this is not always so. It is still uncertain whether this method is suitable for the evaluation of mammograms (and not just specimen radiographs)
GERSHON-COHEN (1970)	Not stated			Not stated	Not stated	Not stated	Not stated	Crystalline; like grains of salt; lie scattered in a unpolarized fashion
GERSHON-COHEN et al. (1966)	Not stated			Not stated	Not stated	For benign lesions	Not stated	Tiny; up to 3 mm in size (rarely longer); usually irregularly shaped; spiculelike; punctate; some may be linear, others curved; but the contours are never smooth
GROS (1963)	Not stated			Not stated	Not stated	For benign lesions	Not stated	Linear; punctate; very faint; dustlike; irregular; very diverse (anarchy). Chainlike, directed toward the nipple

Table 1.1. Survey of the Literature on Breast Microcalcifications (cont.)

Author	Number			Magnification	Histologic localization of microcalcifications	Finer specification of differential diagnosis	Number of lobular neoplasias (LCIS) included among carcinomas	Signs pathognomonic for carcinoma
	Mal.	Ben.	Total					
HOEFFKEN and LANYI (1973)	Not stated			Not stated	Not stated	For benign lesions	Not stated	Dense; crystalline; finely granular; angular or bizarre. Look like a stone that has been shattered by a hammer
INGBLEBY and GERSHON-COHEN (1960)	64	Not stated		Not stated	Yes	For benign lesions	Excluded!	Clustered, fine, tend to be linear like a broken needle tip; larger amorphous calcifications also occur but are not specific
LANYI (1977)	60	111	171	Magnification with hand lens	Yes	Not stated	Excluded	Size, number, extent, density, contours have no major diagnostic significance. Microcalcifications are mainly polymorphous (point, line, teardrop; irregularly shaped, crumbly), rarely punctate throughout. Densely arranged, usually forming a triangular, trapezoidal, or rosette-shaped cluster. Cluster shapes frequently change with radiographic projection
LEBORGNE (1951)	Not stated			Not stated	Yes	For benign lesions	Not stated	Clustered; from convergent arrangement; innumerable; punctate; resemble grains of salt
LEGAL et al. (1976)	27	33	60	Not stated		Listed for benign and malignant cases but disregarded in the evaluation	2	Risk assessment depends on microcalcification shape: see Table 1.2. *Punctate and worm-shaped* calcifications are always found in carcinoma
LEGAL et al. (1984)	101	126[d]	227	Not stated	Yes	For benign and borderline lesions	6	

LEVITAN et al. (1964)	23	13	46	Not stated	Yes. Also demonstrated by micro-radiography	Yes	Not stated	More fine than coarse; irregular; tend to be numerous. Psammomatous microcalcifications are visible microscopically but not on radiographs
MENGES et al. (1973)	13	54	67	Not stated	Yes	For benign lesions	Not stated	The greater the number microcalcifications, the greater the likelihood of carcinoma. More than 5 justify biopsy. Arranged linearly or in clusters
MILLIS et al. (1976)	33	27	60	Micrometer eyepiece and dissecting microscope	Yes	For malignant lesions	1	The relationship of calcification to other radiological features, number, and distribution was studied; density and shape were not recorded as these features have not been found helpful in distinguishing between malignant and benign lesions. Malignant microcalcifications are indistinguishable from benign.
MOSKOWITZ (1979)	Not stated			Not stated	Not stated	Not stated	Not stated	Risk depends on microcalcification shape (see Table 1.2). Risk is particularly high for linear and branched shapes
MUIR et al. (1983)	17	28	45	3–4× magnification with a hand lens	Yes	Not stated	Not stated	Round + elongated + bizarre (comet-shaped, tadpole-shaped, crescent-shaped). But elongated and bizarre shapes are more frequent in benign processes
SIGFUSSON et al. (1983)	70	143	213	Not stated	Yes	Not stated	10	Risk depends on microcalcification shape (see Table 1.2). Indistinct microcalcifications that are not rounded and show no sedimentation ("teacup sign") favor malignancy
WILLEMIN (1972)	Not stated			Not stated	Not stated	Not stated	Not stated	10–1000 μm in size; of variable shape (rounded-to-oval; rod-shaped or vermiform); usually resemble grains of salt; from several to many thousand; grouped in a rounded or oblong area with polycyclic contours

[a] 15 without a palpable mass;   [b] without a palpable mass;   [c] specimen radiography;   [d] 27 borderline cases.

Table 1.2. Risk vs radiographic appearance of microcalcifications as described in the literature

Risk	LeGal et al. (1976, 1984)	Moskowitz (1979)	Sigfusson et al. (1983)
None	Ring-shaped. This type was found exclusively in benign lesions (galactophoritis)	Small (150–200 µm), irregular or smooth, solid or hollow microcalcifications, 5 or more per cluster per cm diameter wide; degree of risk: 1–3, follow-up	Rounded, cloudy microcalcifications with sedimentation; LCIS in 6% of cases biopsied, no carcinoma
Minimal	Regular, larger, punctate. This type had a 60% association with benign lesions, 18% with borderline lesions, and 22% with malignancies	Innumerable, irregular microcalcifications clustered in an area less than 1 cm; degree of risk: 6–8, biopsy	As above, and somewhat irregular; carcinoma found in 17% of cases biopsied (with LCIS: 24%)
Moderate	Fine, punctate; 50% of lesions were benign, 40% malignant	Small, puncate, angular microcalcifications interspersed among larger ones; degree of risk: 7–9, biopsy	Irregular (few) or linear (ductal) arrangement; carcinoma found in 37.9% of cases biopsied (with LCIS: 41%)
High	Punctate, irregular, 66% of lesions were malignant, 23% benign, 11% borderline	Linear, semitranslucent, sharply marginated, arranged in linear or branching arrays; degree of risk: 8–10, biopsy	Irregular (abundant), forming a markedly linear or branching array: carcinoma found in 96% of cases biopsied
Definite carcinoma	Wormlike (100% carcinoma)		

Table 1.3. Number of calcifications seen in 1044 mammograms at the Gummersbach Radiology Institute from 2 January to 3 March 1983

Calcifications of lobular origin		
Calcified microcystic (blunt duct) or sclerosing adenosis (clustered)		9
Milk of calcium cysts		58
Scattered	27	
Solitary	8	
Clustered	23	
Calcifications of intraductal origin		
Calcifications in noninfiltrating ductal carcinomas (clustered)		6[a]
Infiltrating carcinoma with ductal calcifications		1[a]
Calcified secretion as in plasma cell mastitis/comedomastitis		6
Calcifications outside the lobular and ductal system		
Calcified fibroadenomas		19
Calcified liponecrotic cysts		94
Macrocysts	5	
Microcysts		
Scattered	9	
Solitary	73	
Clustered	7	
Unsuspicious calcifications in scar tissue		7
Other innocent microcalcifications of unknown etiology		
Follow-up necessary		33
Arterial calcification		37
Calcified sebaceous glands		30
Scattered	5	
Solitary	8	
Clustered	15	
Scattered and clustered	2	
	Total	300

[a] Histologically confirmed

clustered microcalcifications). This means that while some type of breast calcification is detected in every 4th or 5th examination, clustered microcalcifications are found in every 13th to 14th examination, raising problems of differential diagnosis and, according to EGAN et al. (1980), justifying referral for biopsy in order to detect the six carcinomas. Thus, problems of differential diagnosis in these cases are combined with a very low "cancer yield" in relation to the cost and invasiveness of the diagnostic procedure.

From 1 October 1974 until 30 September 1983, a total of 1037 breast biopsies were recommended at the Gummersbach Radiology Institute for clinically occult and nonoccult changes having various radiographic presentations. Almost 50% of the biopsies were positive for carcinoma. The yield was even higher for clinically nonoccult lesions, in which approximately three out of four biopsies confirmed malignancy (Fig. 1.3). The situation was reversed for clinically occult lesions (independent of radiographic signs), where carcinoma was proved in one out of five cases (Fig. 1.4).

With the nonoccult lesions, it does not matter which radiographic sign prompted the referral for biopsy. As Fig. 1.3 shows, the carcinoma yield is virtually

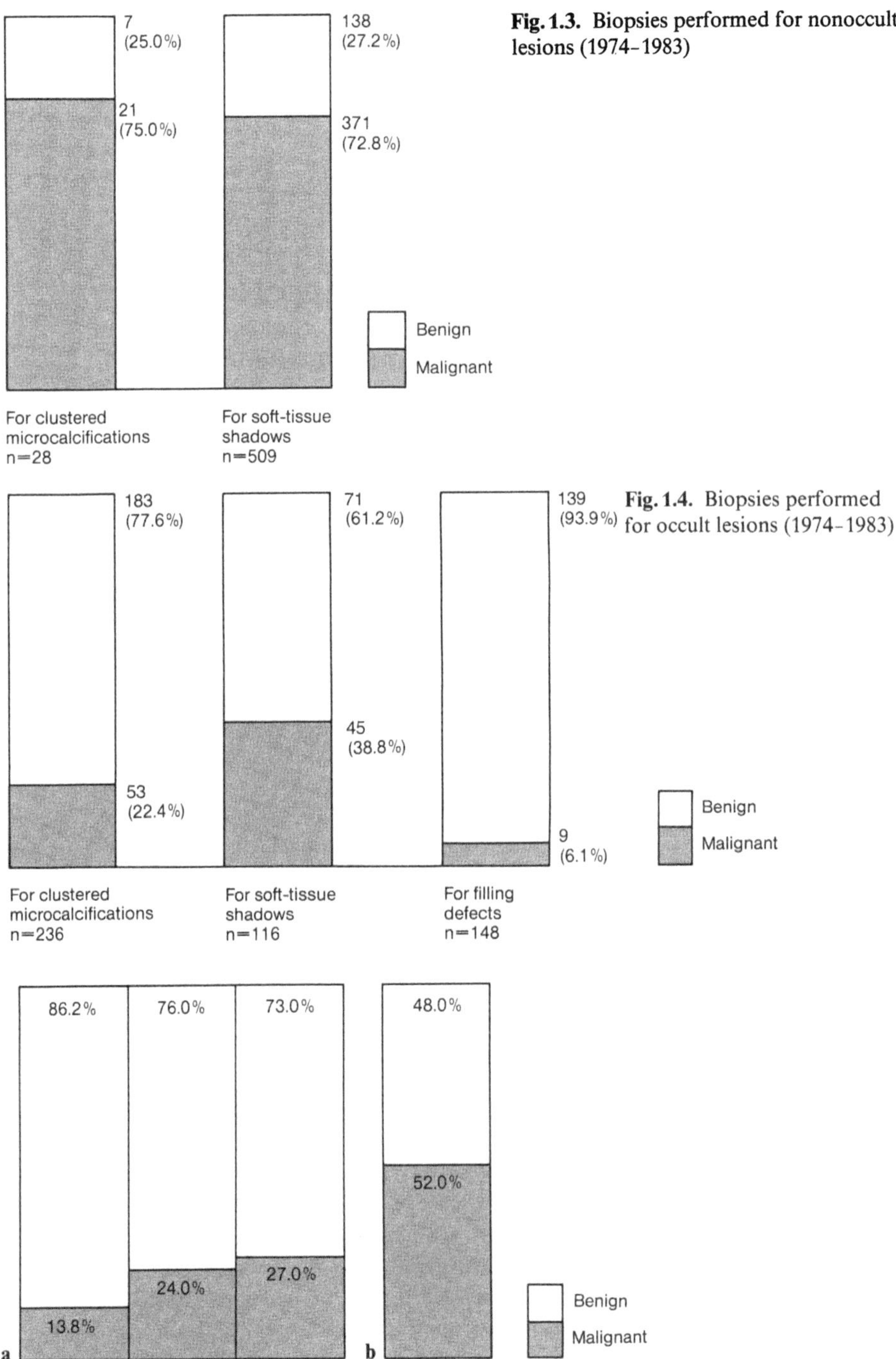

Fig. 1.3. Biopsies performed for nonoccult lesions (1974–1983)

Fig. 1.4. Biopsies performed for occult lesions (1974–1983)

Fig. 1.5 a, b. The evolution of carcinoma yields in microcalcification diagnosis. **a** Gradual improvement is apparent in the early years (3-year periods from 1 October 1974 to 30 September 1983). **b** The improvement becomes dramatic following full implementation of our differential diagnostic system (from 1 January 1983 to 31 March 1985) the same in biopsies recommended for clustered microcalcifications and for other symptoms: 75% vs 72.8%.

Yet analysis of the cases biopsied exclusively for clinically occult radiographic abnormalities (Fig. 1.4) demonstrates that a "filling defect" or "duct amputation" on galactograms leads to the poorest yield, at 6.1%. (This result is almost identical to that reported by GREGL in 1979.) The best yield with occult lesions is provided by round shadows and radial structures, which are positive for carcinoma in every 2nd or 3rd biopsy. Only 1 in every 4–5 biopsies performed to evaluate clustered microcalcifications is positive for carcinoma.

By comparison, SCHWARTZ et al. (1984) found 161 malignant tumors (29%) in 557 breasts with occult lesions (in addition to 14 lobular neoplasias). They found 96 of the carcinomas (30%) in 320 cases where biopsy had been performed for microcalcifications alone. Thus, even in view of this outstanding result, 70% of the biopsies performed for microcalcifications did not yield carcinoma. (On the basis of other radiographic signs 237 cases were biopsied, and clinically occult carcinomas were found in 65 of these, or 27%; thus 73% of these operations were unrewarding as well.)

Is it possible, then, to achieve a better result, especially in the evaluation of microcalcifications? Or are the American authors (EGAN et al. 1980; COLBASSINI et al. 1982; MOSKOWITZ 1979) correct in asserting the futility of this diagnostic approach?

During the period from 1974 to 1983, the author was able almost to double the yield of cases biopsied for microcalcifications from 13.8% to 27%. Between 1983 and 1985 the author completed work on a differential diagnostic system that enabled him to find 12 ductal carcinomas in 23 cases biopsied solely on the basis of clustered microcalcifications (Fig. 1.5). This was the result of a systematic, comparative histologic-radiographic analysis of true-positive and false-positive cases.

It must be asked whether this result was obtained at the cost of undetected carcinomas. This question can be answered if it is assumed that the percentage of carcinomas detected solely on the basis of microcalcifications remains more or less constant in relation to *all* carcinomas.

In our case this percentage was 14.1% (74 of 499) during the "early" period (1974–1983), and it remained virtually unchanged, at 14.3% (12 of 84), in the ensuing period. The percentages of *occult* carcinomas detected on the basis of microcalcifications relative to all carcinomas are also virtually identical: 10.6% (53 of 499) in 1974–1983, and 10.7% (9 of 84) in 1983–1985. Statistically, then, it is unlikely that the fact that a microcalcification cluster did not justify biopsy was the reason that a carcinoma went undetected during the 1.5-year period the diagnostic system was in use.

To test the usefulness of the new differential diagnostic system, the author evaluated the preoperative mammograms of 297 breasts biopsied for clustered microcalcifications, doing so without knowledge of the history, clinical findings, comparison films, or histologic diagnosis (LANYI and NEUFANG 1984). As Table 1.4 shows, it is possible to forego 73% of biopsies when this differential diagnostic system is used. Of 42 carcinomas, only 1 was incorrectly diagnosed as benign. This error probably could have been avoided if it had been known that the patient had undergone previous surgery for contralateral breast cancer, and that the extremely fine microcalcifications had not been visible on mammograms 6 months earlier (Fig. 7.5 d). Similar

Table 1.4. Diagnostic accuracy of mammography

42 Carcinomas	True positive	41
	False negative	1
255 Benign lesions	True negative	187
	False positive	68
Sensitivity:	97.6%	
Specificity:	73.3%	

results were achieved in 1985 at the Institute Curie in Paris. (The material in this series, it should be emphasized, did not only involve cases from that institute, but also consisted of case material collected by Madame Le Gal from other institutions.) In this study, 53 of 54 carcinomas were correctly diagnosed and 63 of 99 benign microcalcifications were determined to be definitely benign.

The purpose of this book is to make public the differential diagnostic system developed by the author in order to aid the correct diagnosis of breast carcinomas and reduce the number of unnecessary biopsies.

2 Technical Prerequisites for the Evaluation of Breast Microcalcifications

The early diagnosis of breast cancer is based upon the radiographic visualization of microstructures on the mammogram. Extremely small fibrotic structures and microcalcifications are each of fundamental importance in this process. Almost half (43%–49%) of clinically occult breast carcinomas are detected from the presence of microcalcifications, 21% of which are less than 0.25 mm in size; many are no larger than 0.1 mm (FRIEDRICH 1983; FRISCHBIER and LOHBECK 1977; LANYI 1977b). But accurate diagnosis hinges not just on the perception of these fine calcium particles, but also on their correct interpretation. Only by a meticulous analysis of the shapes of individual calcifications and their clusters is it possible to differentiate definitely benign clusters from those that are definitely malignant or suspicious. Thus, optimum image quality is a critical factor in both the diagnosis and differential diagnosis of breast microcalcifications.

2.1 Factors Influencing Visualization of Image Details

The visualization of details on mammograms is determined by the factors discussed below.

Image Contrast

Contrast is important because a detail that is large enough to be seen may be imperceptible unless it contrasts sufficiently with the surrounding tissues. Image contrast depends on:
- the anode material of the X-ray tube, or the radiation spectrum produced by the anode;
- filtration of the primary radiation;
- the amount of scatter radiation produced by the size and composition of the breast;
- the characteristic curve of the film or image recording system;
- conditions of film development.

Image Sharpness

Sharpness is important because even if a detail has sufficient size and contrast, it may not be perceived if its margins are indistinct. Image sharpness depends on:
- the size of the X-ray focal spot;
- the amount of magnification (focus-film distance, object-film distance);
- the resolution of the image recording system.

Noise

A detail whose size and contrast place it *at the threshold of perceptibility* may be obscured by the high noise content of an imaging system. Noise depends chiefly on the graininess of the film and on X-ray quantum noise ("quantum mottle"), which is less important in mammography. Screen-film systems (see p. 19) are particularly apt to have a "noisy" background caused by the different grain size and the inherent quantum and structural noise of the intensifying screen.

Sensitivity of the Image Recording System

The sensitivity of an image recording system refers to the magnitude of the radiation dose necessary to produce an optimum density. The best mammographic image is that with the highest contrast and resolution and the least noise. A mammographic imaging system may be regarded as optimal when contrast, sharpness, and noise have an *equal influence* on image quality. The size and nature of the breast being examined also affect the quality of the mammogram (at least for the present time). An important concern besides image quality is the amount of radiation exposure produced by the examination. Optimum image quality and an acceptable level of radiation exposure are not incompatible goals, and an effective compromise can be achieved.

Other technical details affecting mammographic diagnosis are the conditions of film development (composition, temperature, and depletion state of the developer, developing time), the luminous intensity of the viewbox, and the power of the magnifying lens. Below we shall briefly review the most recent discoveries and recommendations for optimizing mammographic imaging, followed by a brief discussion of magnification mammography. This summary is based largely on the works of FRIEDRICH (1983, 1984; FRIEDRICH and WESKAMP 1976a, b, 1984a, b), who has done much in recent years to improve our understanding of the technical problems of mammography, and whose research into the physical and technical prerequisites set the stage for the implementation of grid mammography, which was once considered impractical.

2.2 Image Optimization and Dose Reduction

Tube and Filter

The introduction of the molybdenum tube by GROS (1966) at the first European Breast Symposium in Strasbourg was revolutionary in terms of improving image quality. Within two years, however, it was recognized that the dose-contrast relation of selectively filtered molybdenum radiation was optimal only for thin and fatty breasts (MIKA and REISS 1968).

Thick breasts and predominantly fibroglandular breasts absorb too much of the softer component of the radiation, which is important for contrast. The result is an unfavorable dose-contrast relation; the energy distribution on the film creates relatively poor image contrast. In thick, glandular breasts it would be necessary to replace the molybdenum filter with a 0.5-mm aluminum filter in order to filter out the portions of the radiation which are not useful for imaging, but which compound patient exposure. The other alternative would be a return to the tungsten tube. Studies by JENNINGS and FEWELL (1979) have shown that the energy spectrum from a tungsten tube with rhodium or palladium filtration gives better contrast in thick parts and delivers a lower radiation dose than the molybdenum tube. However, the contrast in *thin* parts is somewhat poorer than with the molybdenum tube.

The Grid Technique

The technique of grid mammography contributes both to improving the quality of the mammogram and reducing the radiation dose to the patient. The function of the grid is to decrease the amount of scatter radiation, which accounts for up to 50% of the radiation emerging from the patient. The relative size of the scatter component depends both on the thickness of the breast and the cross-sectional area of the useful beam. Studies by FRIEDRICH (1983) show that reducing the amount of scatter radiation by "coning" (to reduce the beam cross section) would be effective only if the tube had a cross-sectional area of 1 cm². A tube of this size would not be useful in practice.

A more practical and effective solution in terms of image quality would be to use a special, soft radiation grid. The word "special" is emphasized, because formerly (GAJEWSKI 1973) it was believed that grid mammography was impractical for the following reasons:
a) The grid hardens and attenuates the X-ray beam too much.
b) It would be difficult to image breast regions close to the chest wall unless a grid with a very narrow border were available.
c) The grid increases the object–film distance and degrades image sharpness.
d) It was considered unreasonable to increase the radiation dose in the absence of a dose-reducing film-screen system.
With the advent of grid mammography, all these problems have been overcome.

The majority of grids presently available consist of a carbon fiber plate mounted over a grid of lead strips 16 μm thick (grid ratio 5 : 1, 30 strips/cm). The film-screen system is contained in a cassette or an opaque vacuum bag and is introduced from the side or from behind. The object–film distance is only 6–8 mm, and the increased focus–film distance of 60 cm provides a better imaging geometry for the far half of the breast than the 45-cm focus–film distance in conventional mammography. The phototimer behind the film-screen system must be more sensitive than usual because the intensifying screen absorbs 70% of the radiation and the film-screen combination is seven to eight times more sensitive, together significantly reducing the amount of radiation available for measuring the exposure.

The advantages of grid mammography are:
a) superior contrast;
b) better definition of details, microcalcifications, and fibrous septa;
c) dose reduction by a factor of 2–4.

However, in breasts that have a compression thickness of 2 cm or less, the use of a grid does not appear to be useful because contrast enhancement by the suppression of scatter is effective only in cases where an appreciable amount of scatter radiation is produced, i.e., in thick breasts.

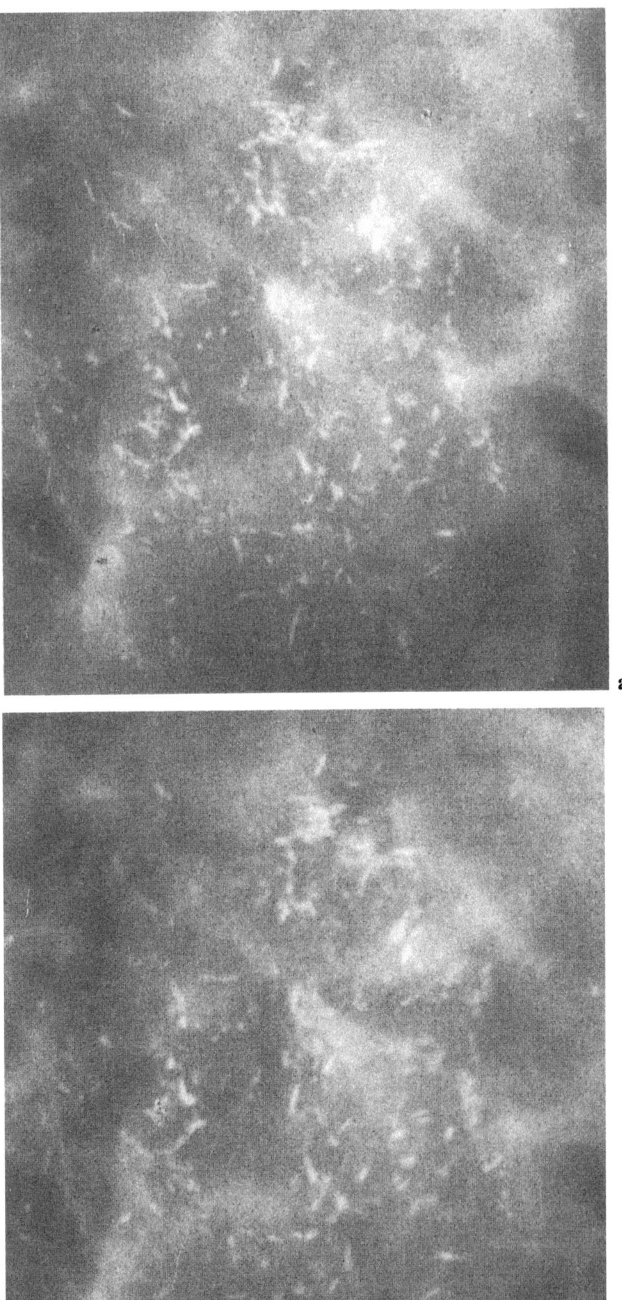

Fig. 2.1a-c. Magnified views of microcalcifications in a breast phantom: Cronex 75 with Lo-Dose I screen (FRIEDRICH 1984). a Diagnost M, b slot Mammomat, c regular Mammomat

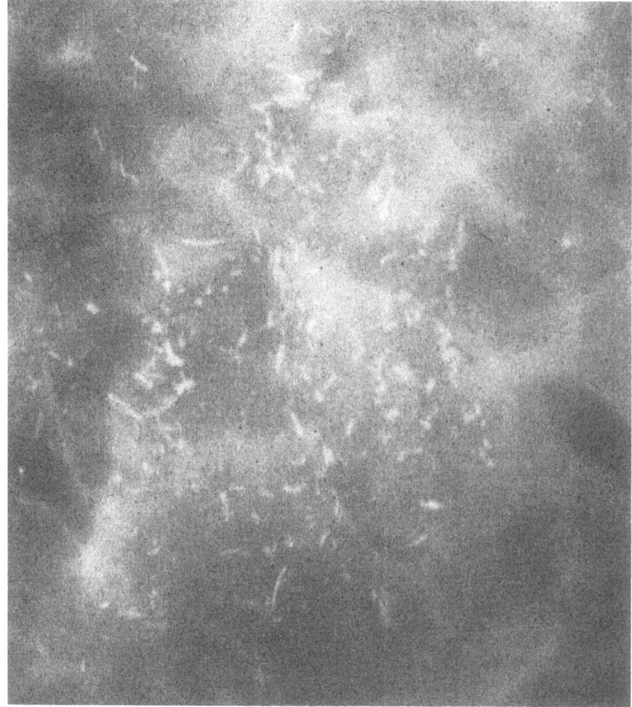

Fig. 2.1c

The advantages of grid mammography have already been confirmed by reports from clinicians (LAUTH et al. 1983) and office practitioners (LAMMERS and KUHN 1979; LENDVAI-VIRÁGH et al. 1983).

The Slit Diaphragm Technique

Studies by FRIEDRICH (1984) show that the "slit diaphragm technique" offers another means of improving image quality by reducing dosage and scatter. The apparatus for this technique (Slot Mammomat, Siemens) incorporates a primary slit above the breast and a protective screen with a single afterslot between the breast and the film-screen system. With this apparatus the radiation dose can be reduced to half that of the conventional grid technique without sacrificing quality (Fig. 2.1 a–c).

Films, Intensifying Screens, Film-Screen Systems

Image quality sufficient to give sharp visualization of features 0.1 mm in diameter cannot be achieved with ordinary, nonscreen radiographic films. An exceptionally fine-grain film is required. Other desirable film properties are high sensitivity, a steep gradient, and a large density range. These properties are present in industrial films, which have a high silver content and a steep characteristic curve (i.e., *image contrast increases with density),* unlike conventional X-ray films with ordinary screens where the characteristic curve and contrast level off at higher densities.

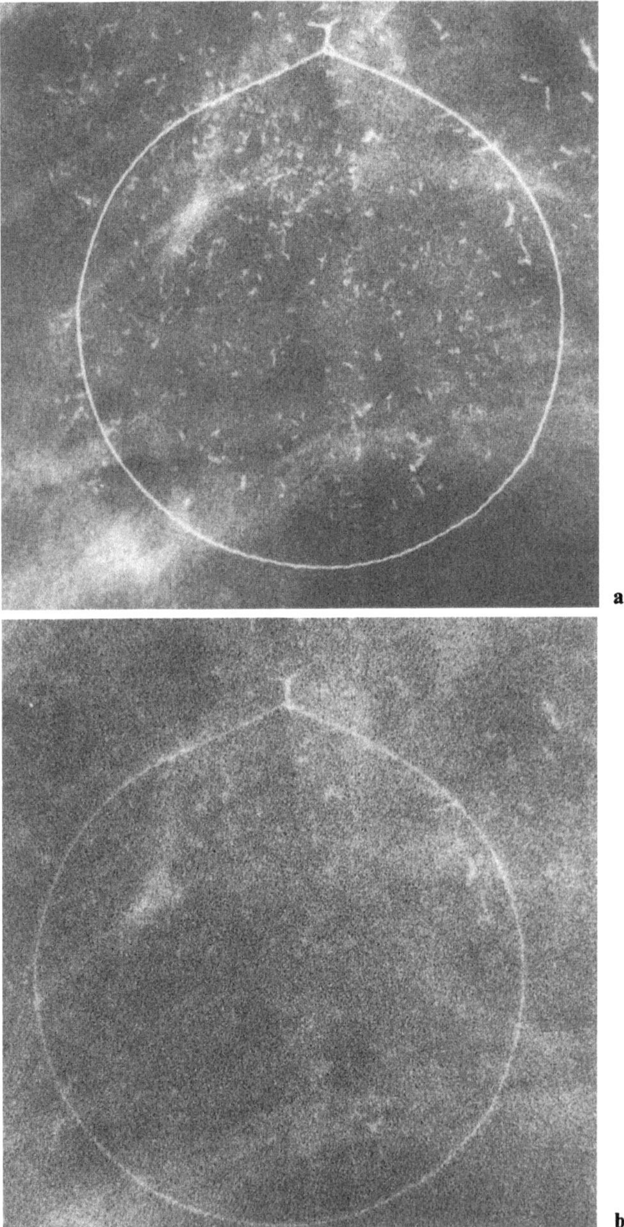

Fig. 2.2 a-d. Magnified views (5×) of the same area of microcalcifications in a breast phantom made by Friedrich (80–300 μm in size, calcium chloride particles embedded in the breast tissue). **a** Mammoray T3 without a screen, relative dose 1; **b** Lo-Dose 1, relative dose 0.13; **c** Cronex 75/Min R 50 film and screen combination, relative dose 0.13; **d** Cronex 70/Min R 50 film and screen combination, relative dose 0.23. While the microcalcifications are almost imperceptible with Lo-Dose 1, they are demonstrated by the film and screen combinations almost as well as by the nonscreen industrial film, but at a much lower dose

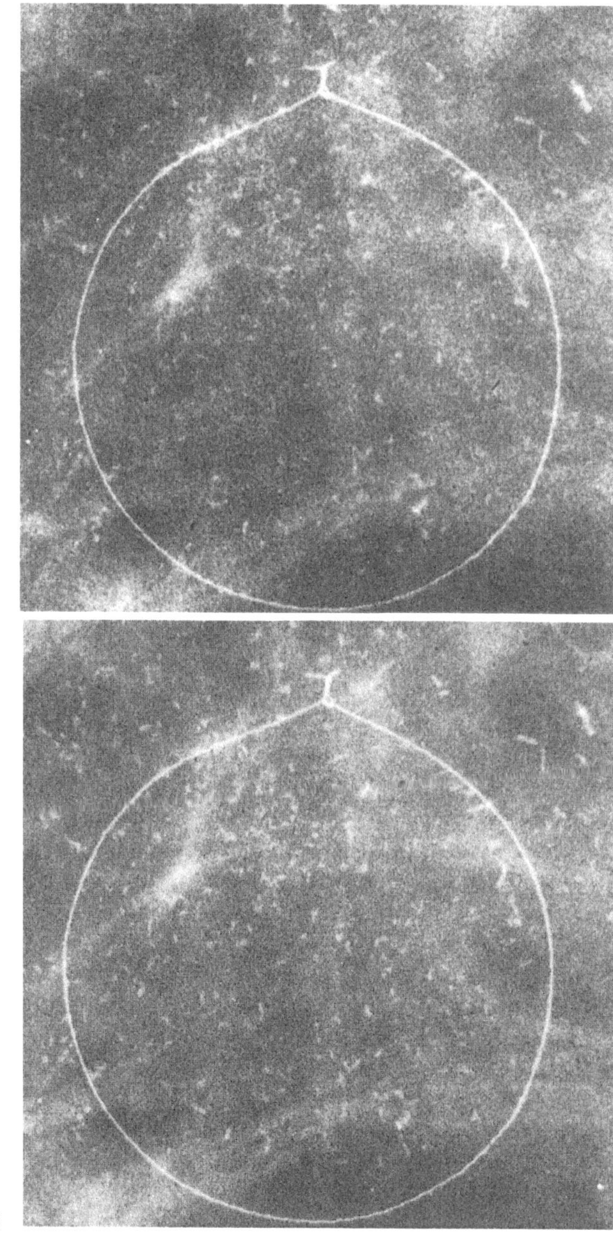

c

d

Fig. 2.2 c, d

The conventional technique (molybdenum anode, molybdenum filtration, 28–41 kV, 45 FFD, industrial film) produces the best images with acceptable dose in small, fatty, easily compressed breasts that have little residual glandular tissue. *Nonscreen* films with a high silver content and a sensitized emulsion layer (e. g., Kodirex, Mammoray M4) have been introduced to offer a lower dose alternative to classic mammographic film. The nonscreen films that process in 90 s (e. g., DuPont Duplex) are recommended for radiologists who do not possess equipment for slow processing.

Intensifying screens have frequently been used in an effort to reduce radiation exposure and tube loading while increasing image contrast. Available combinations consist of single emulsion, relatively *low-silver and low-contrast films* with high-definition intensifying screens. Studies by FRIEDRICH (1983) show that these film-screen combinations are incapable of demonstrating fine microcalcifications. A similar conclusion is reached by HÜPPE and SCHNEIDER (1977). This led FRIEDRICH to develop an alternative concept – that of the "high resolution" film-screen system. This system consists of a double emulsion, high contrast, fine grain, light sensitive industrial film and a mammographic screen. As a result of this combination, the steep gradient of the silver-rich film is preserved, sharpness is reduced, and film graininess is increased somewhat, but there is a marked increase in the sensitivity of the system. In experiments with a phantom made of breast tissue, FRIEDRICH found that very fine structural details and the smallest microcalcifications are most clearly visualized with DuPont Cronex 75 or 70 industrial film combined with an Agfa Gevaert or Cawo MR50 screen. This pairing provides a dose reduction of approximately ⅔–¾ compared with nonscreen industrial film, and the ability to perceive microcalcifications is virtually unchanged (Fig. 2.2 a–d).

Current mammographic film systems are so diverse that they can be compared with one another only by taking into account a range of features. These features are effectively summarized in the signal-to-noise ratio (SNR), which permits a quantitative comparison to be made. FRIEDRICH and WESKAMP (1976 a, b, 1984 a, b) defined the SNR as a quantitative measure of image quality. These authors used the signal–noise matrix as a basis for comparing 18 mammographic film systems. By relating the SNR to the necessary radiation dose ("dose efficiency"), they were able to make a ranking of the systems currently recommended for film mammography.

They found that the best compromise in terms of dose efficiency as well as quality was the double emulsion, silver rich industrial film-screen combination (e. g., Cronex 70/MR50). Among the single emulsion combinations, only the Trimax system yielded comparable results. The single emulsion, 90-s film-screen systems (MinR, Lo-Dose, Agfa NIF) cannot be recommended on the basis of quality or dose efficiency. The double emulsion, 90-s films with a screen (Lo-Dose Plus, Mammoray RP3/MR50) are not significantly better. The sensitized, double emulsion films (Mammoray M4, Kodirex) are markedly better. Recently, firms have introduced improved single emulsion, 90-s film-screen systems (e. g., Kodak MinR screen/OMA film) which are only slightly inferior to the high resolution film-screen combinations, at least in an intermediate density range.

Optimal imaging geometry and correct exposure are essential for good quality. An overexposed or underexposed industrial film may be substantially poorer than a correctly exposed 90-s, single emulsion film-screen system.

Fig. 2.3. Peak anastigmatic with magnification of 4 × lens

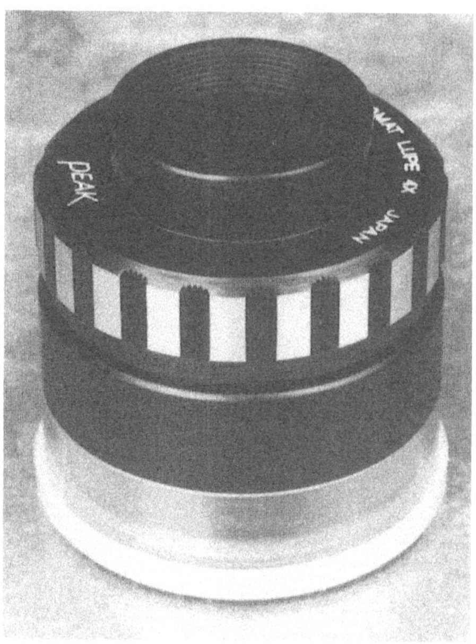

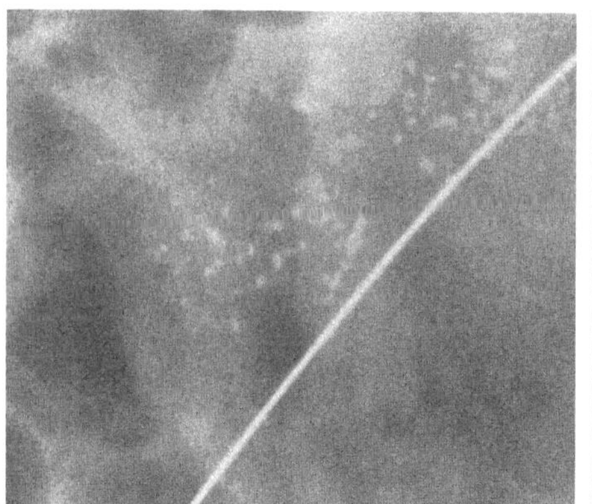

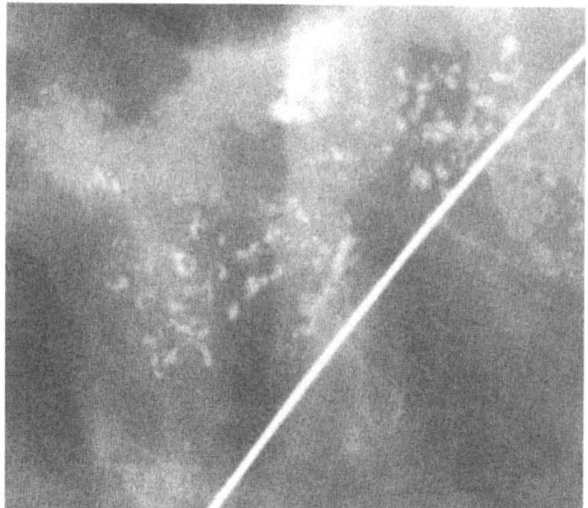

a   b

Fig. 2.4 a, b. Magnification radiographs (4 ×), specimen radiograph with hookwire localization. **a** 0.3 mm focal spot; the microcalcifications are somewhat blurred. **b** 0.1 mm focal spot; the microcalcifications are sharp, and their shapes are more easily evaluated. (J. H. C. L. HENDRIKS, Nijmegen Catholic University, Netherlands)

2.3 Microfocal Spot Magnification Mammography

It is desirable to examine small microcalcification clusters with as much magnification as possible. The simplest (and least costly) solution is to magnify the image secondarily with a hand lens (at least 4 ×) like that shown in Fig. 2.3. However, image

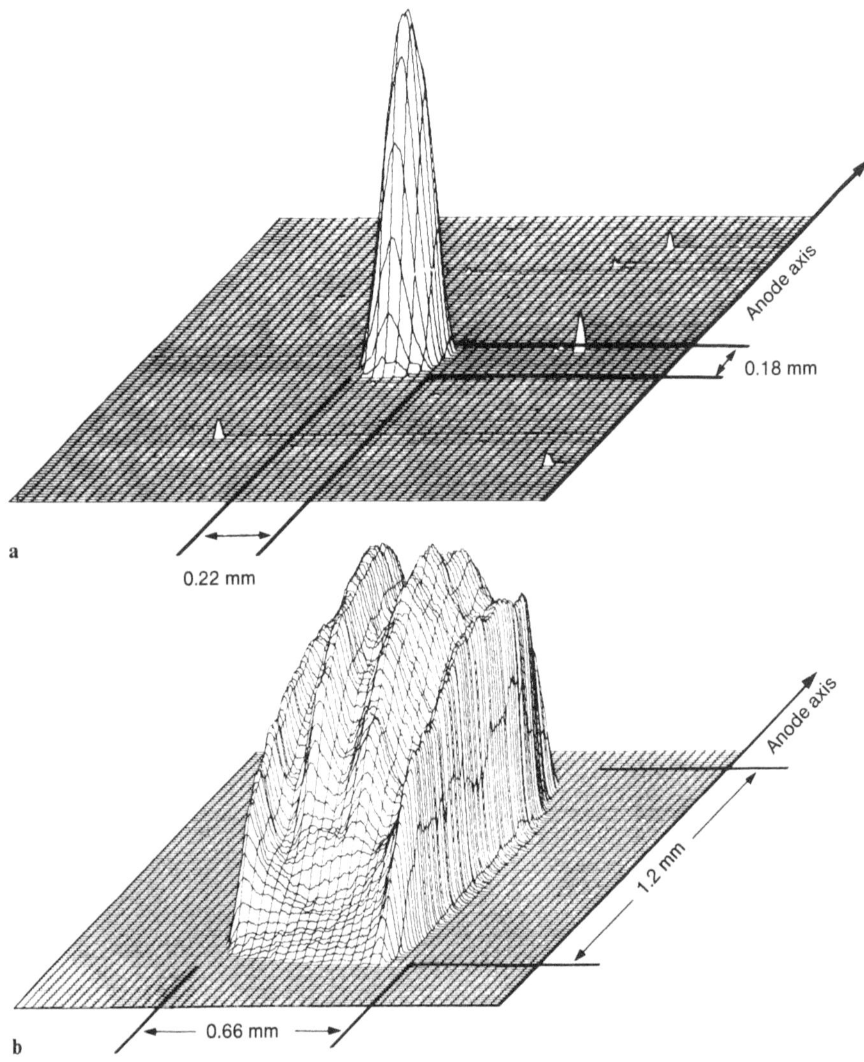

Fig. 2.5 a Density distribution in the 0.22 × 0.18 mm focal spot of the laboratory instrument developed by Philips Mammo-Diagnost for the magnification technique. **b** Density distribution in a 0.66 × 1.2 mm focal spot. The improved image quality of the small focal spot compared with the regular focal spot is apparent. (M. FRIEDRICH, P. WESKAMP)

noise can seriously limit the efficacy of secondary magnification. A better solution is to achieve good primary magnification with the use of a fine X-ray focal spot.

The focal spot should be no larger than the diameter of the smallest detail to be visualized. In mammography, this means a focal spot size of 0.1 mm. To date the author's experience with magnification mammography has been limited to studies of material at the Nijmegen Catholic University in the Netherlands using the Senograph 500. Results with this technique have been very encouraging (Fig. 2.4 a, b).

Even with a focal spot size of 0.2 mm, the almost rotationally symmetric intensity distribution provides a substantially better geometric imaging quality than the conventional 0.6 mm focal spot (Fig. 2.5a, b). In addition, the geometric unsharpness at an object-film distance of 25 cm (2 × magnification) does not degrade image sharpness for a given film-screen combination. The improved image quality of the magnification radiograph is also based on the reduction of scatter radiation. At 2 × magnification the SNR is markedly better than in the contact technique. If now the sharp, high contrast magnification film is viewed through a 4 × hand lens, the resulting 8 × magnification will permit a much better analysis than is possible by examining a conventional mammogram with an 8 × lens.

SICKLES (1982) found in laboratory experiments that the finest aluminum oxide particles (0.15 mm) were perceptible only on magnification xeromammograms. WEGENER (1977) found that the detectability of microcalcifications on xeroradiographs was equivalent to that on optimally exposed molybdenum film mammograms, but that microcalcifications distant from the plate were more easily perceived on xeromammograms.

2.4 Future Developments

The technical evolution of mammography is by no means complete. New imaging systems must have facilities for switching quickly and easily from grid to conventional mammography and back again. They must have a tube with two selectable focal spot sizes for conventional and magnification mammography. Also, more careful attention must be given to selecting the best film or film-screen system, depending on the type of breast being examined, and determining the optimal conditions (filter? with grid? without grid?).

Mammography must be individualized. The examiner should have the first film developed and then modify the imaging conditions accordingly if the image quality is unsatisfactory. In follow-up examinations it is important to assess the composition of the breast from previous mammograms and select the most favorable imaging conditions, taking the compression thickness into account. Daily control of development parameters with test strips is also advised in order to maintain a consistent level of quality.

3 Pathogenesis, Pathophysiology, and Composition of Breast Calcifications

Mammography has drawn attention to a number of different kinds of calcifications that may occur in the human breast. The various etiologic forms of breast calcifications (BRANDT and BÄSSLER 1969, 1972), their morphology (HAMPERL 1968; STEGNER and PAPE 1972), and their composition have been studied by experimental pathophysiologic, histologic, and physicochemical methods. The following briefly summarizes the results of these studies.

The pathogenesis of intramammary calcifications is not uniform. They may develop in association with inflammatory, degenerative, and toxic metabolic processes, or they may result from mechanical injury. The matrix, or starting point, for the calcification process may be inspissated secretions (e.g., in cysts or cribriform carcinoma) or damaged cells (e.g., in comedocarcinoma), where calcification results from the deposition of calcium salts at necrotic foci.

HASSLER (1969) presents the following conclusions drawn from microradiographic studies:
a) the calcifications of malignant disease typically are multiple and are evenly distributed in the tissue;
b) they are granulelike and have a relatively low intensity;
c) they form within dilated lactiferous ducts that contain basophilic cellular debris in an alkaline medium.

On the other hand, ultrastructural studies by AHMED (1975) show that calcium deposits in breast carcinoma occur not only in glandlike spaces among the cancer cells but also within the tumor cells and in the neighboring stroma. According to these observations, the microcalcifications of breast carcinoma would be the result of an active secretory process by the tumor cells rather than the product of mineralization of necrotic debris. A similar hypothesis was advanced by STEGNER and PAPE (1972). According to this theory the permeability of the cell membrane to calcium ions is greatly increased in actively secreting ductal carcinomas, so that a calcium depot can form together with available casein and phosphate protein in an optimal pH environment.

A spectrometric microanalysis of microcalcifications from a breast carcinoma (Fig. 3.1; MAROS et al., quoted in HOEFFKEN and LANYI 1973), performed in 1968, indicated the following composition:

$Ca_3(PO_4)_2$	55.0%
$CaCo_3$	9.7%
$Mg_3(PO_4)_2 \cdot H_2O$	13.3%
Protein	22.0%

An electron beam analysis (ordered by the author and performed at the Engelskirchen Microanalytic Laboratory in 1975) revealed the presence of $Ca_3(PO_4)_2$ par-

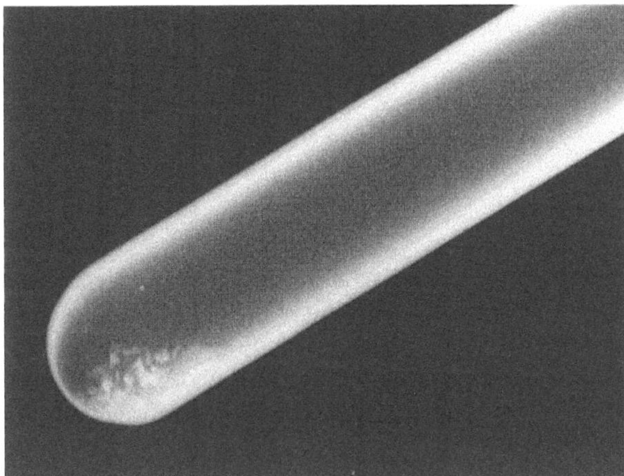

Fig.3.1. Microcalcifications were removed from a histologically confirmed comedocarcinoma and studied by spectrometric microanalysis (Advanced Medical Training Institute, Budapest 1968)

ticles about 5 µm in size and Si-containing particles of equal size embedded in the organic base material (matrix) of the microcalcifications from a comedocarcinoma.

GALKIN et al. (1982), in an electron microscopic and X-ray microanalysis of malignant and benign microcalcifications from 42 breasts, found calcium phosphate as well as calcium particles combined with other elements (Al, Fe, Mg, Si, Cu, Zu, Cr, Ti, Ni, Pb, Am, Ag, Mo, Cl). In 16 of the 42 cases the authors found no calcium, but only the aforementioned elements individually or in combination with one another. They did not establish a composition that was specific for malignant disease. Regardless of the source of the microcalcifications, their compositions tended to be the same or similar. In other experiments (HASSLER 1969; AHMED 1975; TORELL et al. 1984) hydroxylapatite, $Ca_5(PO_4)_3OH$, was demonstrated in addition to calcium phosphate.

BOUROPOULOV et al. (1984) found no difference in the localization or composition of microcalcifications associated with carcinoma or cystic breast disease.

4 Calcifications Within the Lobular and Ductal System of the Breast

Calcifications occurring in the lobular and ductal system of the breast account for 26.3% of all intramammary calcifications encountered in daily practice (see Table 1.3). They account for 24.5% of cases the author has referred for biopsy (281 of 1144 biopsies). These calcifications, whether of benign or malignant etiology, almost always represent casts of the cavities in which they occur, and this determines their shape and arrangement. An accurate knowledge of normal, pathologic, and radiographic anatomy is necessary to establish the localization of the calcifications and make a differential diagnosis.

4.1 Normal Anatomy and Radiographic Anatomy

Lobules

Anatomy

Anatomically, the lobules are the structural unit of the glandular parenchyma. They produce milk and are influenced by hormones. A single lobule in the sexually mature female is about 550 μm in diameter on average and consists of a cluster of 20–40 acini (called alveoli in the lactating breast) and the intralobular segment of the terminal milk duct. The acini are the branching processes of the terminal duct. They are round or oval in cross section and tubular in longitudinal section (Figs. 4.1 and 4.9), and even in the normal state they may contain small amounts of secretion. The acini are lined with epithelium whose outermost row consists of myoepithelial cells (myothelia). These epithelial cells contain bundles of smooth muscle filaments and envelop the acini. The milk is extruded from the alveoli by the contraction of these cells. The basement membrane separates the acini from the loose *intra*lobular connective tissue. This latter mesenchymal structure contains a dense network of capillary vessels. This network is the medium by which, on the one hand, hormones are transported from the bloodstream into the epithelium, and on the other, retained secretions are cleared into the lymphatic system (the "epithelial-stromal junction" of OZELLO, 1970).

The lobule is bound externally – surrounded – by a dense, collagenous supportive tissue.

Radiography

Occasionally the lobules can be visualized by galactography, where the acini present as fingerlike processes at the ends of the ducts, creating a "gloved hand" appearance (Fig. 4.3).

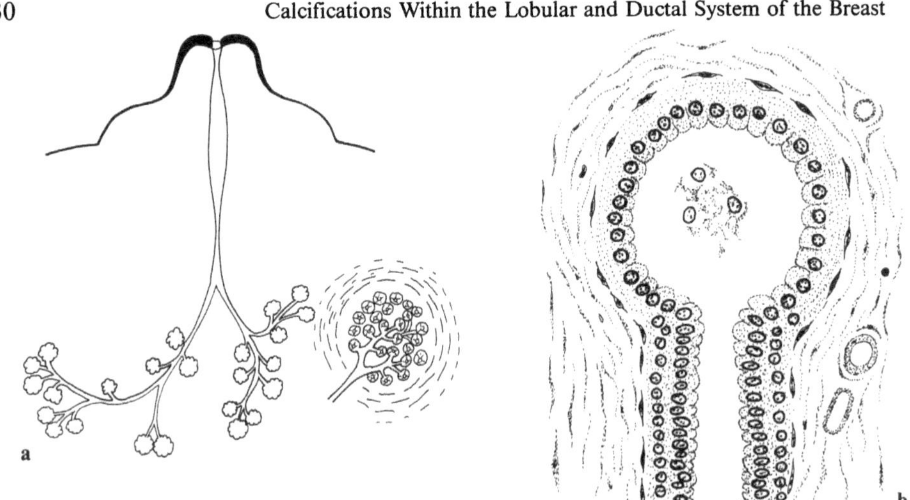

Fig.4.1. a Schematic diagram of the ductal system from the acinus to the excretory pore (after BÄSSLER 1978). **b** Longitudinal section of an acinus (after GROS 1963)

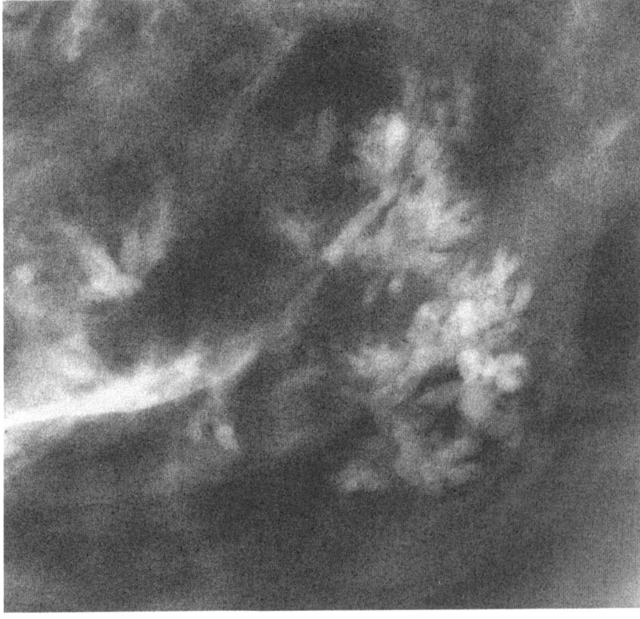

Fig.4.2. Galactogram showing a fingerlike array of slightly hypertrophic acini at the ends of the mammary ducts (highly magnified)

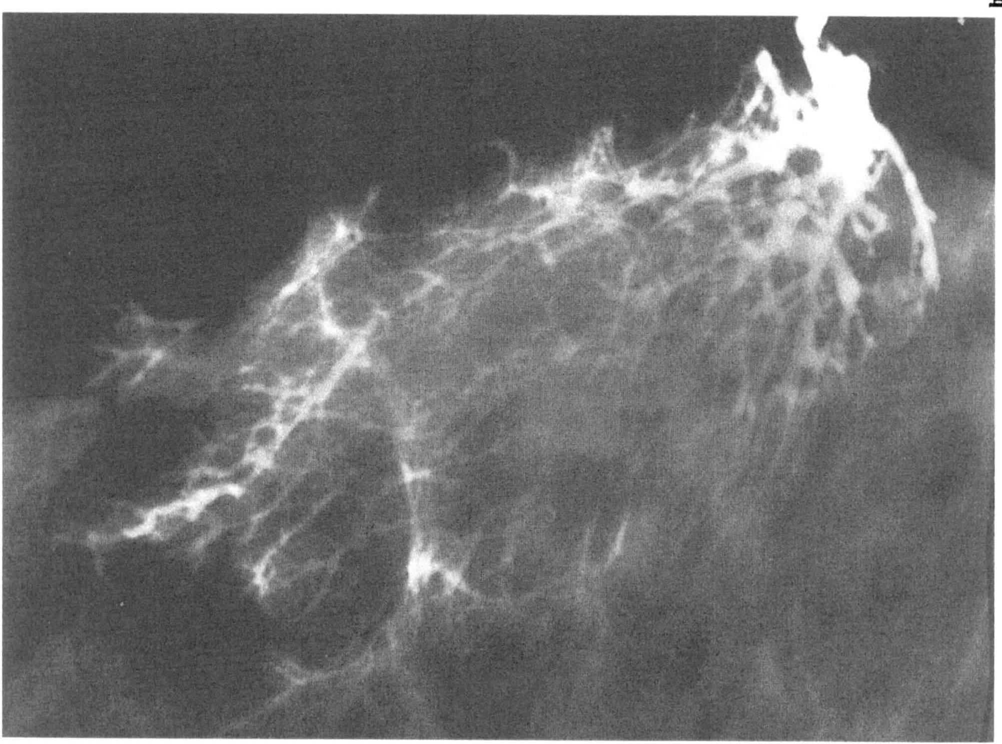

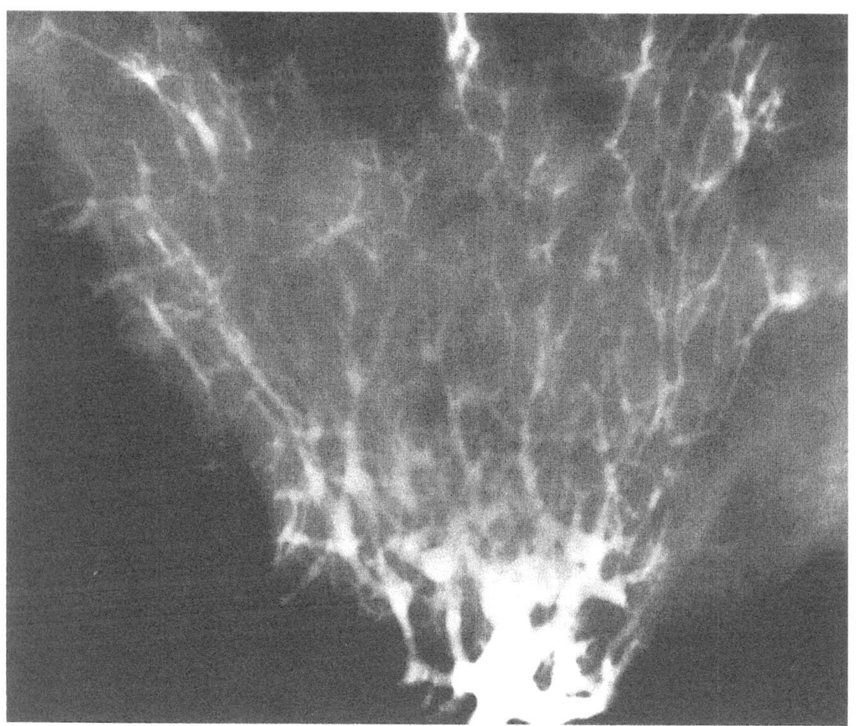

Fig. 4.3a, b. Galactograms: two views. The ductal system has a triangular configuration on both views, but it presents a considerably greater area on the craniocaudad view (**a**) than on the lateral view (**b**). The insular interductal areas devoid of contrast medium are of diagnostic and differential diagnostic importance, as are the wavy outer contours and swallowtaillike notching of the system posteriorly

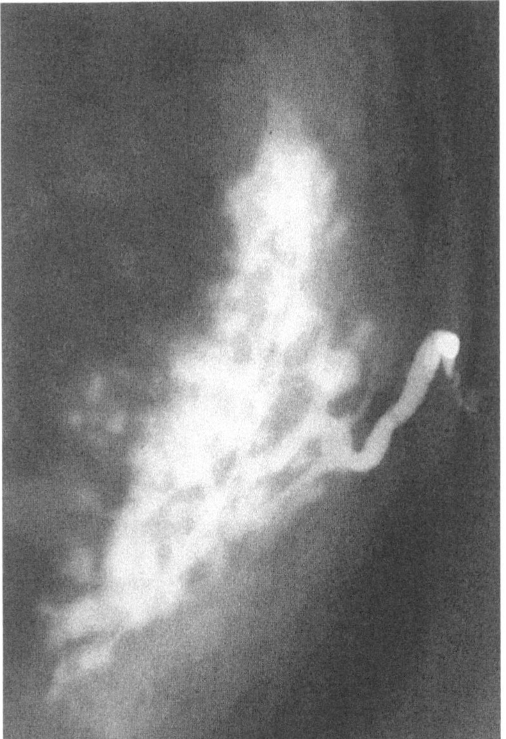

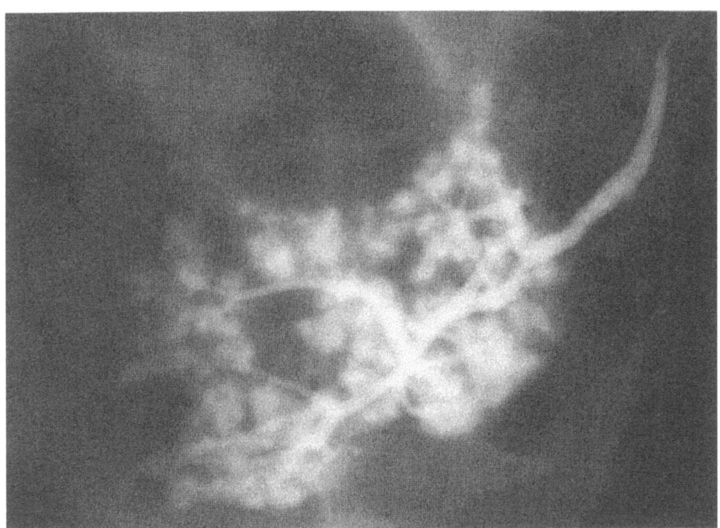

Fig. 4.4a, b. Galactograms showing how the shape of the ductal system varies with the radiographic plane. The system appears triangular on the craniocaudad view (**a**) and rectangular on the lateral view (**b**)

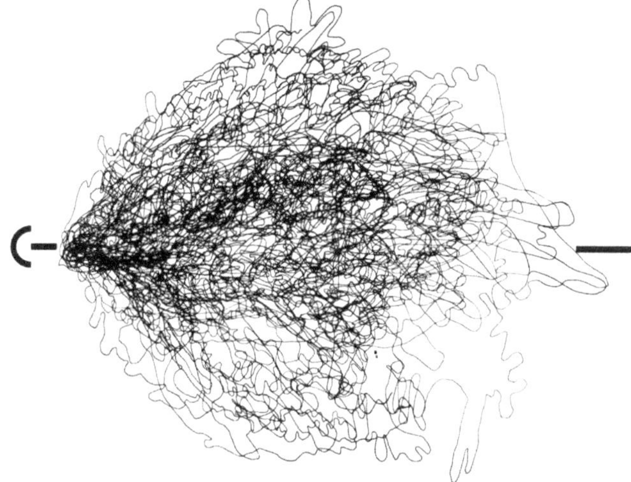

Fig. 4.5. Summation of 60 milk duct contours visualized by galactography in the craniocaudad projection. The contours were traced under a magnifying lens, copied onto transparent sheets, brought to a uniform size with an episcope, and superimposed. Note the triangular, wavy contours and the posterior notches

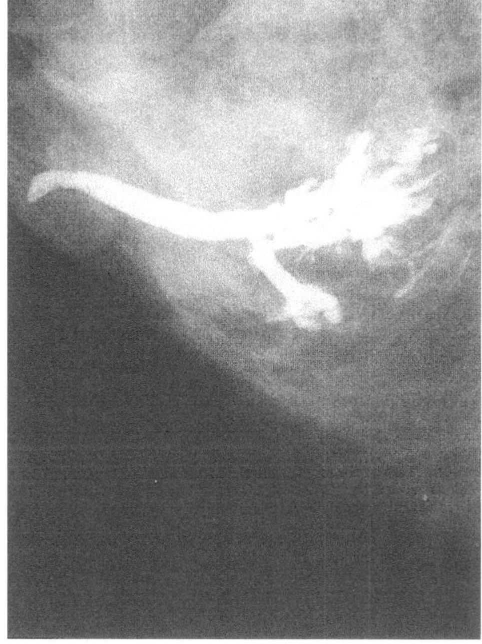

Fig. 4.6. Galactogram showing the antler-like (nontriangular) ramification of the second order ducts – a pattern commonly seen in sialography

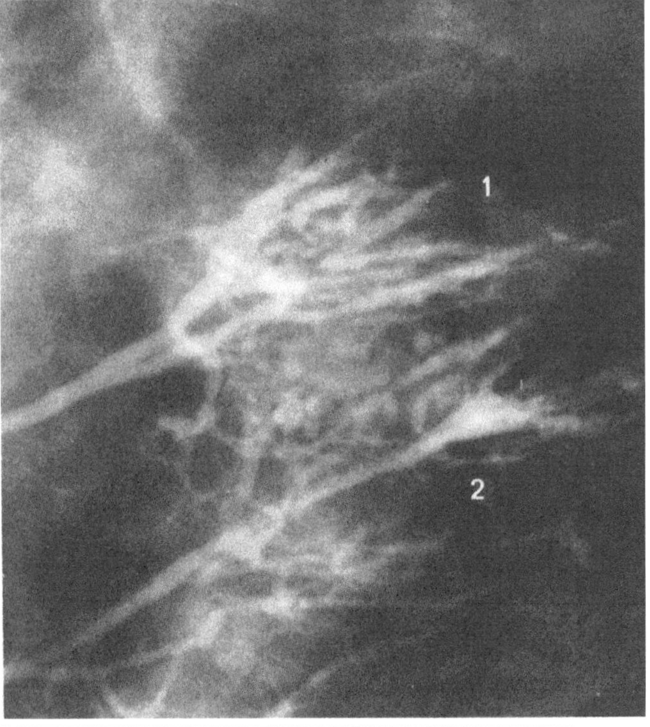

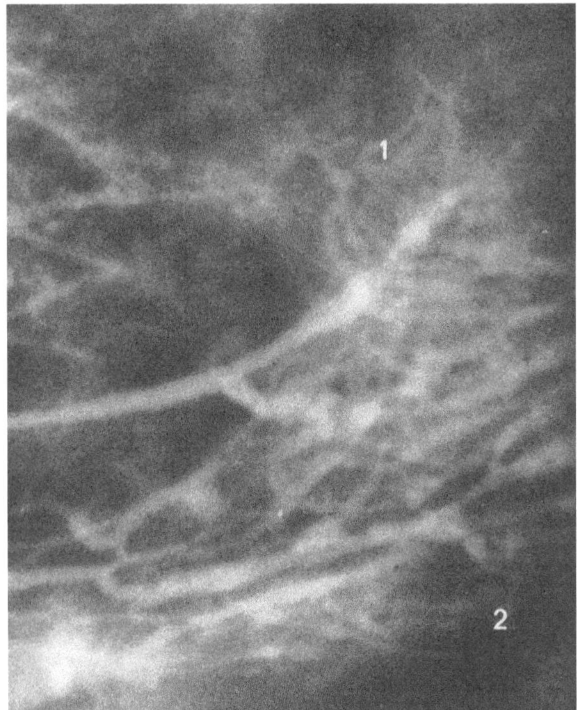

Fig. 4.7 a, b. Alteration in the shape of the smallest ducts. **a** Lateral view: *1* and *2* are triangular. **b** Craniocaudad view: *1* antlerlike ramification, *2* triangular

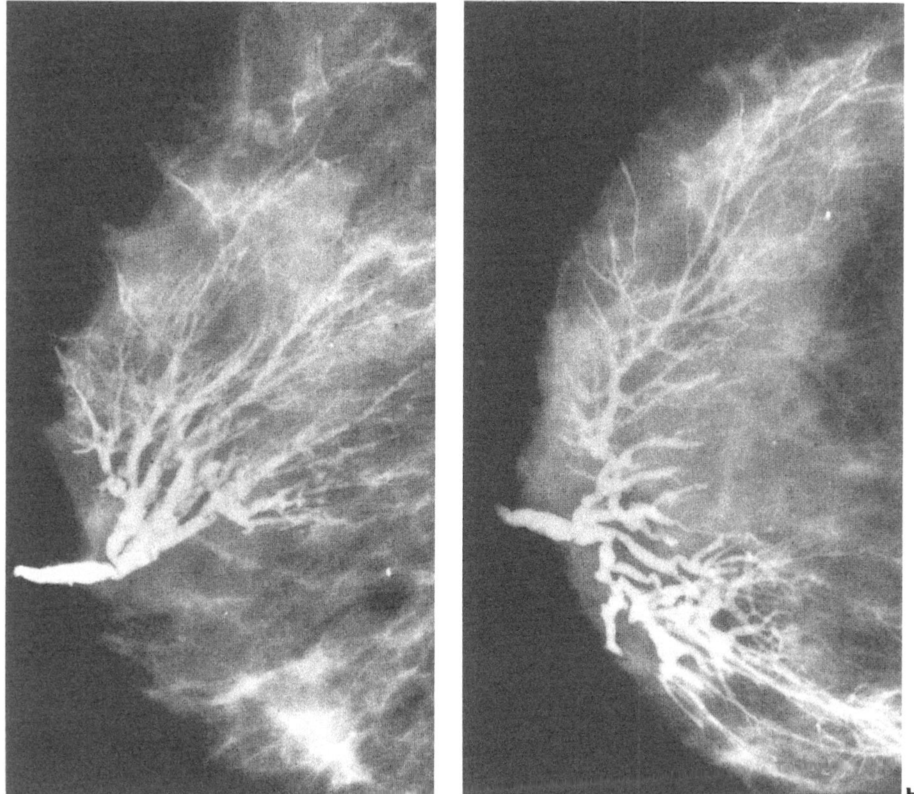

Fig.4.8. **a** The lateral galactogram appears to show one ductal system with a triangular configuration. **b** The craniocaudad view, in contrast, demonstrates two ductal systems that communicate in the area of the lactiferous sinus to form a propellerlike, butterflylike, or antlerlike configuration

Milk Ducts

Anatomy

The terminal *intralobular* duct segments open into the terminal extralobular ducts. These unite to form the lactiferous ductules, which in turn unite to form the 15–25 main lactiferous ducts, each of which drains a lobe of the gland. Each lactiferous duct expands beneath the areola to form a lactiferous sinus and terminates in an excretory pore on the surface of the nipple. The caliber of the ducts increases as they converge toward the nipple. Overall, the mammary ducts form a cavitary system that is arranged concentrically on the nipple, and whose function is to carry milk produced in the lobules to the nipple surface. The ducts are lined by two layers of cubo-columnar epithelial cells, which in the area of the lactiferous sinus are replaced by squamous cells; these give way to the keratinized squamous epithelium of the epidermis at the excretory pore (see Fig. 4.1 a).

Radiography

Contrast material (galactography) is needed to visualize the normal anatomy of the ductal system. Generally the ducts present a triangular pattern on both radiographic planes, possibly with a greater surface area on one projection than the other (Fig. 4.3). The apex of the triangle is toward the nipple or the sagittal axis, and the base is toward the chest wall. Marked variations of the ductal pattern are not uncommon, and a rectangular or even trapezoidal pattern may appear due to changes in duct position or radiographic projection (Figs. 4.4, 4.7, 4.96 b, c).

However, by superimposing drawings of 60 galactographic contours on two planes, it has been demonstrated that the triangular pattern is characteristic (Fig. 4.5). In rare cases the ducts will show an antlerlike ramification (Figs. 4.6, 4.7, 4.96 b) – a pattern commonly seen in sialography.

The communication of two ductal systems is also possible (Fig. 4.8). If the contours of the visualized ducts are outlined as in Fig. 4.5, a roughly triangular pattern is obtained which has wavy contours and one or more "swallowtail" notches posteriorly.

4.2 Pathology and Radiography of Calcifications of Lobular Origin

Calcifications of the lobular region can occur in several pathologic conditions:
1) cystic breast disease
2) lobular neoplasia (LCIS or lobular precancer)
3) "true," infiltrative lobular carcinoma

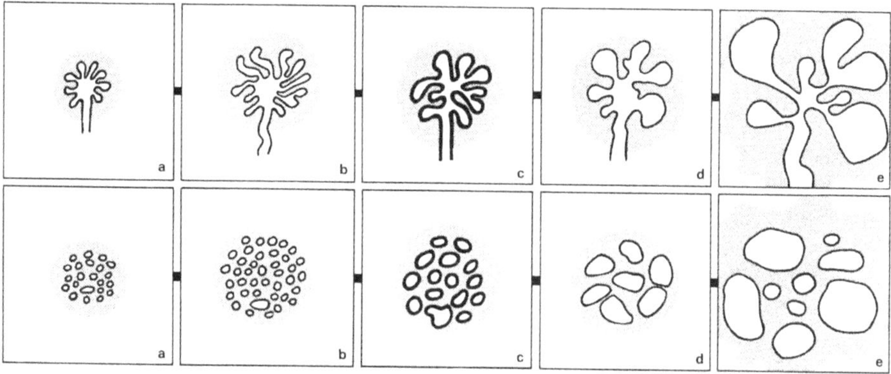

Fig. 4.9. Schematic drawings showing the development of microcystic breast disease. *Top row,* longitudinal sections; *bottom row,* transverse sections. *a* Normal lobule→*b* simple lobular hypertrophy→*c* blunt duct adenosis→*d* microcystic adenosis→*e* microcystic breast disease

Lobular Changes in Cystic Breast Disease

These changes can be differentiated histologically into several forms:
1) microcystic (blunt duct) adenosis
2) sclerosing adenosis
3) microcystic disease with milk of calcium cysts

Microcystic (Blunt Duct) Adenosis

Pathology

The histologic picture of cystic breast disease in general is marked by the combined presence of proliferative and regressive changes in the epithelial *and* mesenchymal elements of the gland. All portions of the "glandular tree" from the acini to the large excretory ducts, and the tissues immediately surrounding them, are affected. The cause is probably hormonal.

The proliferative changes include not only the *proliferation of glandular epithelium,* ranging from simple *epitheliosis* and *hyperplasia* to *papillomatosis,* but also a *dilatation and proliferation of ductal elements* throughout the ductolobular system. When these proliferative changes occur in the lobular region, adenosis is said to be present. Various histologic forms are recognized according to the extent of the proliferative process:

Simple Lobular Hypertrophy. The number of acini are increased up to fourfold, but their lumina and epithelial lining are normal (Fig. 4.9b). The hypertrophied lobule is about 1 mm in diameter.

Blunt Duct Adenosis. This is characterized (FOOTE and STEWART 1945) both by an increase in the *number of acini* and by *epithelial proliferation.* The epithelium of the acini forms *multiple layers,* the cell nuclei are slightly enlarged, and the cytoplasm is relatively abundant and loose textured. The lumina of the acini are somewhat enlarged (the word "duct" in blunt duct adenosis actually refers to the acinus). The lobule in "pure" blunt duct adenosis is approximately 1–2 mm in size (Fig. 4.9 c).

Microcystic Adenosis. The acini have enlarged to the point of cystic dilatation, but they remain within the lobular boundaries. The lobule may reach 3–5 mm in diameter (Fig. 4.9 d). The epithelium of the microcysts is often flattened by the pressure of the cystic contents.

All these forms of adenosis may coexist in the setting of cystic disease, or they may occur in mixed forms. Thus, the different types of adenosis should not be regarded as separate illnesses but as components or variants of cystic breast disease, and they should be interpreted as such by the pathologist.

Radiography

Microcystic (blunt duct) adenosis assumes radiographic importance when calcium deposits in the blunt ducts or intralobular microcysts cause these structures to become visible on mammograms, creating problems of differential diagnosis. This was the case in 12.3% of all microcalcifications in our series (see Table 1.3). Calcifications in areas of microcystic (blunt duct) adenosis may be either *clustered* (circum-

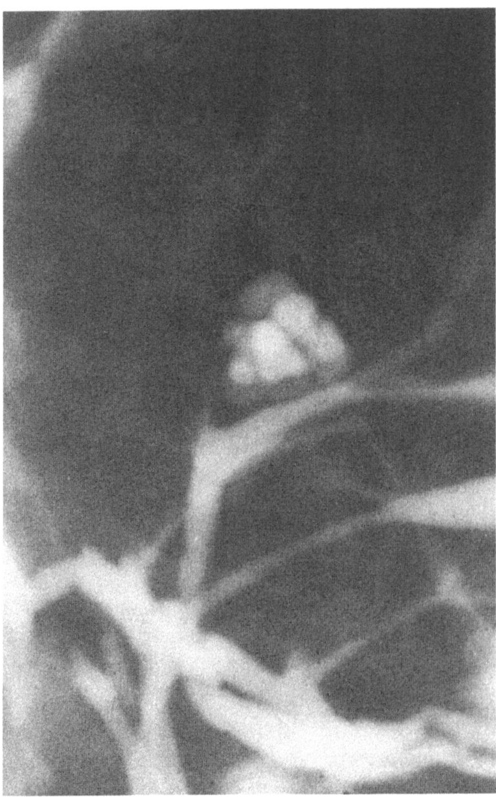

Fig. 4.10. Galactogram showing a cluster of about seven microcysts at the end of a terminal duct. Note the flattening of adjacent sides and the intercystic septation: microcystic adenosis (highly magnified)

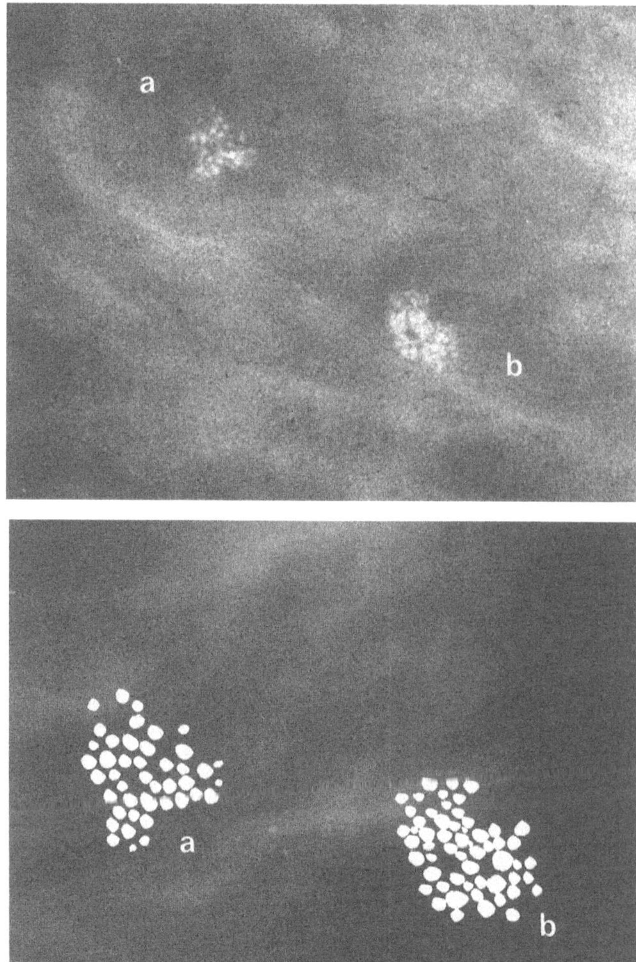

Fig. 4.11. Detail of mammogram with semischematic diagram. Two microcalcification clusters, each 4 mm in size, inside neighboring foci of microcystic adenosis (with incipient sclerosis). Cluster *a* is amorphous or roughly triangular; cluster *b* is round to oval

Fig. 4.12. Summation of the contours of 58 microcalcification clusters in microcystic (blunt duct) and sclerosing adenosis, craniocaudad view. Lines were drawn through the outermost calcifications of each cluster using a 4× magnifying lens. The resulting cluster outlines were traced onto transparent sheets and superimposed. The "core" of the superimposed contours demonstrates the rounded shape that is typical of the clusters in microcystic (blunt duct) and sclerosing adenosis

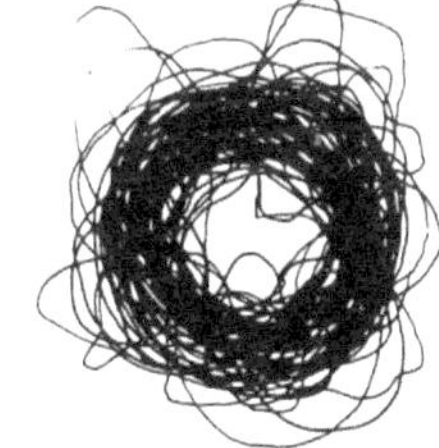

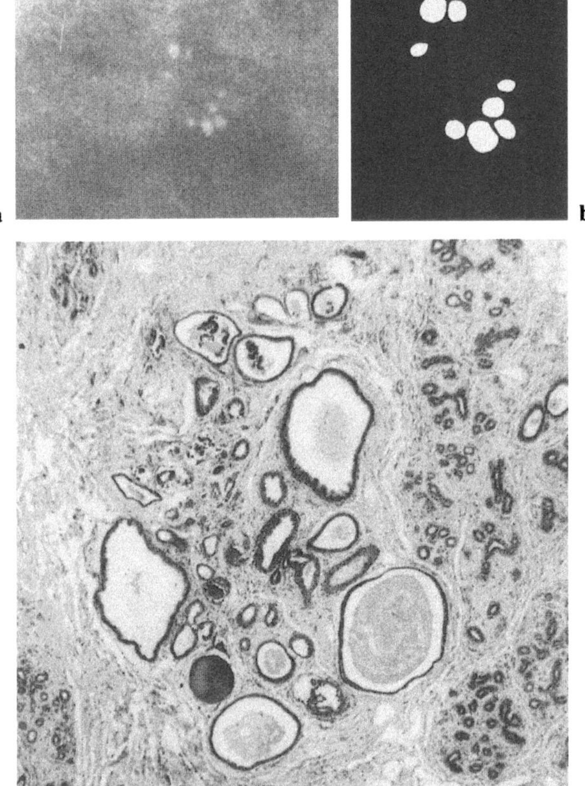

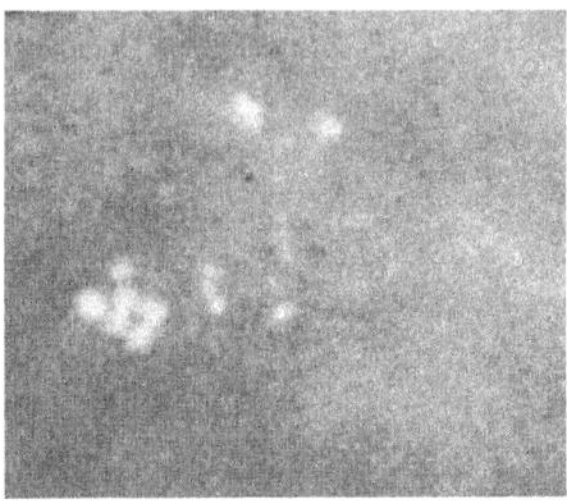

Fig. 4.14. Mammogram (approx. 16 ×): roughly oval cluster of 14 rounded microcalcifications of approximately equal size. Six of the calcifications are grouped very closely together and show fine septation. This morulalike pattern established the preoperative diagnosis of microcystic (blunt duct) adenosis

Fig. 4.13. a, b Mammogram and semischematic diagram: 4 mm ovoid cluster of eight round-to-oval, partly "facetted" microcalcifications. Several fine septa are visible between adjacent calcifications. **c** Histology: microcystic adenosis with psammomatous granules and secretions in the small cysts. The "septa" represent intercystic connective tissue (approx. 30 ×)

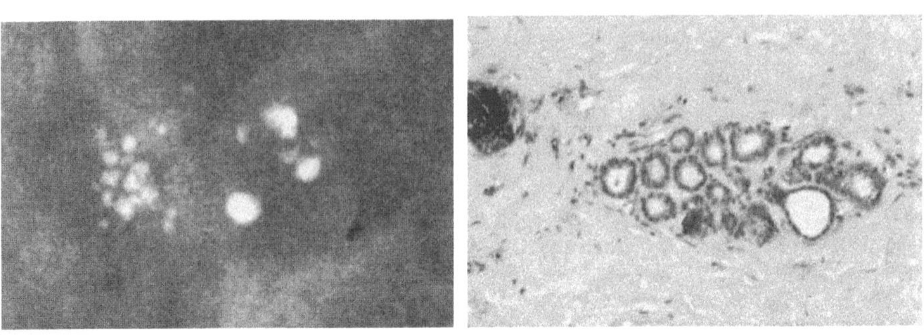

Fig. 4.15. a Detail of mammogram (4.5 ×): oval cluster, 4 mm in size, of about 20 rounded microcalcifications of varying size; note the "facetting" of adjacent calcifications. **b** Histology: microcystic (blunt duct) adenosis (approx. 50 ×)

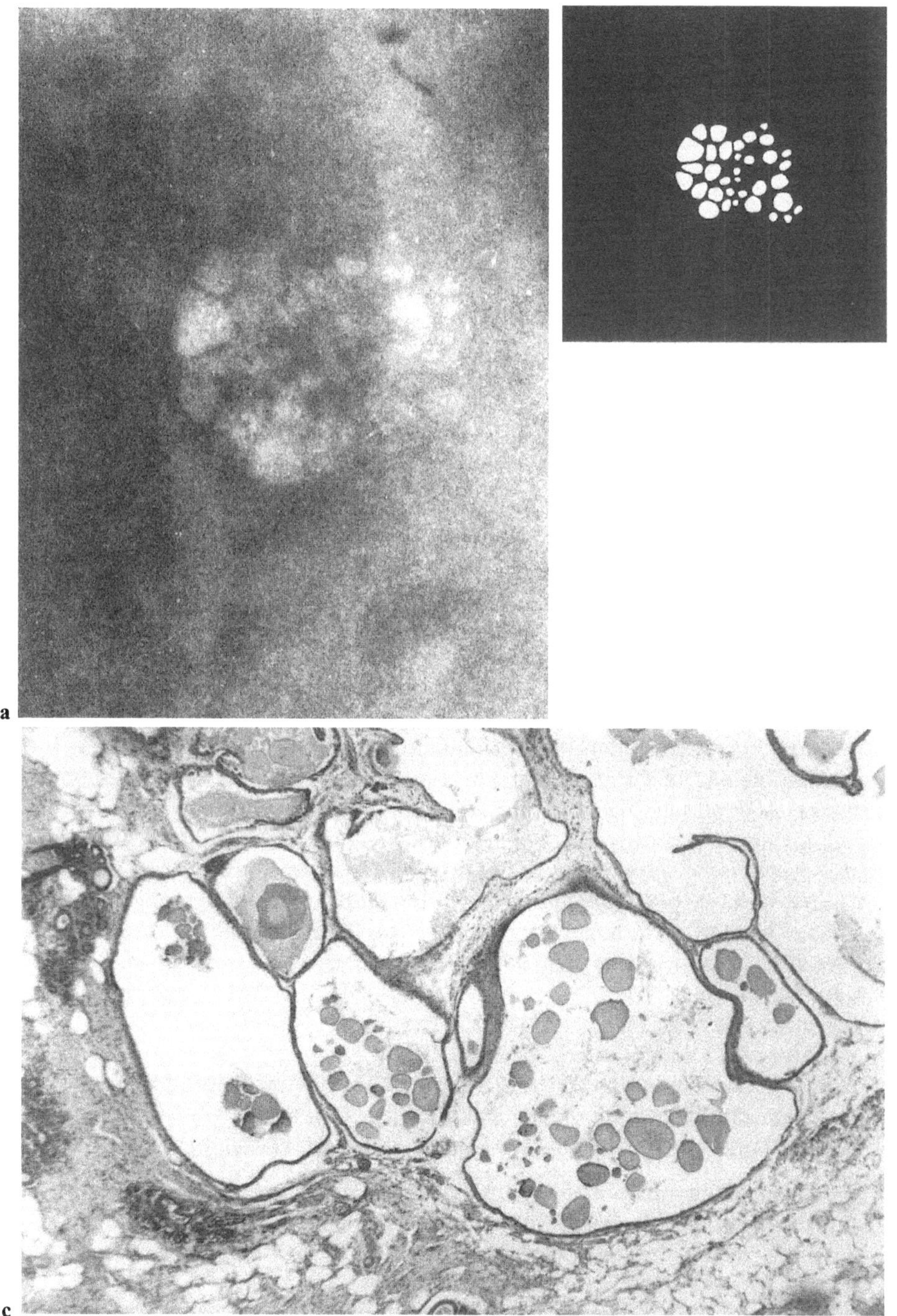

Fig. 4.16. a, b Mammogram and semischematic diagram: approximately 30 rounded, partly facetted, faint microcalcifications with fine septa contained in a cluster 5 mm in size. Note the raspberry- or morulalike appearance of the cluster. **c** Histology: cystic adenosis. The cysts contain numerous psammomatous calcifications; the epithelium is flattened. The narrow spaces between the cysts correlate with the septa on the mammogram (approx. 30×)

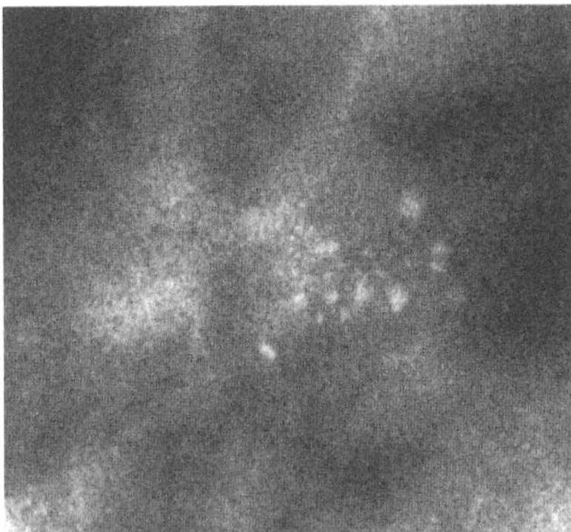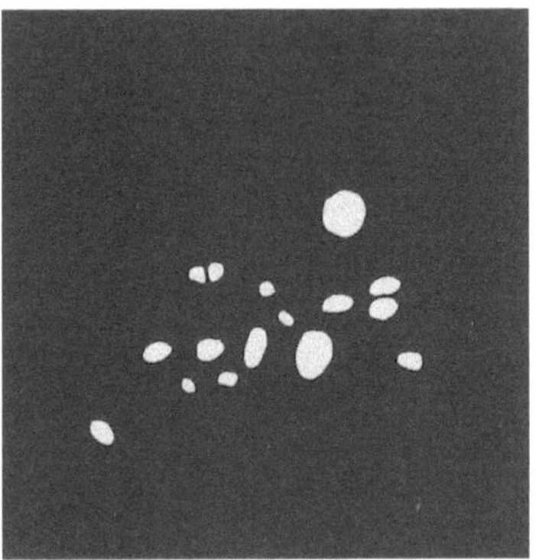

a b

Fig.4.17a, b. Mammogram and semischematic diagram: 3 mm triangular cluster of faint, predominantly punctate microcalcifications. Septation and facetting are visible in two places, creating a diplococcuslike pattern. These signs, together with the small cluster size, are typical of microcystic adenosis. The triangular shape of the cluster results from the incomplete calcification of the otherwise balloon-shaped focus of adenosis. Nevertheless, uncertainty prompted a recommendation for biopsy. Histology: microcystic (blunt duct) adenosis

scribed) or *scattered* (diffuse). Among our own patients who were biopsied for microcalcifications (1974–1983), 12% had a histologic diagnosis of microcystic (blunt duct) adenosis.

Foci of microcystic adenosis are commonly seen on galactograms, where they present at the end of a terminal duct as a dense cluster of tiny cysts resembling a raspberry or a morula (Fig.4.10). The adjacent sides of the cysts are somewhat flattened, giving an impression of "septa," because the tension within the fluid-filled cysts is less than the opposing force of the collagenous capsule bordering the lobule.

LANYI and CITOLER (1981) have shown in comparative radiographic and histologic studies that the radiographic feature characteristic of the microcalcification cluster of microcystic (blunt duct) adenosis is the presence of punctate microcalcifications which are
- 0.1–0.3 mm in size
- uniformly faint or moderately intense
- at least in part densely packed and separated only by fine lines (septations), producing a raspberry- or morulalike pattern (Figs.4.11–4.14)
- collected in round or oval clusters 2–5 mm in diameter (Figs.4.15, 4.16).

The occasional triangular or amorphous cluster shape is probably caused by incomplete calcification of the small intralobular cysts (Fig.4.17). Clusters larger than 5 mm are formed by multiple, densely packed foci of microcystic (blunt duct) adenosis with calcifications (Fig.4.18).

The unpublished studies done in cooperation with HOLLAND and HENDRIKS (Nijmegen Catholic University) and with CITOLER have helped to elucidate the nature of the calcifications in microcystic (blunt duct) adenosis. It was determined that the calcifications were without exception psammomatous, and that they "floated" singly or multiply in milk of calcium contained within the cysts. Apparently these calcifications form by much the same mechanism as pearls do in an oys-

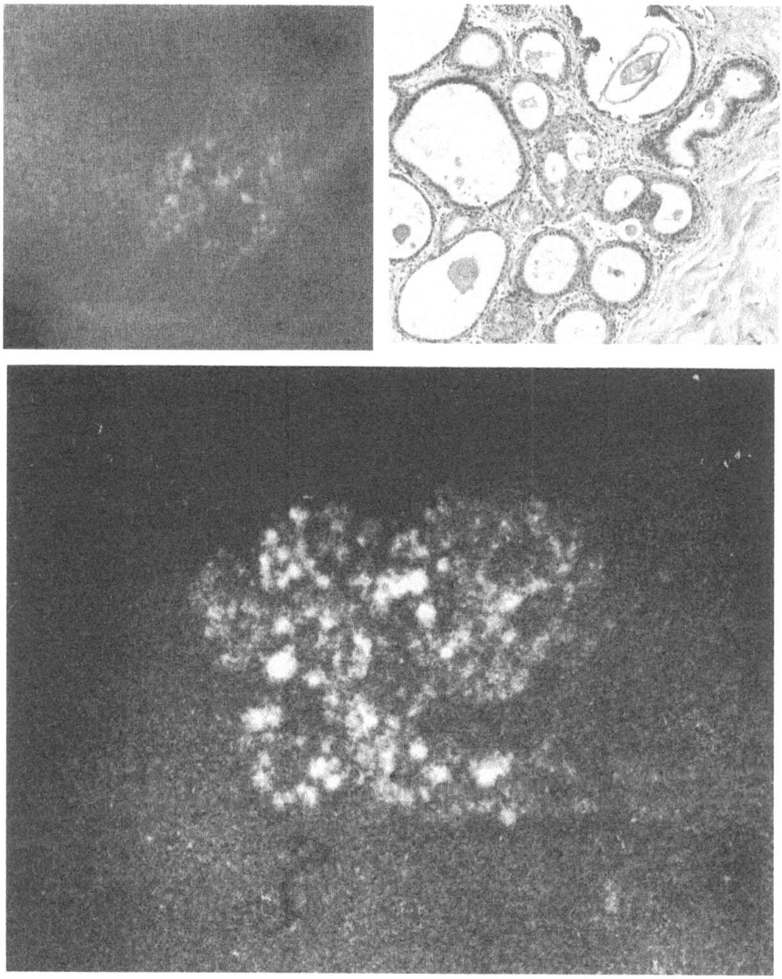

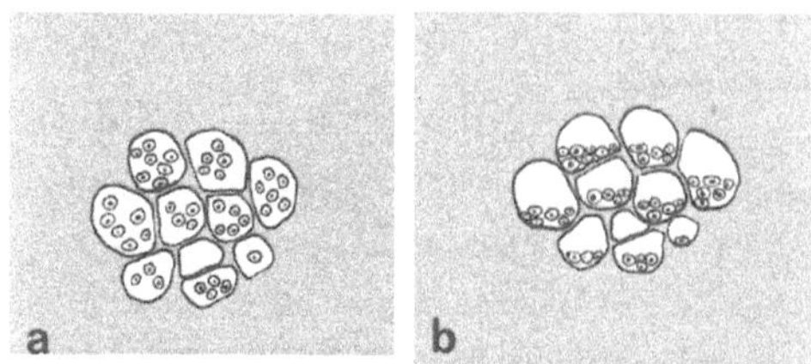

Fig. 4.18. a Mammogram: rounded, dense cluster, 6–7 mm in size, of faint microcalcifications. **b** Specimen radiograph: the cluster is rosette-shaped, appears to consist of several smaller clusters, and shows "septation" between larger calcifications. **c** Histology: microcystic adenosis affecting 2–3 lobules, with calcifications inside the small cysts. There is slight papillary epithelial proliferation. Though the lesion is shrunken by fixation, it corresponds completely to the radiographic picture. Note the septa between contiguous cysts

Fig. 4.19a, b. Schematic drawings of a focus of microcystic adenosis. Milk of calcium and psammomatous granules in the cysts mark the intercystic septa on the mammogram. **a** Craniocaudad view, **b** lateral view

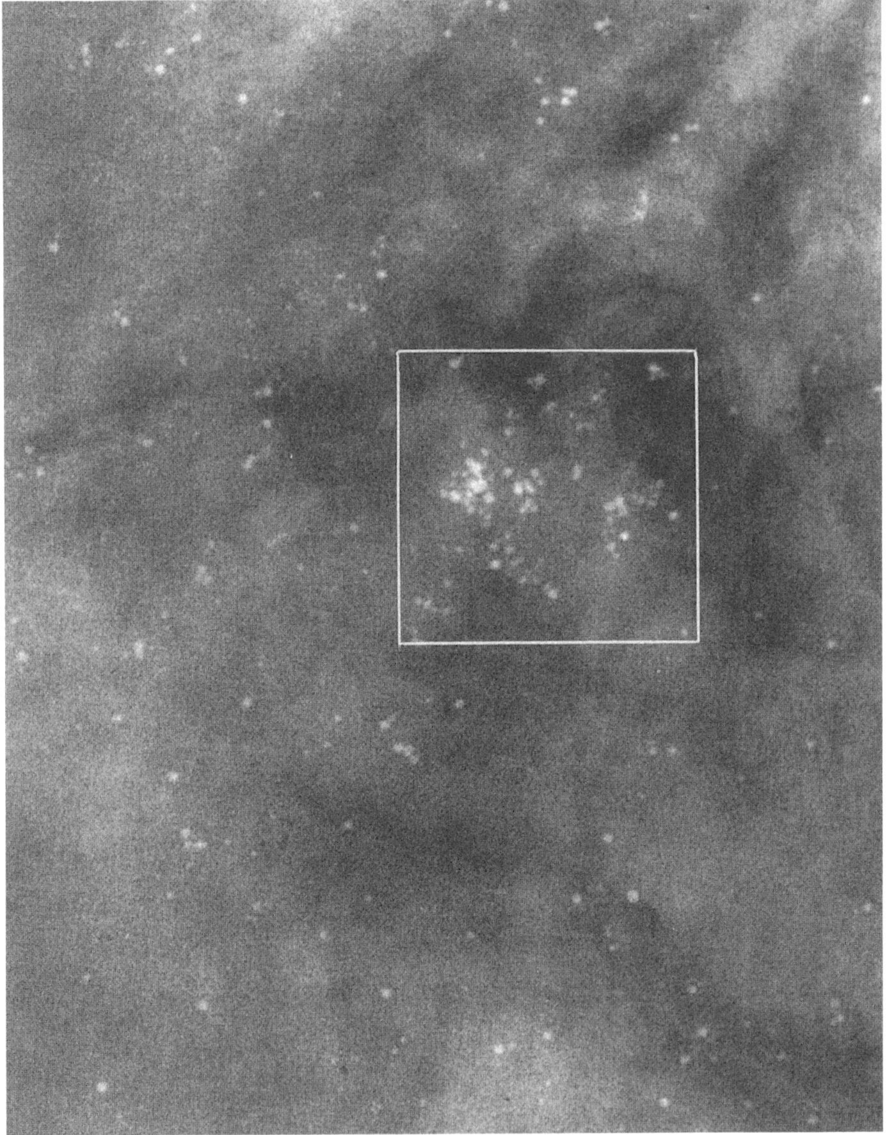

Fig. 4.20. Detail of mammogram (5 ×): scattered, monomorphous, rounded, punctate microcalcifications of uniform size, bilateral. The calcifications are particularly numerous in the boxed area. Previously one spoke of a "clustering tendency" and recommended biopsy on suspicion of carcinoma. But closer analysis reveals the facetting and septation typical of microcystic adenosis. Nowhere is there the polymorphism characteristic of carcinoma. Histology: microcystic (blunt duct) adenosis

ter. On mammograms we do not actually see the tiny psammomatous granules themselves, but the histologically undetectable milk of calcium contained within the cysts. This substance provides a "contrast medium" that delineates the cyst contours and intercystic septa (Fig. 4.19). In some cases, however, large psammomatous calcifications may be seen filling an entire cyst (Fig. 4.13 c).

The diffuse calcifications of microcystic (blunt duct) adenosis form by a similar mechanism, but here the calcification process is not confined to one lobule or a few closely adjacent lobules; it occurs throughout an entire lobe or several lobes of one or both breasts. The punctate microcalcifications are monomorphous and of a uniform size. Clustering is occasionally seen, but the septation establishes the benignity of the condition (Fig. 4.20).

Sclerosing Adenosis

Pathology

Sclerosing (fibrosing) adenosis (FOOTE and STEWART 1945; HAMPERL 1939; INGLEBY and GERSHON-COHEN 1960; URBAN and ADAIR 1949) is a special form of adenosis in which proliferation of the fibrous tissue and myoepithelium surrounding the acini causes compression and deformation of the lobular lumina (Fig. 4.21). This lesion, known also as myoid sclerosis, is a feature of many forms of cystic breast disease. It may also occur in proximity to, yet completely independent of, carcinoma.

In 1144 cases studied histologically from October 1974 to September 1983 at the Gummersbach Radiology Institute, the area surrounding the main abnormality was satisfactorily described in 762 cases. The pathologist found sclerosing adenosis in 143 cases (18.7%), describing it in 12.7% of carcinomas and 23% of benign conditions (Tables 4.1–4.3). Elsewhere in the literature, SANDISON (1958) stated that the overall prevalence of this lobular lesion was 7%, FOOTE and STEWART (1945) found it in 12.5% of benign leisons and 7% of carcinomas, and HOFMANN and BOSBACH (1970) found it in 2.8% of women with breast disease. In our patients biopsied for *clustered* milk of calcium cysts ($n = 52$), sclerosing adenosis was described as a satellite lesion in 15 cases (28.8%), and it was found in 19 out of 38 cases (50%) biopsied for *diffuse* milk of calcium cysts (with or without a "clustering tendency").

Presumably this high association of sclerosing adenosis with milk of calcium cysts led to the false belief that such cysts were the characteristic calcification of sclerosing adenosis (GERSHON-COHEN et al. 1966; HOEFFKEN and LANYI 1973).

Sclerosing adenosis has no clinical significance as long as the sclerosing process – fibromyoepithelial proliferation – does not cross the lobular boundaries and form a palpable mass through pseudoinfiltration. This tumorlike form of sclerosing adenosis is quite difficult to diagnose and is easily mistaken for carcinoma microscopically, especially on frozen sections.

Radiography

Microcalcifications, radial structures, and combinations of the two are the cardinal radiographic features of sclerosing adenosis (Figs. 4.22 and 4.23). The microcalcifications of sclerosing adenosis show considerable polymorphism compared with the uniformly punctate calcifications of microcystic (blunt duct) adenosis. This polymorphism develops as the lobular cysts containing milk of calcium and psammoma bodies become "distorted" by the proliferating myoepithelium and fibrous tissue (Figs. 4.22 and 4.23). As the more recent (unpublished) studies together with CITOLER and with HOLLAND and HENDRIKS indicate, these deformations almost

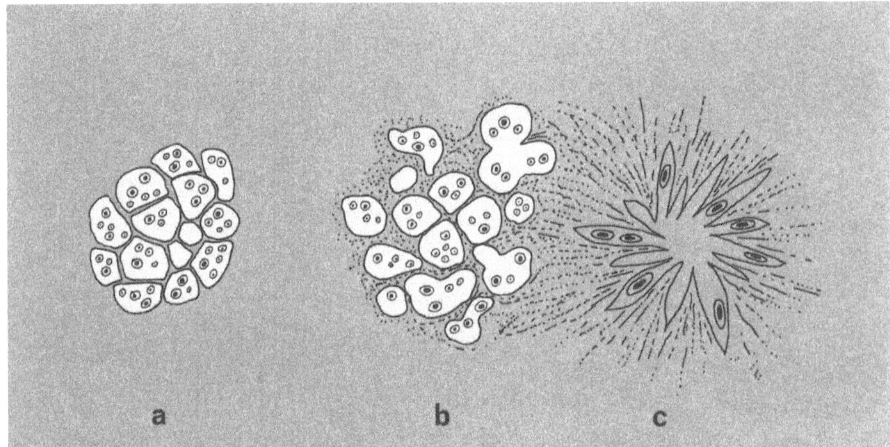

Fig. 4.21 a–c. The evolution of polymorphous microcalcifications associated with sclerosing adenosis. **a** Microcystic (blunt duct) adenosis. **b** Fibromyothelial proliferation occurs around the focus, deforming the lobular cysts, which are filled with milk of calcium and contain psammomatous granules. **c** A completely sclerosed lobule with narrowed acini; occasionally the acini contain microcalcifications, but usually they are not visible radiographically

Table 4.1. Associated histologic findings in 762 cases in which the area surrounding the primary abnormality was adequately described by the pathologist. Proliferative processes ranging from type 2 cystic disease to lobular neoplasia are evenly distributed among malignant and benign lesions, with 36.3% and 36.5% respectively. Lobular neoplasia occurred regularly, regardless of the nature of the primary abnormality. Sclerosing adenosis in the vicinity of carcinoma was noted in almost 13% of the malignant cases

	Malignant (315/499)[a]	Benign (447/645)[a]
Sclerosing adenosis	12.7%	23%
Type II cystic disease	1.6%	13%
Papillomatosis without atypia	16.2%	13%
Papillomatosis with atypia	7.9%	1.8%
Type III cystic disease	0.6%	2.2%
Lobular neoplasia	10.5%	7%

[a] Numbers in parentheses represent the number of cases with accurate histologic description of surrounding area and the total number of cases examined.

always occur in close proximity to the sclerosing adenosis in an adjacent focus of microcystic adenosis, or when a larger focus of microcystic adenosis itself becomes partially sclerosed.

In a lobule that is completely sclerosed, the lumina of the acini become so narrow that they are no longer visible radiographically, even if they contain microcalcifications. It should be remembered that radiographs do not demonstrate the individual psammoma bodies, but rather the cavities that contain *milk of calcium and psammoma bodies*. With CITOLER, the author found on careful histologic study of 26 foci of sclerosing adenosis that, although the radiographic diagnosis had been made on the basis of clustered microcalcifications, there was only one case where

Table 4.2. The malignant lesions (see Table 4.1) were broken down by radiographic features (soft-tissue shadow, soft-tissue shadow + microcalcifications, microcalcifications only). The proliferative processes are evenly distributed in the first two groups (34.9% and 33.8%, respectively). A striking number of lobular neoplasias were found in the cases biopsied on the basis of microcalcifications alone. The incidence of sclerosing adenosis, at more than 26%, also is remarkably high in these cases. The surrounding area was probably examined more carefully in the cases biopsied for microcalcifications alone

	Soft-tissue shadow (194/316)[a]	Soft-tissue shadow + microcalcifications (59/109)[a]	Microcalcifications alone (62/74)[a]
Sclerosing adenosis	9.8%	6.8%	26.6%
Type II cystic disease	2.0%	0%	1.5%
Papillomatosis without atypia	15.5%	20.3%	14.0%
Papillomatosis with atypia	8.2%	5.0%	9.0%
Type III cystic disease	0%	0%	3.0%
Lobular neoplasia	9.3%	8.5%	16.1%

[a] Numbers in parentheses represent the number of cases with accurate histologic description of surrounding area and the total number of cases examined.

Table 4.3. The benign lesions (see Table 4.1) were broken down by radiographic features. From left to right: soft-tissue shadow, clustered milk of calcium cysts, scattered milk of calcium cysts, microcystic (blunt duct) adenosis and sclerosing adenosis detected from microcalcifications, calcified fibroadenoma, calcified secretions, and liponecrotic microcysts. The proliferative processes are rather evenly distributed in the first six groups regardless of radiographic signs (33%–47%). The lobular neoplasias showed virtually the same association with calcified secretions as with clustered milk of calcium cysts; this was considerably higher than their association with scattered milk of calcium cysts or with the adenoses. Sclerosing adenosis was associated with all benign lesions except liponecrotic cysts, showing the highest association with clustered and scattered milk of calcium cysts (28.8% and 50%, respectively). But this also means that no sclerosing adenosis was found in about ⅔ of the clustered and ½ of the scattered milk of calcium cysts

	Soft-tissue shadow 237/402)[a]	Clustered milk of calcium cysts (52/68)[a]	Scattered milk of calcium cysts (38/44)[a]	Micro-cystic adenosis, sclerosing adenosis 70[a]	Calcified fibro-adenoma (20/28)[a]	Calcified secretions (23/25)[a]	Lipo-necrotic microcysts (7/8)[a]
Sclerosing adenosis	19.4%	28.8%	50.0%	27.1%	5.0%	17.3%	0%
Type II cystic disease	10.1%	17.3%	15.8%	17.1%	15.0%	8.6%	14.2%
Papillomatosis without atypia	10.5%	15.4%	21.0%	12.9%	10.0%	26%	0%
Papillomatosis with atypia	2.9%	0%	0%	1.4%	0%	0%	0%
Type III cystic disease	3.4%	0%	2.6%	1.4%	0%	0%	0%
Lobular neoplasia	5.5%	13.5%	7.9%	4.3%	5.0%	13%	0

[a] The numbers in parenthesis represent the number of cases with accurate histologic description of surrounding area and the total number of cases examined.

microcalcifications within the narrowed, compressed acini were present histologically in a size that could be seen on mammograms. On the other hand, the picture was always the same: small, deformed cysts of microcystic adenosis adjacent or peripheral to an area of sclerosis (Figs. 4.21 and 4.23). The small, deformed cysts filled with milk of calcium may appear linear, curvilinear, or v-shaped on radiographs and thus mimic the calcification shapes of intraductal carcinoma (see p. 108) (MacErlean and Nathan 1972). This raises the danger of misinterpretation by the radiologist. Fortunately, there will almost always be undeformed microcysts with septation that will enable a correct diagnosis to be made. This "diplococcuslike" pattern is hardly ever seen with intraductal carcinoma! The variations in the calcification shapes of sclerosing adenosis can be substantial; however, when the cluster is rounded or rosette-shaped, a correct mammographic diagnosis is facilitated. The cluster may range from 3 to 8 mm in size. Extensive, diffuse sclerosing adenosis like that shown in Fig. 4.24 is rare.

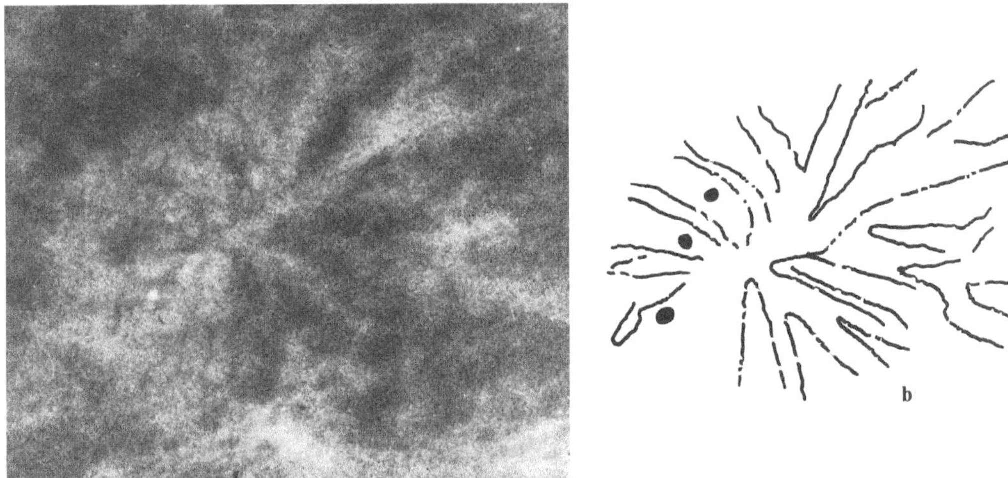

Fig. 4.22. a Detail of mammogram (3.5 ×); **b** schematic drawing. Radial feature with three microcalcifications. Although the radial structure is not typical of carcinoma, the development of a small scirrhus on the basis of a comedocarcinoma cannot be ruled out. Histology: sclerosing adenosis with fibromyothelial proliferation

Fig. 4.23 a–d. Two cases of sclerosing adenosis biopsied on the basis of clustered microcalcifica- ▷ tions. **a** Specimen radiograph (approx. 5 ×): dense, round-to-oval, rosette-shaped cluster of numerous punctate, comma-, and v-shaped (polymorphous) microcalcifications. Closer analysis shows that the cluster is probably made up to four or five smaller clusters. **b** Histology: lobule with areas of fibrotic proliferation. Most of the originally rounded lobular cysts are elongated and deformed (approx. 80 ×). **c** Section from an adjacent lobule, also fibrotic, showing the deformed cystic cavities with psammomatous granules. It is reasonable that milk of calcium in these cavities would present radiographically as in **a** (approx. 150 ×). Case from the Nijmegen Cathologic University, the Netherlands (Dr. Holland, Dr. Hendriks). **d** Detail of mammogram, magnified approx. 5 ×. This picture from the Gummerbach Radiology Institute is almost identical to **a.** Histology: sclerosing adenosis (Professor Citoler, Cologne)

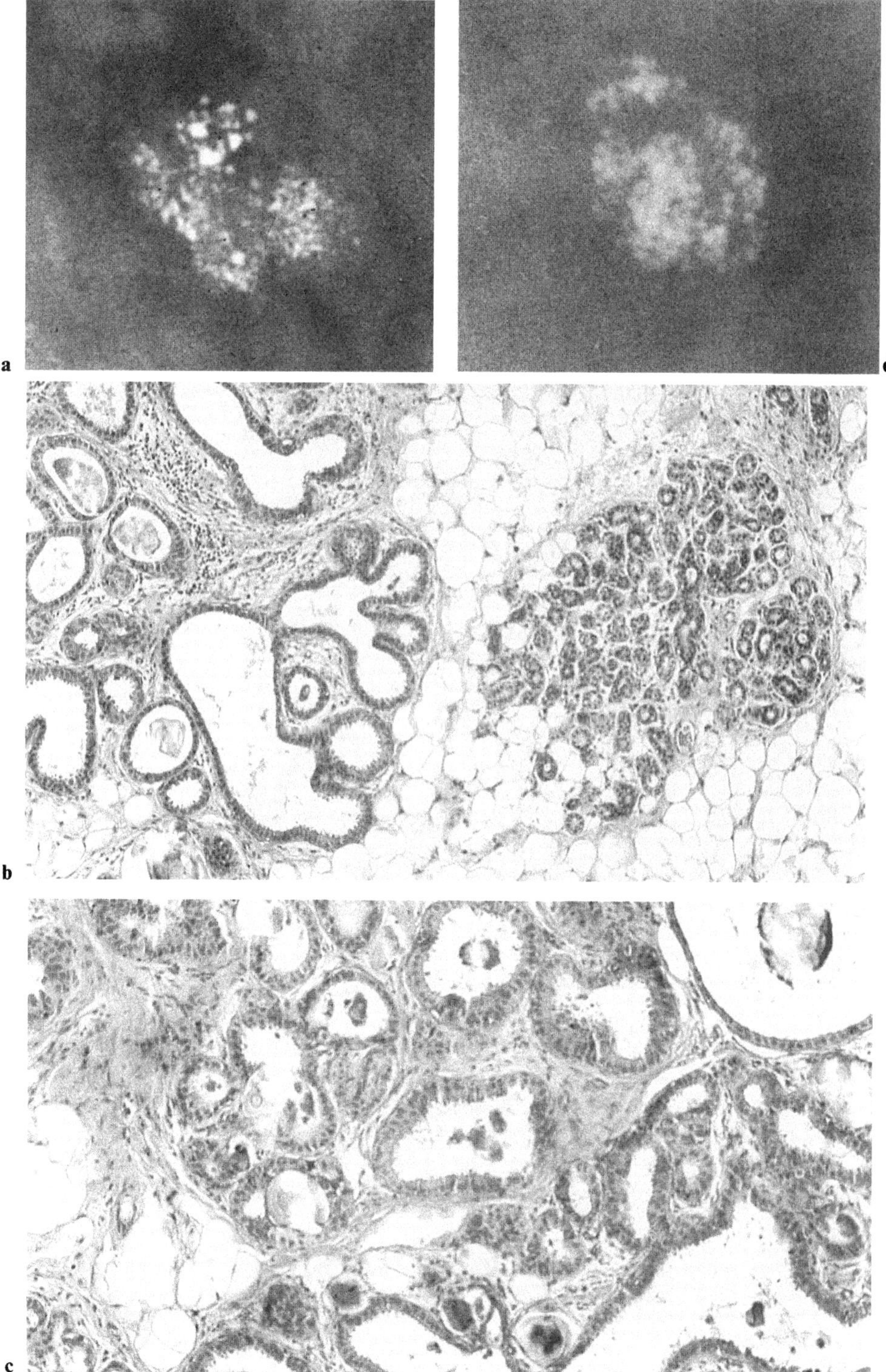

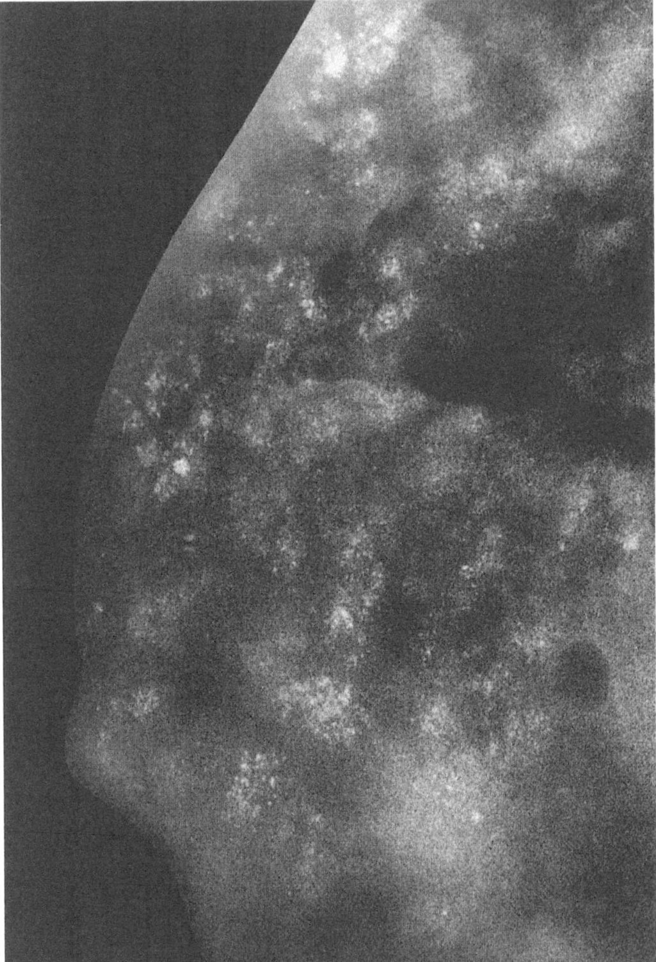

Fig. 4.24. Detail of mammogram (4×): numerous oval, amorphous, partly coalescent clusters of predominantly rounded, punctate, occasionally polymorphous microcalcifications. Similar but less pronounced changes were visible in the opposite breast. Histology: extensive sclerosing adenosis

Besides the cases of microcystic (blunt duct) and sclerosing adenosis identified in cases where the area surrounding the principal lesion was adequately described by the pathologist, there were 12 cases of type 2 cystic disease[1] (17.1%), 1 case of type 3 cystic disease (1.4%), 9 of papillomatosis without atypia (12.9%), 1 of papillomatosis with atypia (1.4%), and 3 of LCIS (4.3%). In 44 cases no proliferative changes were seen in proximity to these microcalcifications of lobular origin (Table 4.3).

---

[1] In the classification commonly used in Germany for describing the risk of malignant transformation – similar to the classifications of KIAER (1954) and INGLEBY and GERSHON-COHEN (1960) – type 1 is cystic disease without epithelial proliferation, type 2 with epithelial proliferation but without atypia, and type 3 proliferation with moderate atypia. The practical utility of such a classification is very questionable.

Microcystic Disease with Milk of Calcium Cysts
Pathology

Cystic breast disease originates in the lobules. Recalling the pattern of progression mentioned earlier (lobular hypertrophy→large acini→blunt duct adenosis→microcystic adenosis), it is apparent that the cysts will enlarge beyond the lobular boundaries when the pressure of the cystic contents becomes greater than the resistance of the collagen capsule surrounding the lobule (Figs. 4.9 and 4.25). The multilocular cysts do not lose their original character, and they are really nothing but oversized adenosis cysts. When they are seen to communicate with their terminal milk duct on the pneumocystogram, the evidence is conclusive (Fig. 4.26).

The simple (uncomplicated) cysts are lined by flat, cuboidal epithelial cells. If the secretion contains calcium, psammoma bodies will form as previously described ("mammolithiasis" after FRANTZ et al. 1951) (Figs. 4.28 c and 4.38 c). Knowing the lobular origin of breast cysts, it is correct to say that cysts containing milk of calcium probably contain psammoma bodies from the outset, and that only the number of bodies increases as the cyst becomes larger. BÄSSLER (1978) claims that cysts of this type are extremely rare, but in the author's material 112 cases of clustered or diffuse milk of calcium cysts were confirmed histologically; they represent 46.0% of all cases biopsied for microcalcifications. As a rule these cysts contain psammoma bodies, but usually they are not detected or reported by the pathologist because they do not contribute to the histologic diagnosis.

Another type of calcification is the circumscribed cyst wall calcification resulting from the deposition of calcium salts in the fibrous capsule.

Radiography

The following mammographic signs of milk of calcium cysts were first described by LANYI in 1977 and confirmed by SICKLES and ABELE in 1981. This type of calcification was once considered pathognomonic for sclerosing adenosis (GERSHON-COHEN et al. 1966; HOEFFKEN and LANYI 1973), but actually the cyst itself has nothing to do with this process. We are dealing, rather, with the incidental concurrence of two components of cystic disease on two entirely different levels of examination: milk of calcium cysts on the mammogram, and sclerosing adenosis on the histologic section (Tables 4.1–4.3).

On mammograms, the milk of calcium cyst may appear as a rounded, calcium dense feature 1–2 mm in diameter in both views (Fig. 4.36 a). Alternatively, it may appear as a rounded smudge of variable density 2–5 mm in size on the craniocaudal view (Fig. 4.28 a), and as a superiorly flattened, teacup-shaped density on the lateral view (Figs. 4.27, 4.28 b, 4.37). The explanation for this phenomenon is simple: on the mediolateral projection in the standing patient, the calcific psammomatous granules, with their higher specific gravity, settle out of the lighter components of the secretion (protein and fat) and form a visible sediment on the bottom of the cyst. This stratification is not apparent in the craniocaudal projection. (In the past this phenomenon was not seen on lateral mammograms taken in the supine position.) Similarly, fluid levels are sometimes seen in cysts visualized by galactography when the cyst fluid does not mix well with the water-soluble contrast medium (Figs. 4.27 b, 4.30 a, b and 4.31). Histologic examination generally will confirm the presence of

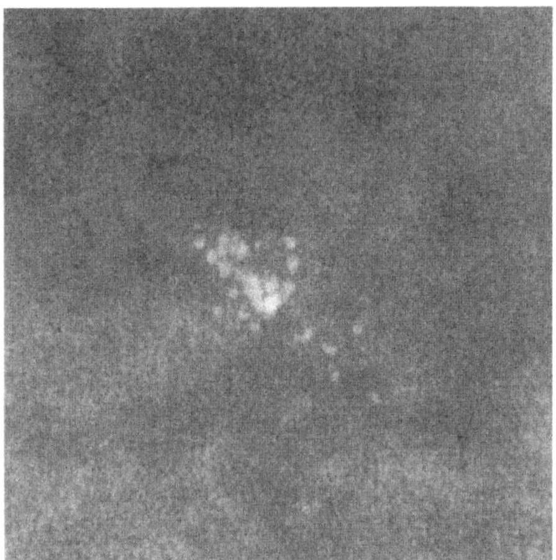 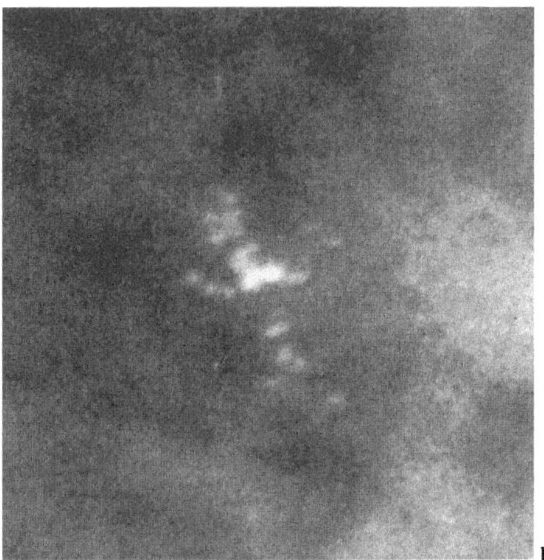

a   b

Fig. 4.25 a, b. Details (4 ×) from lateral mammograms showing the development of milk of calcium cysts from a focus of microcystic adenosis. **a** Amorphous, triangular cluster of about 30 densely grouped microcalcifications, 2 of which are amorphous (comma-shaped?); all others are punctate, some facetted with multiple septa. Radiographic diagnosis: despite the cluster configuration and minimal polymorphism, the facetting and septation are strongly suggestive of microcystic adenosis. Follow-up is advised. **b** One year later, the small cysts have enlarged, and almost all show "teacup signs" with occasional septa; the former questionable polymorphism is no longer apparent

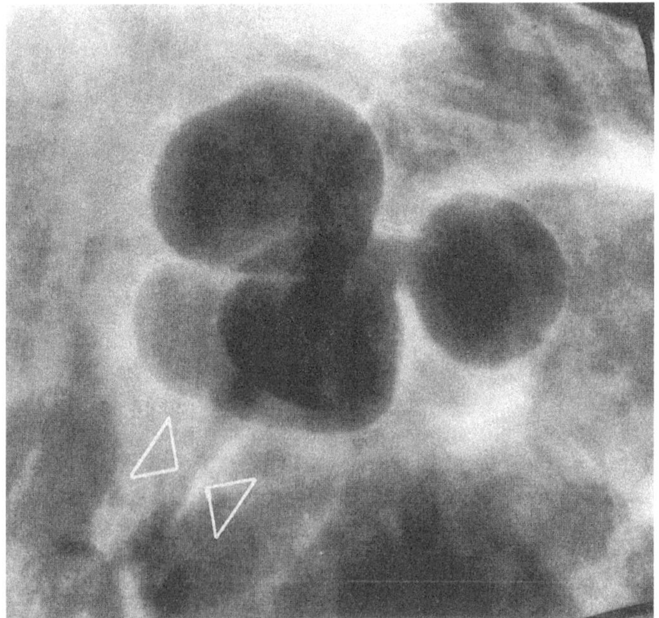

Fig. 4.26. Pneumocystogram: multilocular cyst 2 cm in size, with air delineating the associated terminal duct *(arrows)*. This is an extraordinarily large cystic adenosis

---

Fig. 4.27. a Lateral mammogram: multiple punctate, predominantly linear or "teacup" calcifica- ▷ tions. **b** Lateral galactogram of the involved segment: associated with the microcalcifications are small cysts, some of which appear teacup-shaped, indicating that the cystic contents have not mixed with the contrast medium (2 ×)

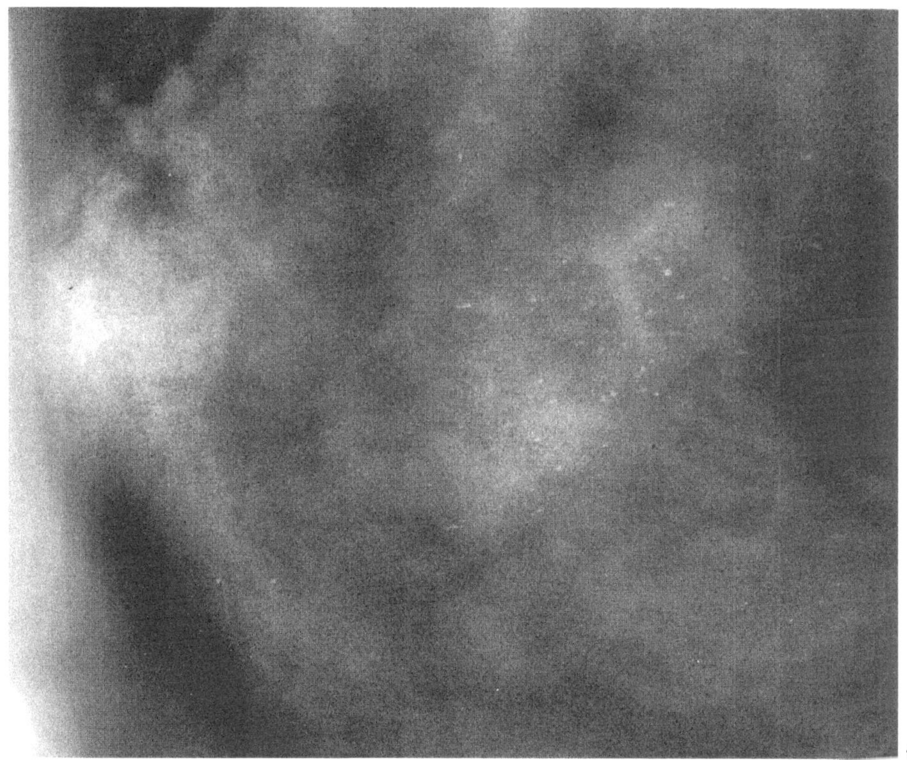

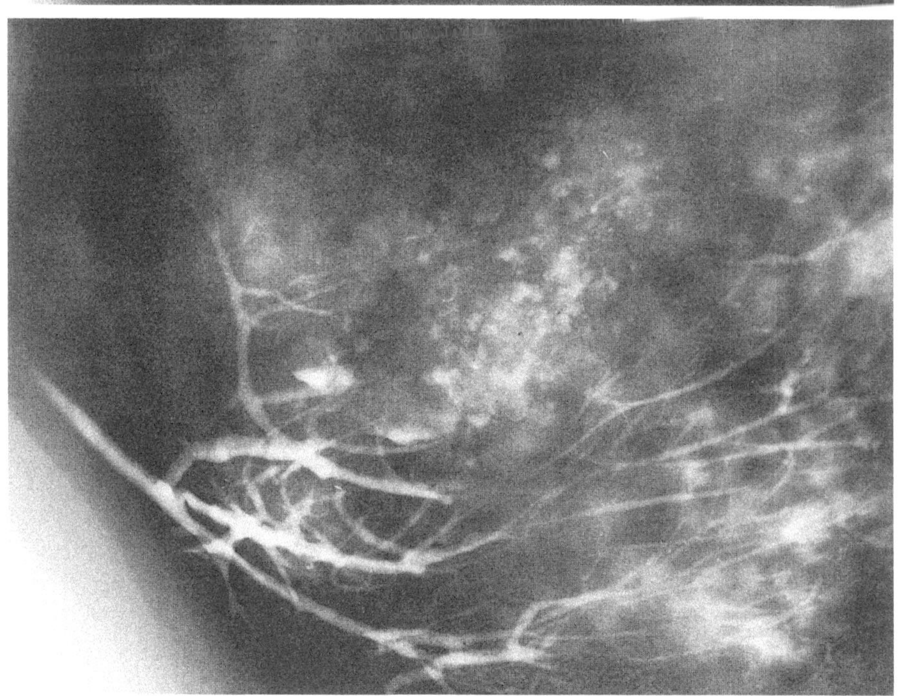

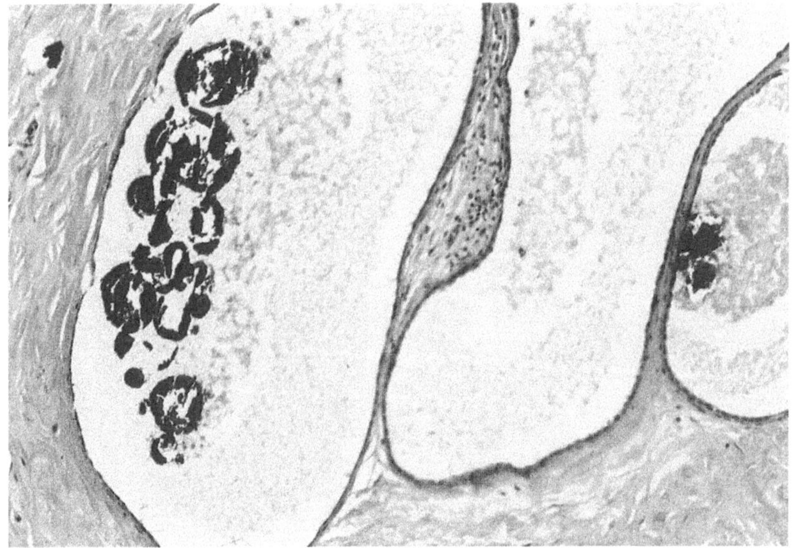

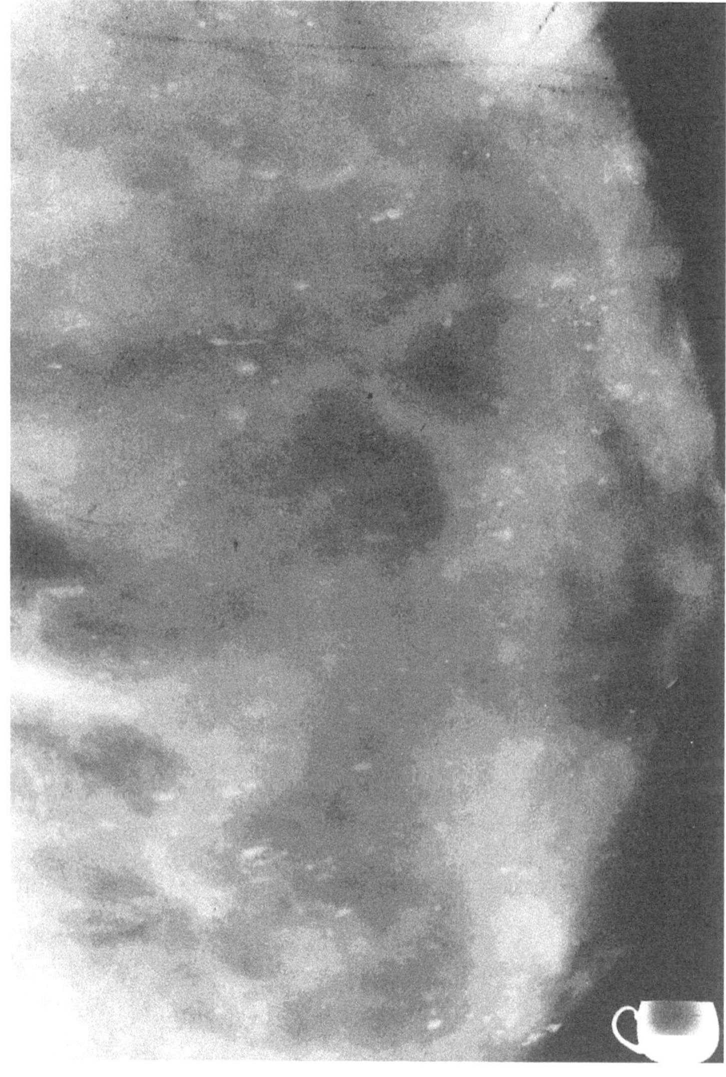

b

Fig. 4.28 a-c. Details of mammograms (3 ×). **a** Craniocaudad view: numerous scattered, predominantly faint, rounded microcalcifications. **b** Lateral view: here the calcifications appear teacup-shaped due to the presence of fluid levels. The contralateral picture is identical. **c** After bilateral subcutaneous mastectomy, careful histologic examination showed ubiquitous cysts with flattened epithelium and secretions or with psammomatous beads, which proved to be calcium granules on Kossa staining (approx. 50 ×)

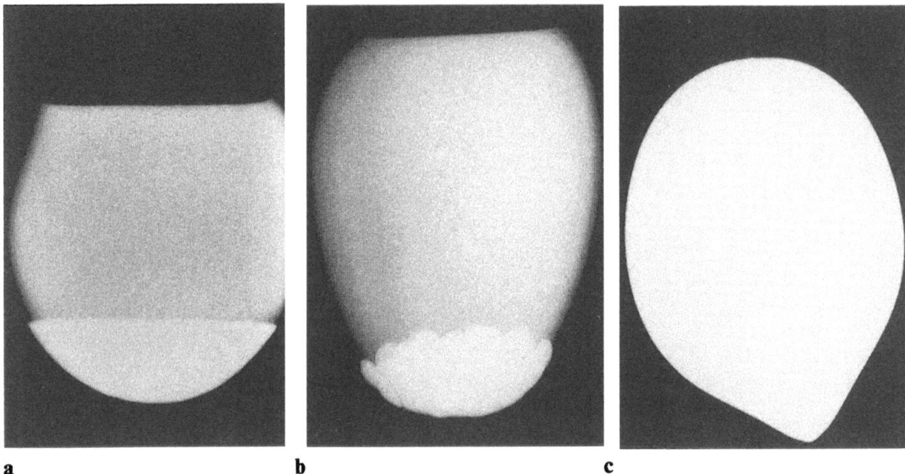

a   b   c

Fig.4.29a-c. In an experiment, an air balloon was filled with barium sulfate and with calcium tablets. Lateral radiographs were taken without compression (**a**) and with compression (**b**) and a craniocaudad film (**c**) was taken. While the calcium tablets exhibit the teacup sign without compression (**a**), the "bottom sediment" becomes heaped up when compression is applied (**b**)

psammoma bodies in the cyst lumen (Figs. 4.28 c and 4.38 c). Sometimes milk of calcium cysts present a fusiform shape on lateral mammograms. This is most likely caused by the compression of the breast, which heaps the loose sediment into a pile (Fig. 4.29 b). Milk of calcium cysts may be clustered or scattered. Clustered milk of calcium cysts that are demonstrable on two views may well belong to a single terminal duct (Fig. 4.30), whereas scattered cysts belong to an entire duct system or to multiple duct segments (Fig. 4.31). If the secretion is not calcified in all cysts, but several cysts within a larger area contain calcified secretions, a "pseudocluster" is created. This occurs when the plane of the projection creates the illusion of a cluster where none exists (Fig. 4.32). Pseudoclusters often are visible only on one plane, because the cysts do not belong to the same terminal duct.

Milk of calcium cysts tend to occur bilaterally, but they may be more numerous in one breast than the other. Clusters of these cysts are usually rounded or amorphous (Figs. 4.33 and 4.34); triangular and propeller configurations are rare (Fig. 4.35). Together with other radiographic signs of cystic disease, they are found in association with a large, palpable cyst or calcified fibroadenoma. Milk of calcium cysts and microcystic (blunt duct) or sclerosing adenosis often coexist.

In 90 histologically examined cases of clustered and scattered milk of calcium cysts in which the area surrounding the main abnormality was satisfactorily described, we found 15 cases of type 2^2 cystic disease (16.7%), 1 of type 3 cystic disease (1.1%), 16 of papillomatosis without atypia (17.8%), and no papillomatosis with atypia. Lobular neoplasia was described in 10 cases (11.1%). There was no appreciable difference between clustered and scattered milk of calcium cysts in

---

[2] See footnote 1 on p. 50.

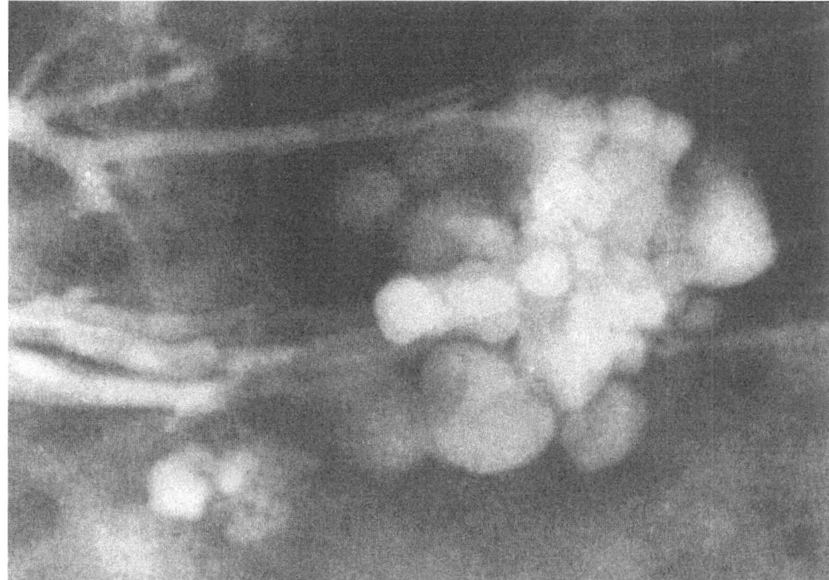

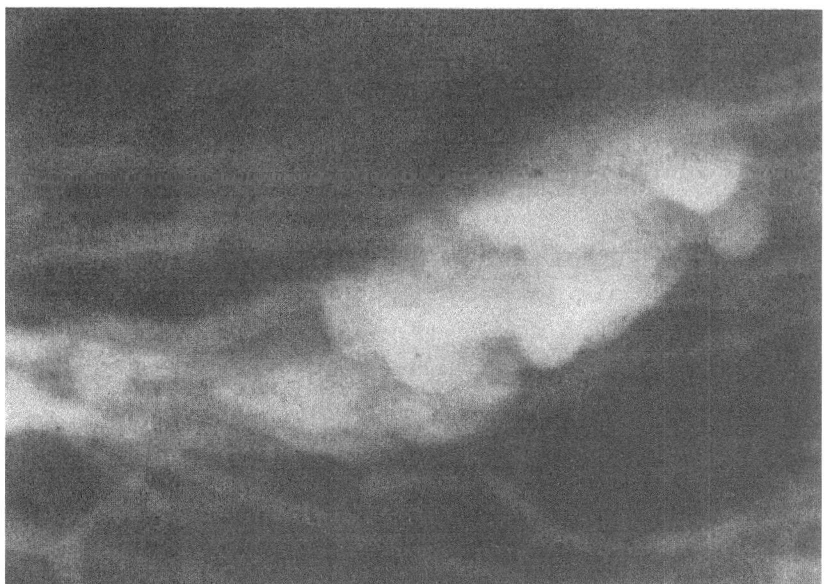

Fig. 4.30a, b. Galactogram (approx. 4×). **a** Craniocaudad view: extensive, round-to-oval cluster of cysts at the end of a duct. **b** The same cluster appears oval on the lateral view, and some cysts show fluid levels ("teacups"). If such cysts contained milk of calcium, the picture of clustered milk of calcium cysts would appear

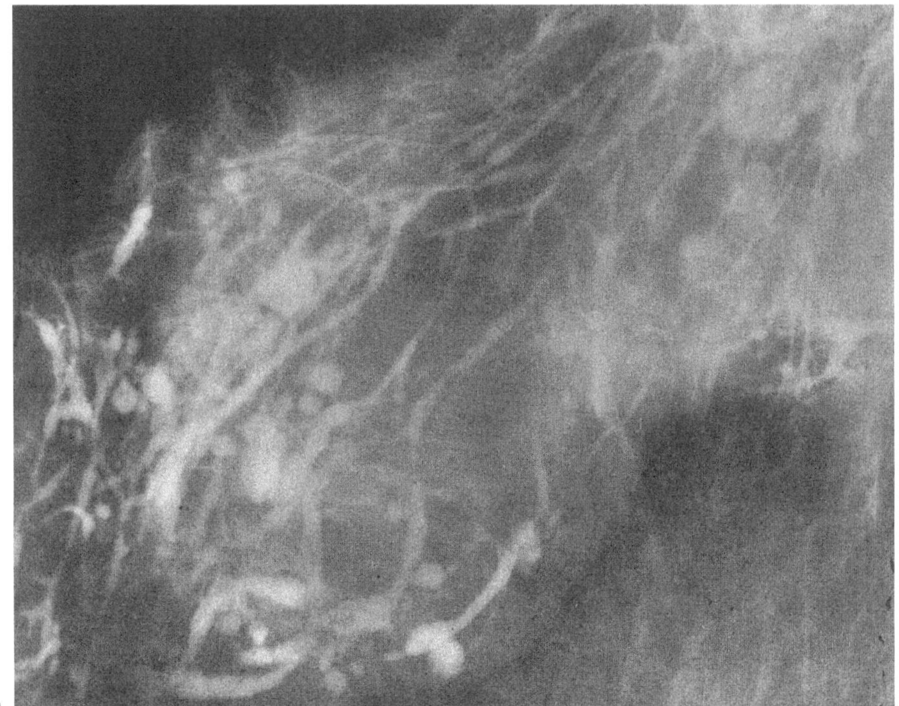

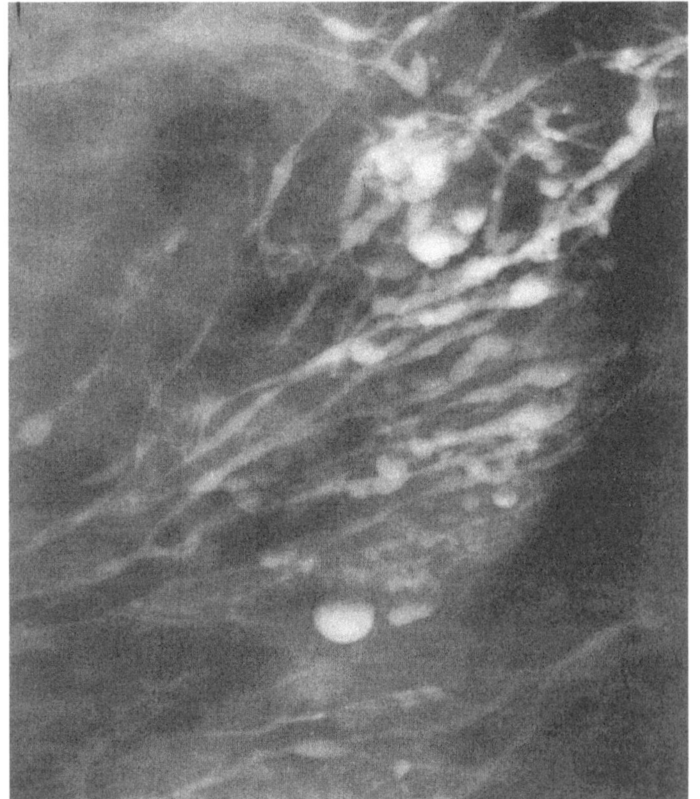

Fig. 4.31 a, b

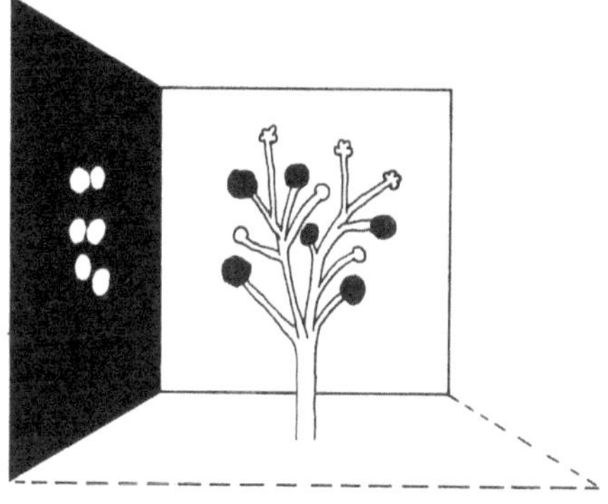

Fig. 4.32. Drawing showing how a "pseudo-cluster" of milk of calcium cysts *(black spots)* is created. These cysts do not belong to the same duct, but their projection simulates the appearance of a clustered array (*white spots* on black background)

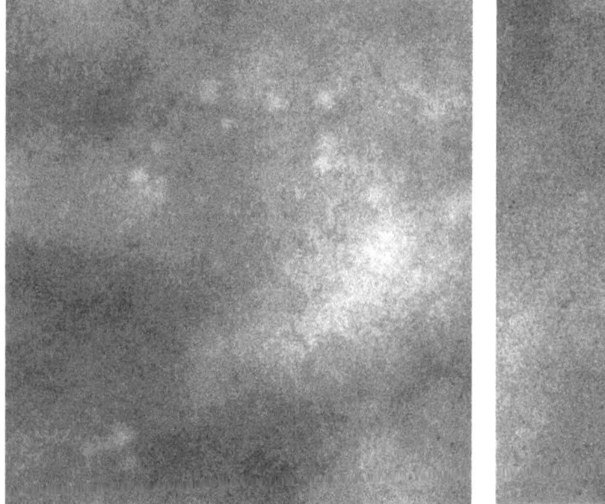

a

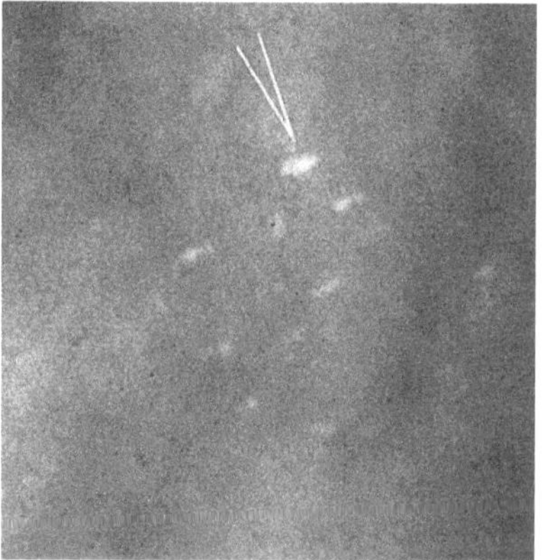

b

Fig. 4.33 a, b. Details of mammograms (4 ×). **a** Craniocaudad view: round-to-oval cluster of about 15 faint, rounded microcalcifications. **b** The cluster also appears rounded on the lateral view. The calcifications, however, are streaklike, teacup-shaped, and hill-shaped (one at the top, *arrow)*

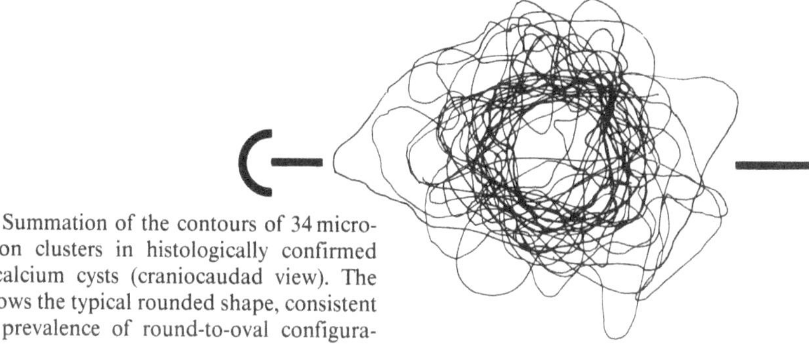

Fig. 4.34. Summation of the contours of 34 micro-calcification clusters in histologically confirmed milk of calcium cysts (craniocaudad view). The "core" shows the typical rounded shape, consistent with the prevalence of round-to-oval configurations

◁ **Fig. 4.31 a, b.** Galactogram (low magnification). **a** Craniocaudad view: numerous cysts are demonstrated at the ends of the ducts. **b** Lateral view: fluid levels are visible in some of the cysts. If these cysts contained milk of calcium, the picture of scattered milk of calcium cysts would appear

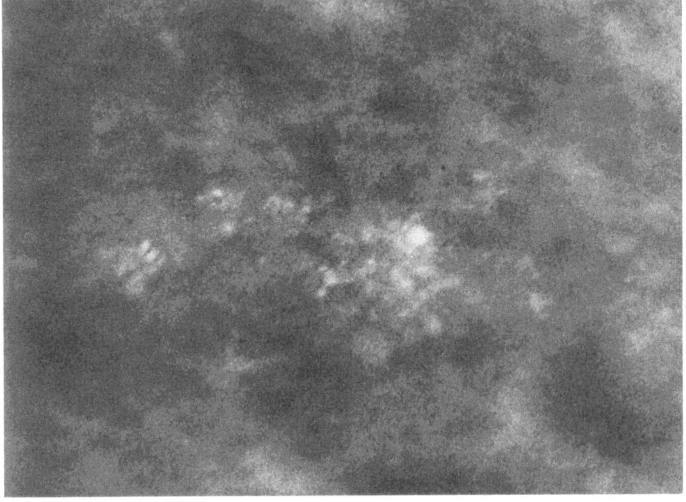

a

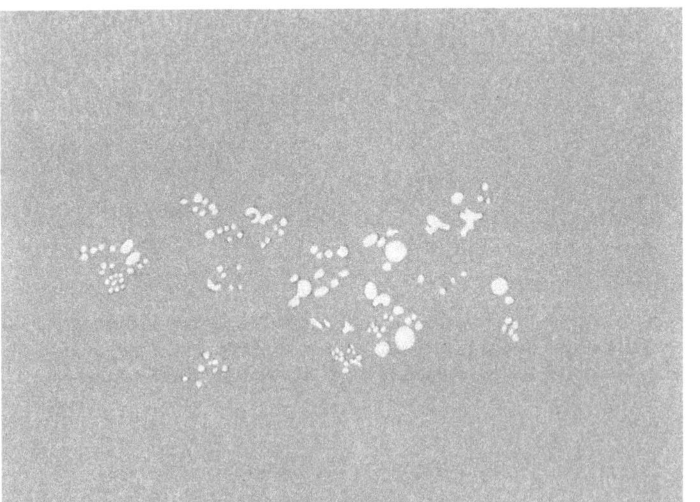

b

Fig. 4.35 a–d. Details of mammograms with accompanying semischematic diagrams (4×). **a, b** Craniocaudad view shows a roughly propeller-shaped cluster of predominantly faint, rounded, occasionally comma-shaped or branched microcalcifications. Smaller clusters typical of microcystic adenosis are also seen. **c, d** On the lateral view the cluster shape is approximately rectangular. Several microcalcifications show teacup signs. Histology: milk of calcium cysts

terms of proliferative processes (see Tables 4.1–4.3). Thus, like microcystic (blunt duct) adenosis and sclerosing adenosis, milk of calcium cysts are unrelated to proliferative processes in their environment (Fig. 4.36).

Milk of calcium cysts are rarely found in association with breast carcinoma. The author has seen such an association only twice. One case involved large, unilateral milk of calcium cysts coexisting with a mammographically occult, clinically pal-

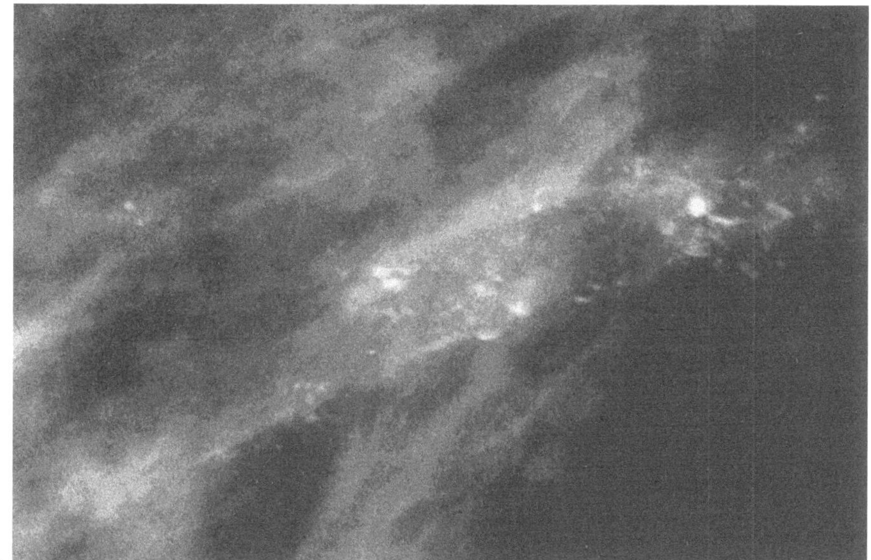

c

d

Fig. 4.35 c, d

pable carcinoma (Fig. 4.37). In another case a tubular carcinoma was found adjacent to clustered milk of calcium cysts, which also were visible histologically (Fig. 4.38). No causal relationship existed between the cysts and the malignancies, and their coexistence was purely coincidental.

Calcifications of the cyst wall are crescent-shaped (Fig. 4.39) or consist of multiple punctate, ringlike, or amorphous microcalcifications (Fig. 4.40).

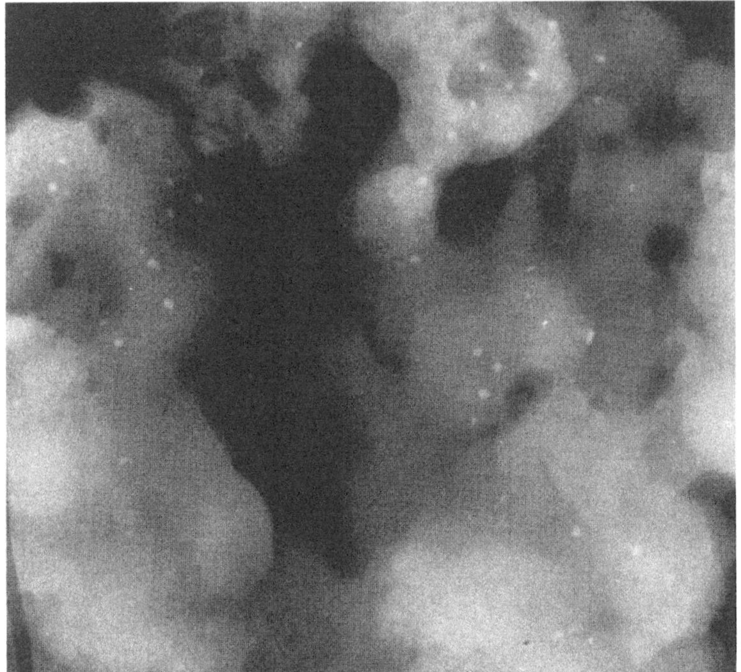

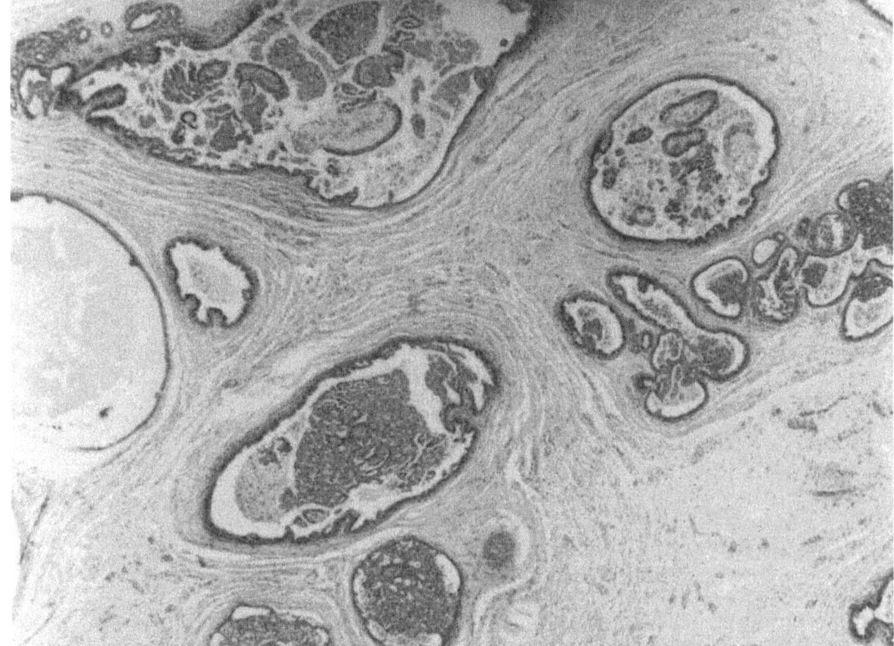

Fig. 4.36a, b

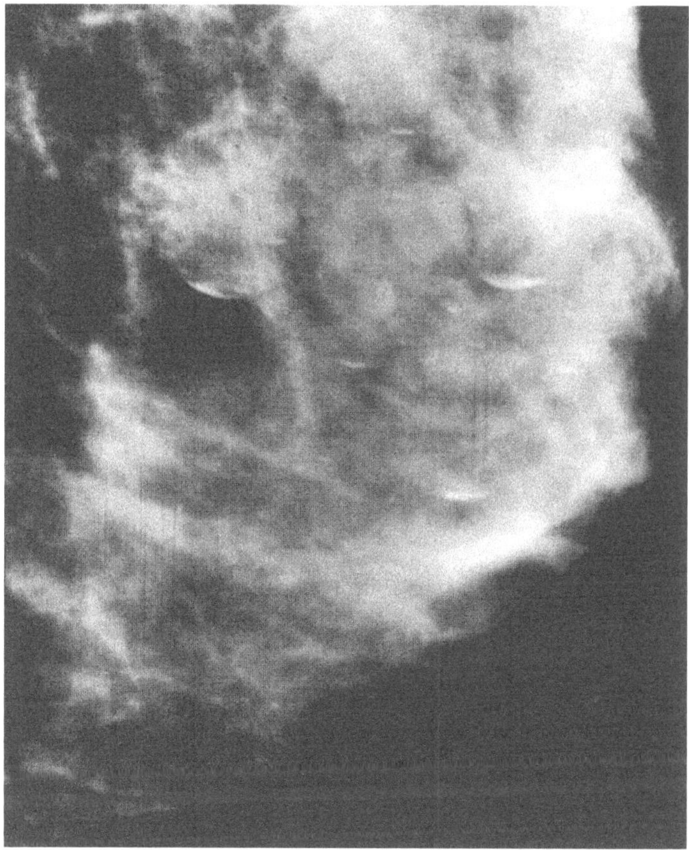

Fig.4.37. Detail of lateral mammogram (original size): unusually large milk of calcium cysts with teacup signs in the setting of gross cystic disease. The clinical finding suggests carcinoma (palpable behind the nipple), which is mammographically occult

◁ **Fig.4.36. a** The specimen radiograph shows rounded, monomorphous microcalcifications of uniform size occupying an area of about 2 cm in a 17-year-old girl. No teacup signs were visible on the lateral film. Because milk of calcium cysts are unusual at this age, biopsy was recommended. Histology (Professor CITOLER): relatively severe juvenile papillomatosis with milk of calcium cysts. The calcifications were located within the cysts; the intraductal papillomas were free of calcifications. **b** The photomicrograph shows a typical section (approx. 30 ×). The patient has been followed clinically for 7 years and is well

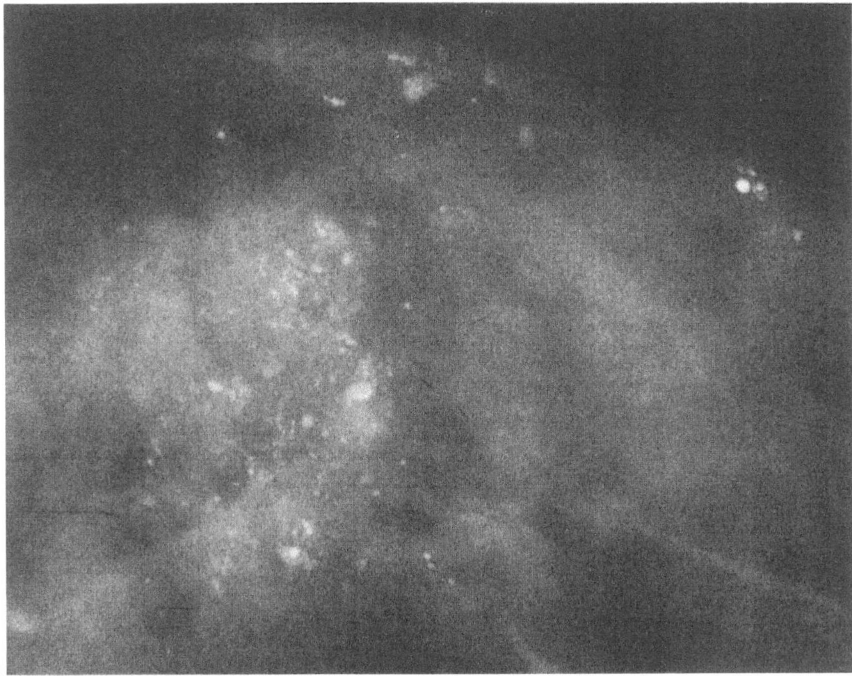

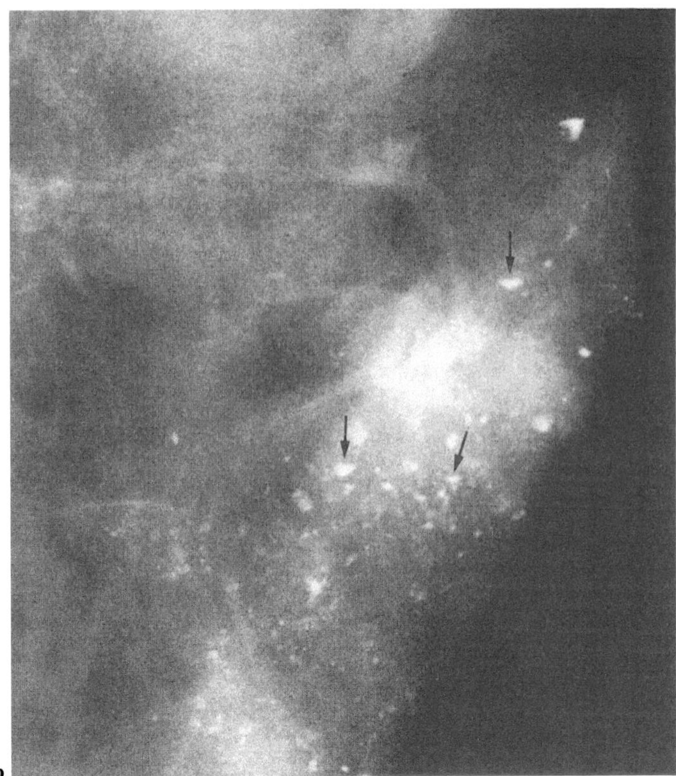

Fig. 4.38 a, b

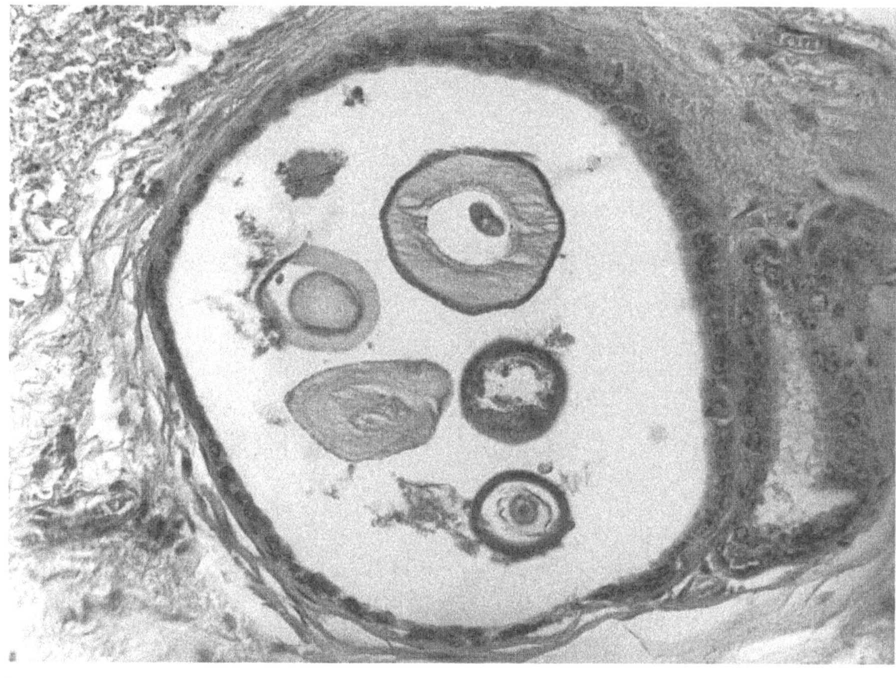

c

Fig. 4.38. a Detail of craniocaudad mammogram (4×). Rounded calcifications of varying size coexist with several fine, linear microcalcifications and microcalcifications arranged in small clusters, characteristic of microcystic (blunt duct) adenosis **b** The lateral view shows several teacups *(arrows).* **c** Histology (Professor CITOLER, Cologne): numerous milk of calcium cysts with psammoma bodies (approx. 300×); a tubular carcinoma 8 mm in size was noted separately

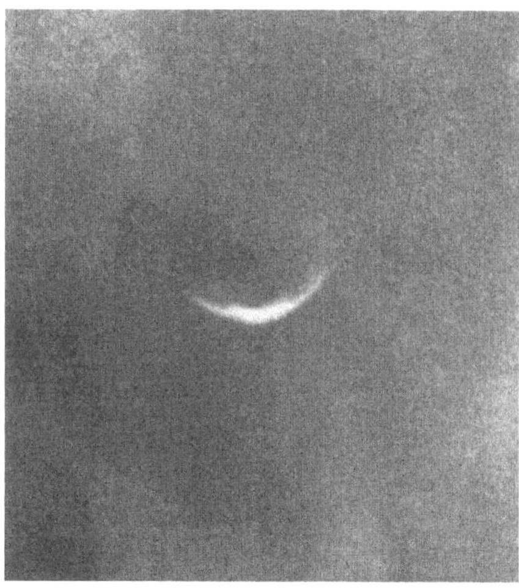

Fig. 4.39. Crescent-shaped calcification of the cyst wall (4×)

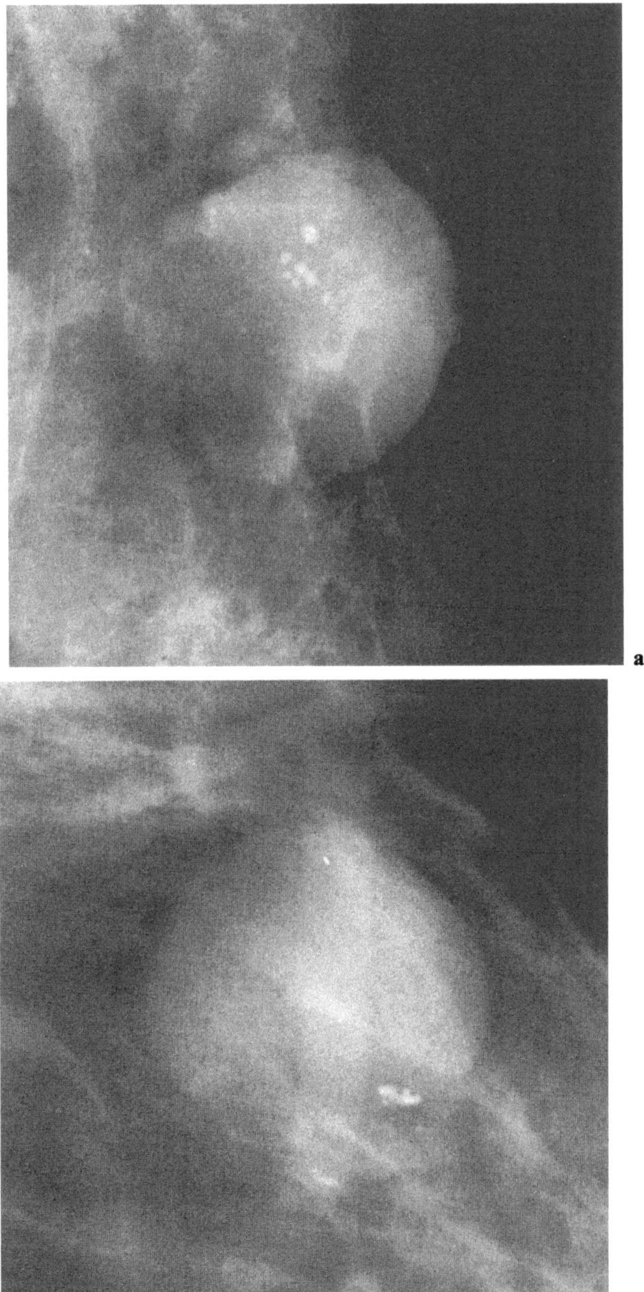

Fig. 4.40 a, b. Details of mammograms (4 ×). **a** Craniocaudad view: round, slightly lobulated shadow with smooth margins containing a cluster of 9 or 10 rounded microcalcifications. These appear at the periphery of the lesion on the lateral view **b**. Cyst with mural calcifications

Lobular Neoplasia, Lobular Precancer or Lobular Carcinoma In Situ

Pathology

Lobular neoplasia, so-called lobular carcinoma in situ, represents the most difficult chapter in current breast pathology, because it is the most contradictory. The problems began with the naming of the lesion. The correct name for a disease should not only express its etiology but should also suggest an appropriate choice of treatment.

A number of names have been suggested over the years for lobular carcinoma in situ. These are, in chronological order: acinar carcinoma (CORNIL 1908; MUIR 1941); lobular carcinoma in situ, abbreviated LCIS, CLIS, or LCS (FOOTE and STEWART 1941); lobular neoplasia (HAAGENSEN 1962); and lobular precancer (BÄSSLER 1978). Interestingly, the names for the lesion have become milder over time, and the use of "so-called" with lobular carcinoma in situ represents an attempt at compromise.

The main problems are:

1) The histologic features are not uniform.
2) The role of lobular neoplasia in carcinogenesis is obscure.
3) The choice of treatment is controversial.

Histologic Features of Lobular Neoplasia

The histologic features of lobular neoplasia (LCIS) are not uniform. The term "carcinoma in situ" generally denotes a process that is *clearly malignant cytologically* (nuclear polymorphism, polychromatophilia, a shift of the nucleocytoplasmic ratio in favor of the nuclei, numerous mitoses), but which is *preinvasive,* meaning that it has not yet broken through the basement membrane.

In the case of lobular neoplasia, HAAGENSEN (1971) states that there are two basic types that may occur simultaneously. In *type A* the lumina of the lobule and possibly of the terminal duct are filled with small, *monomorphous* epithelial cells with a pale cytoplasm. The nuclei are round and show no *mitoses* or *hyperchromatism,* although very rarely these cytomorphologic features of malignancy may be noted (Fig. 4.41 a). In *type B* the cells are larger and less uniform than in type A, and the nuclei are hyperchromatic (Fig. 4.41 b). Thus the cells show certain characteristics of atypia. The more pronounced this atypia, the greater the likelihood that a true carcinoma exists.

According to FISHER and FISHER (1977) and HAAGENSEN (1971) these lesions are as difficult to distinguish from innocent lobular hyperplasia as they are from true carcinoma. ROSEN (1984) similarly states that the minimum criteria for a histologic diagnosis of LCIS have not been established, so that the different statistics on malignant transformation are not comparable with one another.

CITOLER (personal communication, 1984) points out that the type A form of the disease is losing much of its former significance. Increasingly, reviews of earlier "type A" cases are showing that the lesion actually was a simple lobular hyperplasia. An unpublished study done by the author in collaboration with ZIPPEL and NEUFANG has shown that lobular neoplasia in proximity to "true" carcinomas are predominantly of the polymorphous type (type A + B→intermediate type→type B), but that type A lesions tend to occur in proximity to benign processes (Table 4.4).

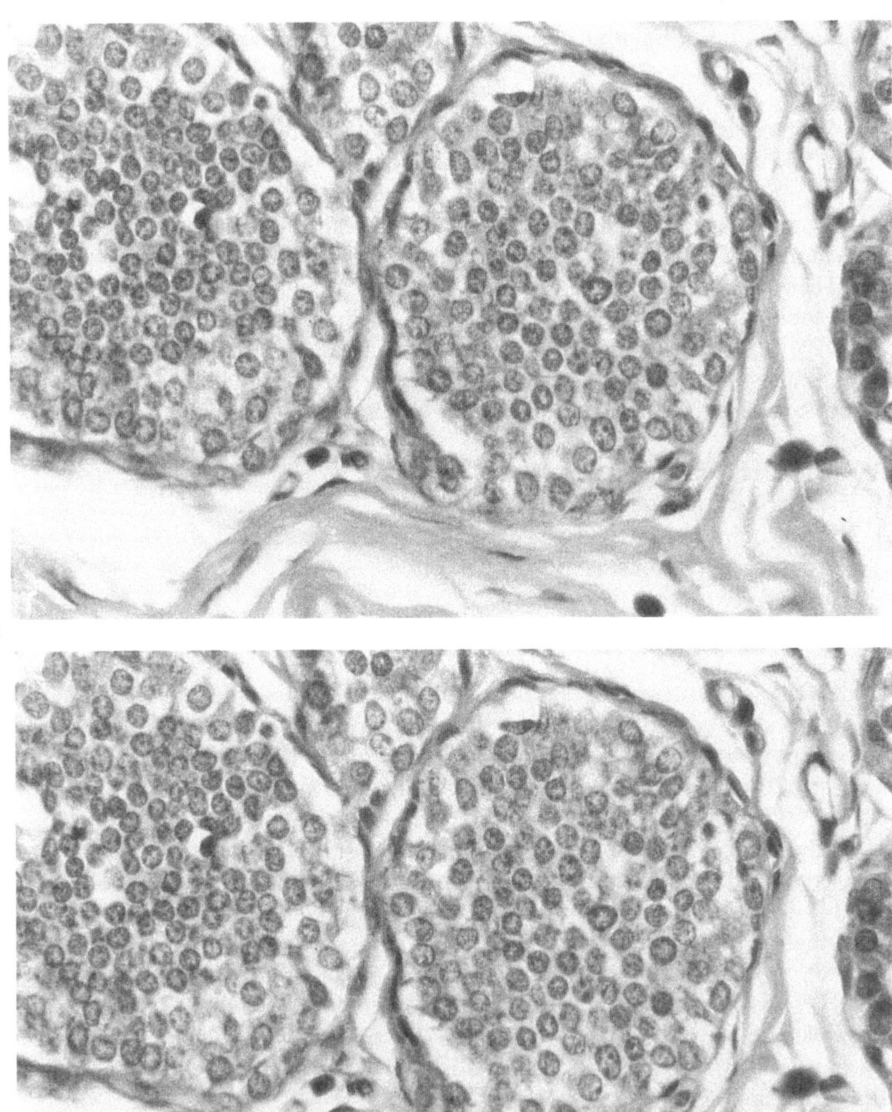

Fig. 4.41 a, b. The main histologic types of lobular neoplasia. **a** Haagensen's type A: small, regular epithelial cells with pale cytoplasm and round nuclei without mitoses or hyperchromatism. **b** Haagensen's type B: the cells are larger, less regular, and have hyperchromatic nuclei (approx. 400 ×) (Professor CITOLER, Cologne)

Though one should be careful in interpreting these figures, they nevertheless show that while lobular neoplasia with polymorphism may well play a role in the development of carcinoma, the significance of type A lobular neoplasia, which appears to be less common than other types, is at least questionable. This means, however, that most of the earlier "risk statistics" are invalid!

Lobular Neoplasia and Carcinogenesis

The role of lobular neoplasia (LCIS) in carcinogenesis has been discussed for almost 80 years. The cardinal question is whether and how often lobular neoplasia can evolve into a true carcinoma.

It is a fact that the transformation of lobular neoplasia into a true infiltrating lobular carcinoma is seen only incidentally in histologic examinations. We know that 50%–60% of carcinomas later detected in follow-ups are of intraductal rather than lobular origin (HAAGENSEN 1971; ROSEN et al. 1978). It is also a fact that pathologists find foci of lobular neoplasia in proximity to breast carcinoma in only 6%–20% of cases.

One question addressed in the study with ZIPPEL and NEUFANG was whether lobular neoplasia occurs significantly more often in association with carcinoma than with benign lesions. In a total of 1144 *histologic reports* (Gummersbach Radiology Institute, 10-1-1974 to 9-30-1983), there were 762 cases where the area surrounding the lesion of interest was described by the pathologist in a detailed manner. (mainly Professors P. CITOLER and K. J. LENNARTZ) (see Tables 4.1–4.3). A total of 63 lobular neoplasias (LCIS) were found in this series: 33 in association with 315 carcinomas (10.5%), and 30 in association with 447 benign lesions (6.7%). The frequencies of lobular neoplasia were *not significantly different* ($p = 0.05$). Thus, the occurrence of lobular neoplasia in this series was completely independent of the principal histologic finding.

A number of follow-up studies have been done in an effort to clarify the role of lobular neoplasia in carcinogenesis and determine the risk of malignant degeneration (ANDERSEN 1977; HUTTER and FOOTE 1969; ROSEN et al. 1978; CITOLER and ZIPPEL 1975; ZIPPEL et al. 1975). All these studies followed the same scheme:
1) Large numbers of old sections were surveyed, and previously unrecognized cases of lobular neoplasia (LCIS) were selected.
2) It was determined what percentage of the selected patients developed an *ipsilateral* and/or a *contralateral* (?) carcinoma within a period of 4–28 years.
3) The data were statistically evaluated, and the risk was determined in relation to the risk of carcinoma in the population at large.

The results determined the risk of developing carcinoma within a maximum of 31 years to be 14.5%–22% for the ipsilateral breast and 6%–15% for the contralateral breast. However, a critical analysis of these publications shows that:
a) The number of cases was small; except for the study of HAAGENSEN et al. (1978), case numbers were well below 100.
b) The number of sections examined was small (e.g., ROSEN et al. 1978 report an average of 1.4 sections per case), and the size of the biopsy specimens was limited.

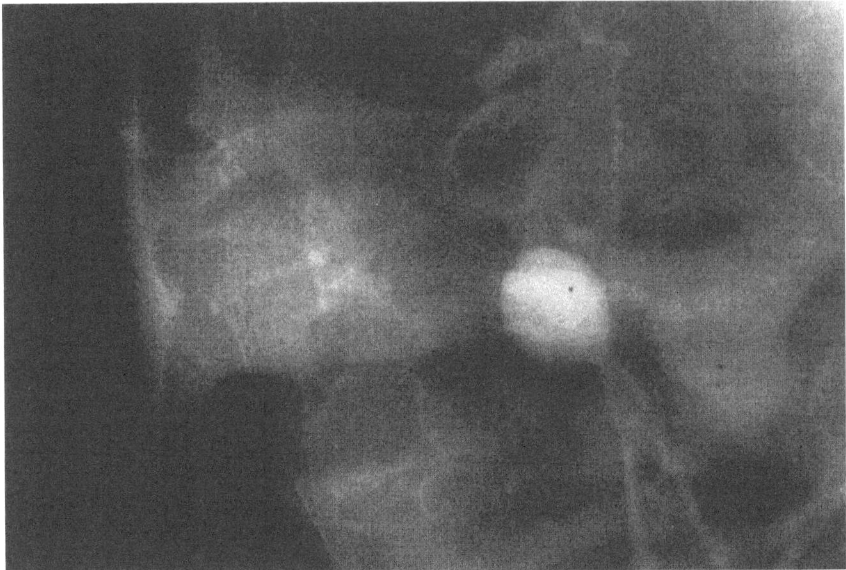

Fig. 4.42. Detail of mammogram (2 ×). A round shadow with smooth margins is seen behind the nipple, at the inner extremity of a cordlike density. Absence of secretion precludes galactography. The mammographic picture is suspicious for papilloma. Histology: papilloma with comedomastitis; type A lobular neoplasia is present as an associated finding

c) Other coexisting lesions that might predispose to carcinoma (e.g., papilloma, papillomatosis with or without atypia) were not taken into account.

Yet these intra*ductal proliferative* processes *are* important because they could explain why the infiltrating carcinomas that develop in association with lobular neoplasia (LCIS) tend to be *intraductal* rather than *lobular.*

With ZIPPEL and NEUFANG the author determined that in 22% of the cases where lobular neoplasia (LCIS) coexisted with benign lesions, papillomatosis or type 3 cystic disease[3] was present. This raises the suspicion that subsequent *ductal* carcinomas developed not from the mostly innocuous type A lobular neoplasia, but from these intraductal proliferative processes. Our percentage of intraductal proliferations is smaller than that reported by ROSEN et al. (1978), who demonstrated coexisting papillomatosis or atypical papillomatosis histologically in 50% of cases. ZIPPEL et al. (1975) found coexisting papillomatosis and lobular neoplasia in 38.1% of cases.

BÄSSLER (1978) states that lobular precancer (or lobular neoplasia) is a lesion that develops in the premenopausal breast but is inconsequential in 77%–85% of cases because it may regress after the menopause. On the other hand, observations by CITOLER (personal communication, 1984) indicate that foci of lobular neoplasia found in women over 60 years of age are associated with a very high risk of carcinoma.

---

[3] See footnote 1 on p. 50

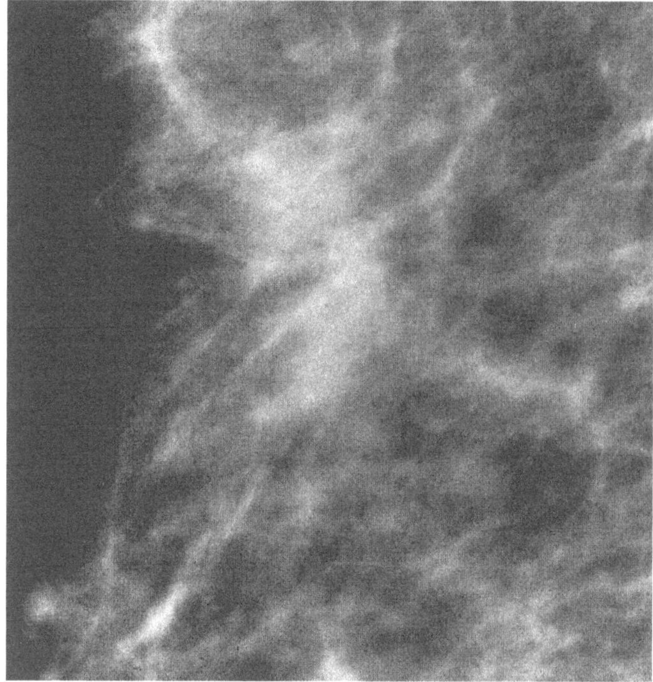

Fig. 4.43. Detail of mammogram (2 ×): with a radiating feature of this type, scirrhous carcinoma cannot be excluded. Histology: fibrosis and lobular neoplasia without nuclear atypia

Therapeutic Implications

A range of treatments for lobular neoplasia (LCIS) have been advocated:
- *bilateral* mastectomy (since bilaterality is presumed)
- mastectomy of the affected side (LEWISON and FINNEY 1968; FARROW 1968) with or without axillary dissection, or subcutaneous mastectomy as described by BOH-MERT and BAUMEISTER (1975), GOLDWYN (1977), or PILGRAM et al. (1980)
- segmental mastectomy accompanied by a low axillary dissection (axillary "sampling"; FISHER and FISHER 1977)
- frequent clinical follow-ups with self-examination (ANDERSEN 1977).

Today we face a situation that is contradictory and at times even grotesque: while some physicians attempt to manage true infiltrating carcinomas up to 1 or even 2 cm in size entirely by segmental mastectomy and irradiation ("nonmutilating therapy"), others routinely treat lobular neoplasia by bilateral mastectomy or subcutaneous mastectomy - often with poor cosmetic results - to prevent the development of a true carcinoma in the future (usually after a 20-year interval). On the other hand, Haagensen and others claim that mastectomy is the treatment of choice for cases of *highly atypical* type B lobular neoplasia. (The question of *how atypical* a given lobular neoplasia is must be answered by a pathologist experienced in this area.)

Radiography

SNYDER (1966) and later HUTTER and FOOTE (1969) were the first to try to prove the value of mammography in the diagnosis of lobular neoplasia. They reasoned that while the finding of punctate microcalcifications on mammograms is not specific, it is associated with LCIS frequently enough to justify biopsy.

The following questions, then, remain to be answered:

1) Are there radiographic signs specific for lobular neoplasia?
2) What is the role, if any, of microcalcifications in the diagnosis of lobular neoplasia?

In the above-mentioned study with ZIPPEL and NEUFANG, a total of 106 cases of lobular neoplasia were analyzed in an effort to answer these questions. Of these cases, 63 were taken from the material of the Gummersbach Radiology Institute and 43 from the Cologne University Women's Clinic.

In the Gummersbach material microcalcifications of varying type and extent ($n=331$) and soft-tissue shadows of varying shape and prominence ($n=431$) led to the diagnosis of the 63 lobular neoplasia. Mammograms and histologic reports were evaluated (Table 4.5).

In the Cologne material the author evaluated 43 lobular neoplasia that had been diagnosed entirely by biopsy performed for clustered microcalcifications, and for which specimen radiographs were available. He attempted to establish the localization of the microcalcifications and determine their relationship to the foci of the lobular neoplasia on the histologic sections. As the tissue blocks containing the microcalcifications had been removed from the considerably larger biopsy specimens and separately embedded prior to histologic study, and the residual specimens were also examined histologically, he wished to know whether lobular neoplasia was present in the blocks containing the microcalcifications, in the residual tissue, or in both. We also wished to learn whether the *radiographically* visible microcalcifications were detectable histologically inside or outside the foci of lobular neoplasia (Table 4.6).

Are There Radiographic Signs Specific for Lobular Neoplasia?

As shown in Tables 4.5 and 4.6, radiographic signs appear to be of no value in the detection of lobular neoplasia in this material. With a probability of error of $p=0.05$, we find that there is no significant difference in the frequency of detection of lobular neoplasia in the following cases:

- In carcinomas with microcalcifications compared with carcinomas without microcalcifications (12.4% vs 9.3%)
- In carcinomas with microcalcifications compared with microcystic (blunt duct) adenosis, sclerosing adenosis, or milk of calcium cysts with microcalcifications (12.4% vs 8.1%)
- In the various histologically benign diseases without microcalcifications compared with benign diseases of the lobular system with microcalcifications (5.5% vs 8.1%)
- In benign lesions without microcalcifications compared with carcinomas without microcalcifications (5.5% vs 9.3%)

Table 4.4. Occurrence of lobular neoplasia in association with 63 benign and malignant lesions

	Malignant	Benign
Type A	7	21
Type B	4	2
Type A + B	2	2
Intermediate	10	0
Unknown	9	5
In regression	1	0
Total	33	30

- In benign and malignant diseases without microcalcifications compared with malignant lesions with microcalcifications and benign lobular changes with microcalcifications (7.25% vs 10.0%)

In contrast, lobular neoplasia is found significantly more frequently in proximity to carcinomas with microcalcifications than in proximity to benign lesions without calcifications (12.4% vs 5.5%). The most probable explanation is that the area surrounding carcinomas with microcalcifications was studied more carefully than that surrounding *benign lesions without* microcalcifications. This explanation is reasonable, since the pathologist who originally examined most of the cases in this series (Professor CITOLER) usually had more sections prepared for intraductal carcinomas detected on the basis of microcalcifications than for benign fibroadenomas, cysts, fibrosis, or mastitis. More careful histologic examination increases the frequency with which lobular neoplasia is diagnosed (FARROW 1968).

Four cases of lobular neoplasia that were discovered among 50 cases of microcalcifications of nonlobular origin (20 from fibroadenomas, 17 from intraductal proliferations, 6 from plasma cell mastitis, 5 from scar calcifications, 2 from liponecroses) that were diagnosed were not evaluated further because of the small number per histologic diagnosis. But the fact that lobular neoplasia also occurred with these conditions demonstrates its ubiquitous character.

What Is the Role of Microcalcifications in the Diagnosis of Lobular Neoplasia?

Aside from carcinomas accompanied by intraductal microcalcifications, for which lobular neoplasia (LCIS) has been described as an associated finding (10.4% in Gummersbach material, 4.65% in Cologne material), microcalcifications are no more important than any other radiographic symptom in the diagnosis of lobular neoplasia (Figs. 4.42 and 4.43, Table 4.5).

a) Of the 30 lobular neoplasia found in association with benign lesions in the Gummersbach material, only 17 were biopsied for microcalcifications, and of these only 13 for microcalcifications of lobular origin.

b) Of the 43 lobular neoplasia in the Cologne series (Table 4.6), 6 were found outside the specimen containing the microcalcifications - i.e., in the residual specimen 2-3 cm from the calcific focus - and 23 were found both inside and outside the specimen tissue. Hence there were 29 cases where foci of lobular neoplasia were identified outside the microcalcification clusters that prompted the biopsy.

Table 4.5. Analysis of 762 cases with various radiographic symptoms in which 63 cases of lobular neoplasia were found (Gummersbach Radiologic Institute). Signs specific for lobular neoplasia could not be identified

Radiographic symptoms and histologic diagnoses	Number of cases	Lobular neoplasia (LCIS)						
		Number	%	Type A	Type B	Inter-mediate	Type A + B	Un-known
Benign lesions with calcifications	**210**	**17**		**11**	**1**	–	–	**5**
Milk of calcium cysts								
scattered	38	3						
clustered	52	7	8.1	7	1	–	–	5
Microcystic (blunt duct) and/or sclerosing adenosis (clustered or scattered)	70	3						
Fibroadenoma	20	1	5	1	–	–	–	–
Intraductal microcalcifications with varying degrees of proliferation	17	2	11.7	2	–	–	–	–
Plasma cell mastitis	6	1	16.6	1	–	–	–	–
Other	7	–	–	–	–	–	–	–
Benign lesions without calcifications	**237**	**13**	5.5	**10**	**1**	–	**2**	–
Papilloma								
Papillomatosis	91	3	3.3	3	–	–	–	–
Papillomalike intraductal projections								
Galactophoritis (comedomastitis)	25	1	4	–	–	–	1	–
Cystic disease	68	6	8.8	4	1	–	1	–
Other (e.g., fibroadenoma, increasing stellate figure)	53	3	5.6	3	–	–	–	–
Carcinomas without microcalcifications	**194**	**18**	9.3	**3**	**3**	**5**	–	**7**[a]
Carcinomas with microcalcifications	**121**	**15**	12.4	**4**	**1**	**5**	**2**	**3**
Soft-tissue shadow with microcalcifications	59	5	8.5	1	–	2	–	2
Soft-tissue shadow without microcalcifications	62	10	16.1	3	1	3	2	1

[a] 1 in regression.

Table 4.6. Analysis of the spatial relationship between clustered microcalcifications and lobular neoplasia, and an analysis of type distribution (Cologne University Women's Clinic)

Mammographic diagnoses	Number of cases	Lobular neoplasia (LCIS)			Histologically demonstrable microcalcifications				Type A	Type B	Type A+B	Intermediate
		In area of specimen containing microcalcifications	In area containing microcalcifications *and* in rest	Only in rest of specimen	In area of lobular neoplasia and surrounding tissue	Only in area of lobular neoplasia	Only in area surrounding LCIS	Neither in area of LCIS or in surrounding tissue				
Microcalcifications of lobular origin (microcystic/blunt duct adenosis, sclerosing adenosis, milk of calcium cysts)	31	9	19	3	14	0	14	3	22[a]	3	4	2
Microcalcifications of lobular and intraductal origin; ductal carcinoma cannot be excluded	5	3	2	0	2	1	2	0	4	0	0	1
Ductal carcinoma *and* microcalcifications of lobular origin	1	0	1 (!)	0	1	0	0	0	0	0	1 (!)	0
Ductal carcinoma	1	0	0	1 (!)	0	0	1	0	0	1 (!)	0	0
Uncharacteristic	5	2	1	2	2	1	1	1	2	2	0	1
Total	43	14	23	6	19	2	18	4	28	6	5	4

[a] 1 LCIS in regression.

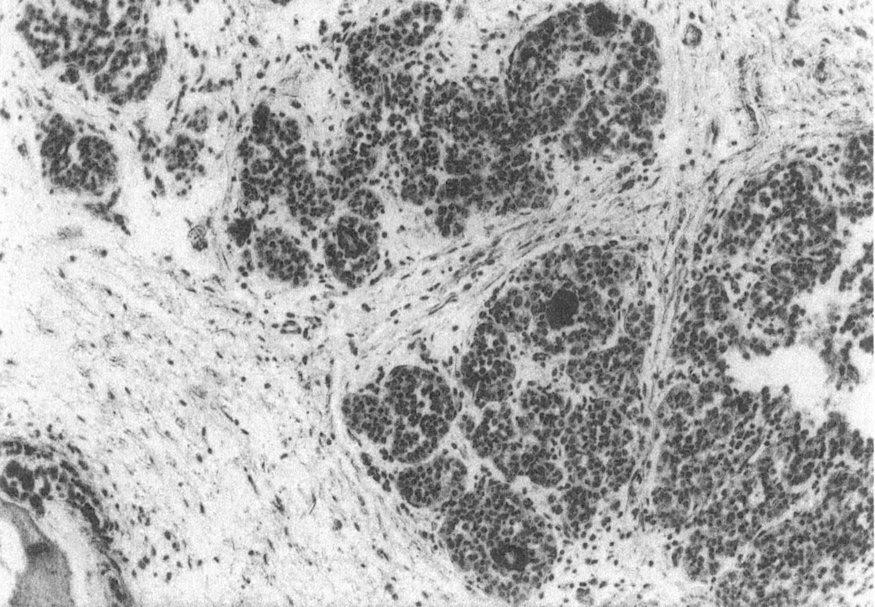

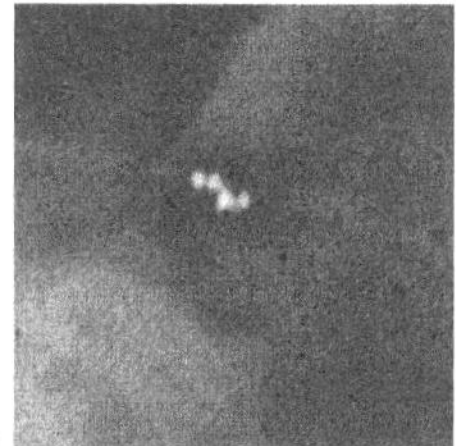

Fig. 4.45. **a** Detail of mammogram (4×) showing four adjacent, rounded microcalcifications with fine septa, corresponding to the row of small cysts seen on the histologic section (approx. 125×). **b** Adjacent to the cysts is an area of ductal lobular neoplasia without microcalcifications (Professor ZIPPEL, Marburg)

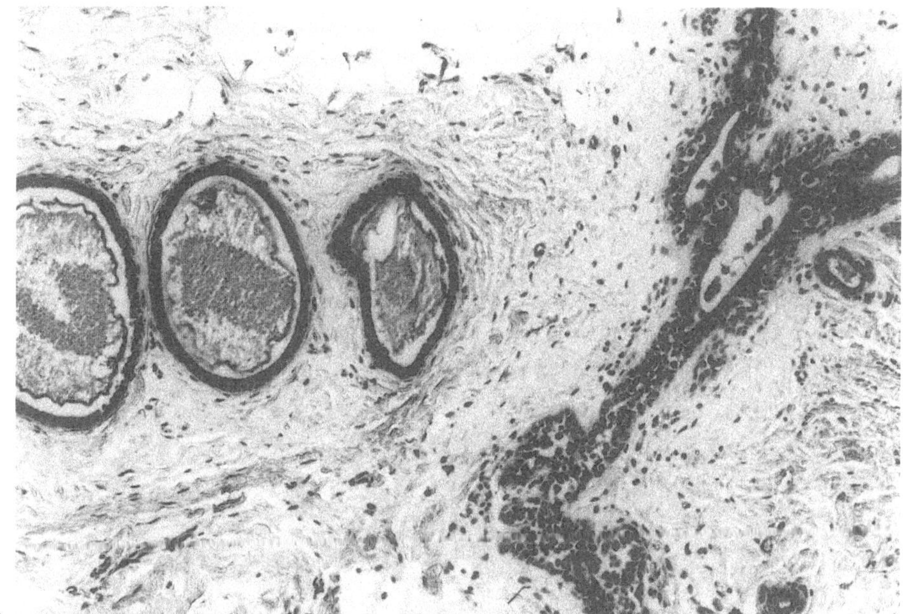

◁ **Fig. 4.44. a** Specimen radiograph (4×): partly clustered, partly scattered, rounded microcalcifications of approximately equal size, as in microcystic (blunt duct) adenosis; the larger, rounded calcifications represent milk of calcium cysts. Histology: multicentric lobular neoplasia (type A). **b** Histologic section (approx. 100×): necrobiotic calcium inclusions are found within the LCIS foci; these are far too small to be visible mammographically (Professor ZIPPEL, Marburg)

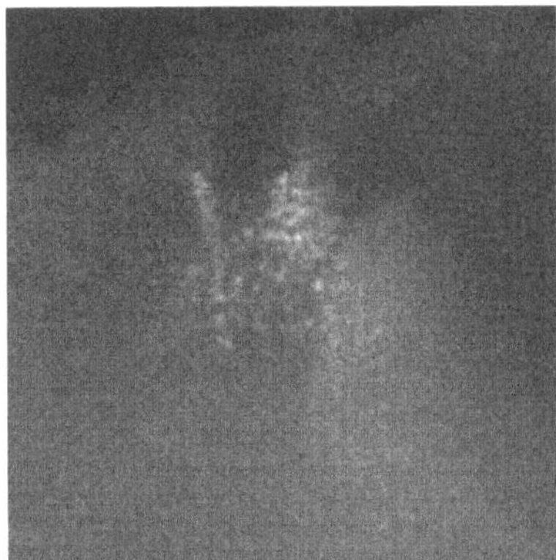

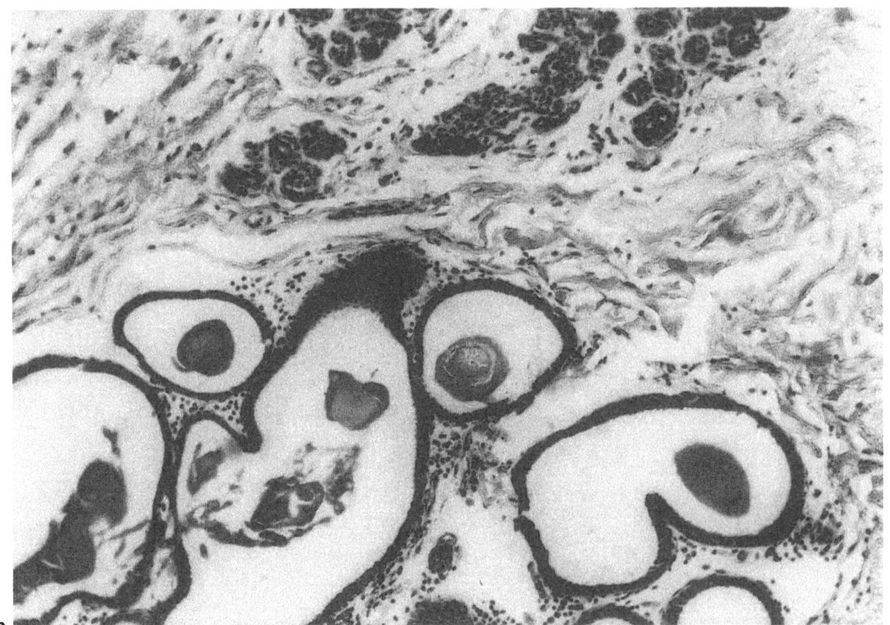

Fig. 4.46. a Detail of mammogram (4 ×): rounded, dense, somewhat rosette-shaped cluster of polymorphous microcalcifications, typical of sclerosing adenosis (see also Fig. 4.23). **b** Histologic section (approx. 125 ×): at the bottom is part of the area of sclerosing adenosis seen on the radiograph (deformed cysts with psammomatous granules); adjacent to it, at the top, are extensions of LCIS. The areas of LCIS are devoid of microcalcifications (Professor ZIPPEL, Marburg)

c) Microcalcifications within the foci of lobular neoplasia were confirmed histologically in only 21 of the 43 cases in the Cologne series. All were too small to be detected radiographically (Table 4.6, Fig. 4.44). In 18 cases microcalcifications were found only outside the foci of lobular neoplasia on histologic sections (Figs. 4.45 and 4.46, Table 4.6).

By comparison, CITOLER (1978) found microcalcifications within the LCIS foci in only 10 of the 30 cases that were studied histologically.

Of the 43 cases of lobular neoplasia in the Cologne material, 7 were detected entirely from intraductal calcifications, 31 from lobular calcifications, and 5 from both lobular and intraductal calcifications. This seems to support the claims of SNYDER (1966) and HUTTER and FOOTE (1969) that microcalcifications of lobular origin play an important role in the diagnosis of lobular neoplasia.

However, if the number of cases of lobular neoplasia detected from lobular mi-microcalcifications is related to the number of biopsies performed for that finding, it becomes clear that we are dealing with a coincidence rather than a true diagnosis. In 182 biopsies (Gummersbach) performed for radiographically visible microcalcifications of lobular origin, a total of 13 cases of lobular neoplasia were found (7%). A "yield" of this size contraindicates biopsy for microcalcifications of obvious lobular origin! It is no longer appropriate to evaluate calcifications histologically on the chance that lobular neoplasia (LCIS) may be associated with them. It is irresponsible needlessly biopsy 93 women in order to confirm lobular neoplasia (predominantly type A) in only 7.

To summarize, the diagnosis of lobular neoplasia (LCIS) is not the task of the radiologist. FARROW (1968) is correct to attribute the increasing recognition of lobular neoplasia to the more "careful microscopic examination of more tissue sections, wider and more frequent diagnostic local excisions, and the usefulness of mammograms in a few selected cases." ROSEN (1984) adds that mammography may be able to identify benign lesions like sclerosing adenosis that can accompany LCIS, but it cannot find the LCIS itself. The author agrees completely with LEWISON (1964), who says, "Some enthusiastic radiologists ... claim that (lobular) carcinoma in situ can be recognized by mammography. In my opinion this is the 'triumph of hope over experience'."

Infiltrative Lobular Carcinoma

Pathology

Infiltrative lobular carcinoma can arise *primarily* from the lobular epithelium or *secondarily* through the centripetal spread of a ductal or ductular carcinoma (Fig. 4.47). Histologically the primary type infiltrative lobular carcinoma is a uniformly small-cell carcinoma with a characteristic circular arrangement of the cancer cells around the lobule ("target" or "Indian file" pattern). In carcinomas that have invaded the lobule secondarily, we see the picture of ductal carcinoma with solid formations as well as papillary and cribriform structures. Histologically there is a polymorphic large-cell hyperplasia with anisomorphism and hyperchromatism of the nuclei. The affected lobule is distended with ductal carcinoma cells, with the result that it loses its original treelike structure and acquires a balloon shape. Reportedly, primary lobular small-cell infiltrative carcinomas account for 3.7%–5.8% of all breast carcinomas (BÄSSLER 1978).

Radiography

Ten small-cell infiltrative lobular carcinomas and ten ductal carcinomas with lobular invasion (3% of all breast carcinomas) were found at the Gummersbach Radiology Institute between 1 October 1974 and 30 September 1983. Characteristic radiographic features could not be established for either of the two variants (Figs. 4.48 and 4.62 a, b). Only one of the ten small-cell infiltrative lobular carcinomas showed the radiographic symptom of microcalcification. There was one other case in which microcalcifications and infiltration were found to coexist.

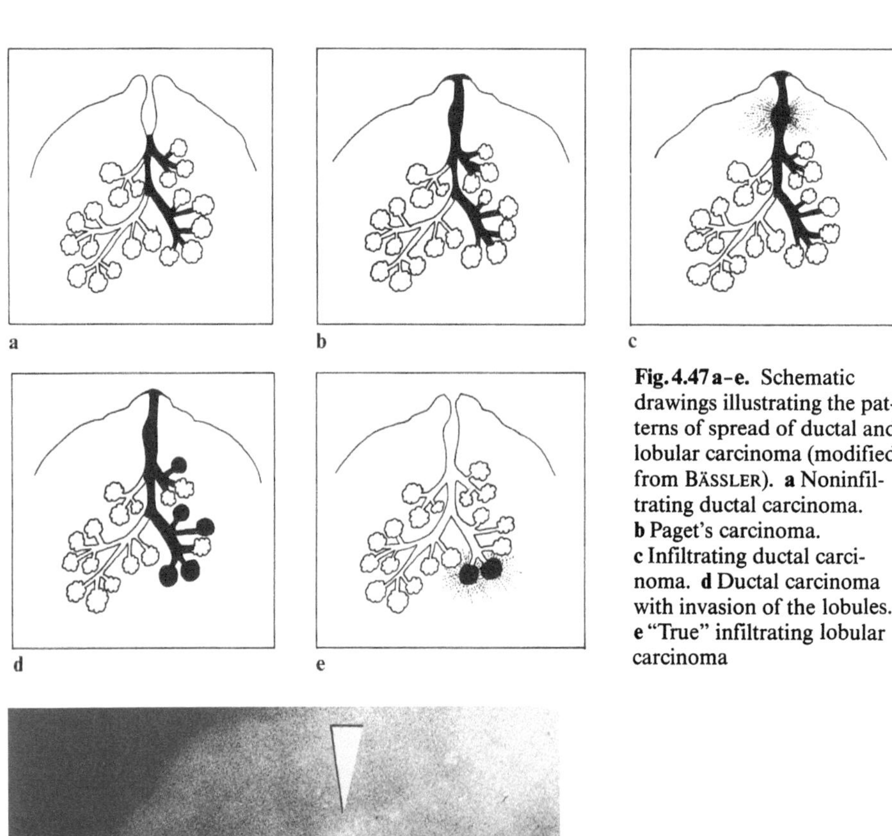

Fig. 4.47 a–e. Schematic drawings illustrating the patterns of spread of ductal and lobular carcinoma (modified from BÄSSLER). **a** Noninfiltrating ductal carcinoma. **b** Paget's carcinoma. **c** Infiltrating ductal carcinoma. **d** Ductal carcinoma with invasion of the lobules. **e** "True" infiltrating lobular carcinoma

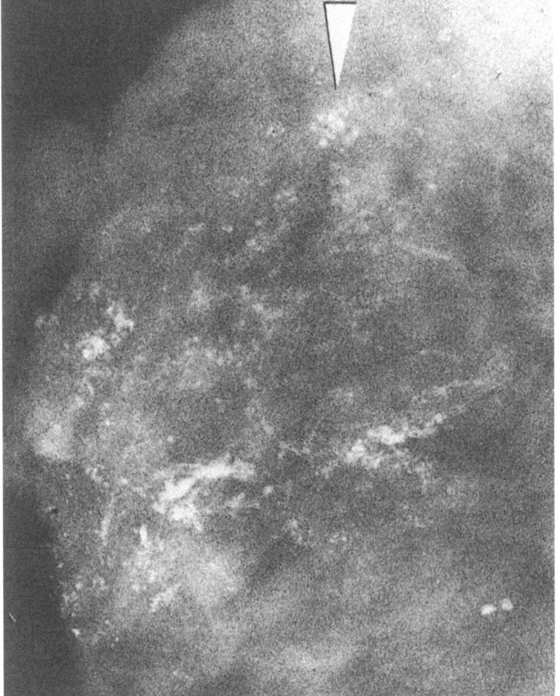

Fig. 4.48. Detail of mammogram (4.5 ×): polymorphous microcalcifications arranged in a ductal pattern. The arrow points to a rounded cluster of punctate, slightly facetted microcalcifications with septa, typical of lobular calcifications. Additional punctate calcifications are seen at other peripheral sites. Histology: ductal and lobular carcinoma. It cannot be determined whether the "lobular microcalcifications" formed in association with the lobular carcinoma

4.3 Pathology and Radiography of Calcifications of Intraductal Origin

The following processes may be associated with the formation of calcifications in the mammary ducts:
a) Ductal carcinomas of varying histologic types, papilloma or papillomatosis that has undergone malignant transformation.
b) Retention of secretions with or without epithelial proliferation or with galacto-phoritis (plasma cell mastitis)
c) Hyalinized, sclerosed intraductal papilloma or fibroadenoma

Ductal Carcinomas of Varying Histologic Types; Malignantly Transformed Papilloma or Papillomatosis

Pathology

According to the literature approximately 95% of all malignant breast disease develop from the epithelium of the milk ducts (and according to my own data, as much as 98.5%). The ductal (intraductal) carcinomas may be differentiated histologically as comedo (solid), papillary, or cribriform. A fourth type, papilloma that has undergone malignant transformation, is discussed as a separate entity.

a) Ductal Carcinoma of the Comedo Type (Comedocarcinoma)

The involved ducts are *densely* filled with solid, atypical epithelial cell masses that show pronounced cellular and nuclear polymorphism. The tumor tissue becomes *necrotic* at the center of the duct, and the necrotized tumor mass may later calcify. Thus, this type of calcification occurs at the *center* of the tubular or branching ducts (Figs. 4.49 and 4.50). When specimens are cut, the calcified cylinders can be pressed from the cut ducts like comedones, hence the name "comedocarcinoma" (BLOOD-GOOD 1934) (Fig. 4.51).

b) Ductal Carcinoma of the Papillary Type (Papillary Intraductal Carcinoma)

This type of carcinoma usually exhibits a typical branching papillary structure (Fig. 4.52a), or one finds multiple, small, short papillary processes that line the wall of the duct (BÄSSLER 1978) and display the cytologic features of carcinoma (Fig. 4.52b). (The initially benign papilloma that has undergone malignant transformation is discussed below.)

c) Ductal Carcinoma of the Cribriform Type

Essentially, this lesion is a highly advanced form of papillary carcinoma in which the minute fingerlike papillary processes become so elongated that they fuse together (HAAGENSEN 1971; Fig. 4.52c, *arrow*). This gives the carcinoma tissue a *spongelike structure* in three dimensions, and its sievelike appearance on histologic sections gives the lesion its name (Latin *cribrum* = "sieve") (Fig. 4.52c). Unlike the solid comedocarcinoma, the papillary and cribriform carcinomas usually show little cellular polymorphism. The cavities of the cribriform carcinoma (the "pores of the

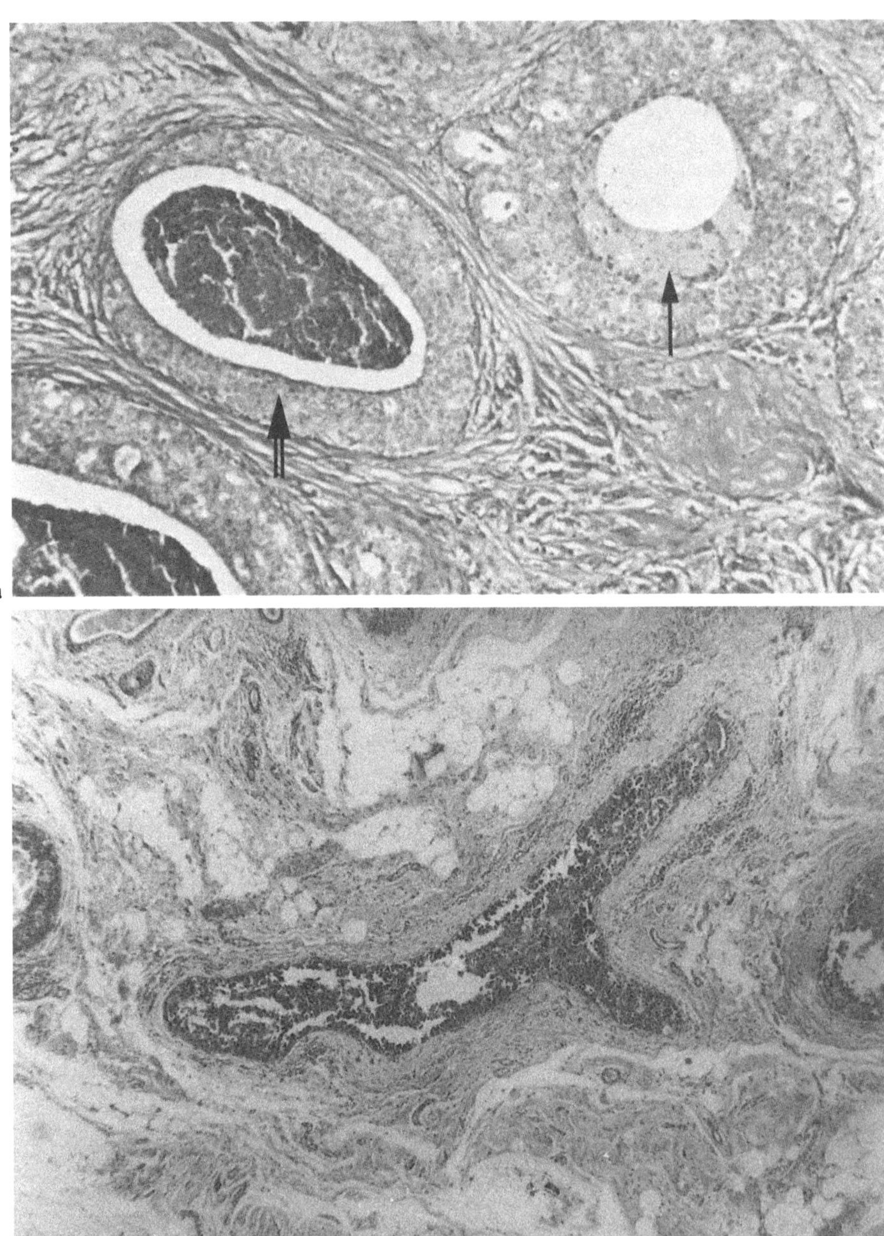

Fig. 4.49. a Histologic section of an intraductal carcinoma of the comedo type (approx. 125 ×). The transversely cut ducts are filled with solid, atypical cell masses. One duct shows partial *(arrow)* and another complete *(double arrow)* central necrosis with calcification (Professor LENNARTZ, Düsseldorf). **b** Histologic section of an intraductal carcinoma of the comedo type (approx. 40 ×). Here the duct is cut longitudinally and shows a branched shape. Note the central calcifications (Professor CITOLER, Cologne)

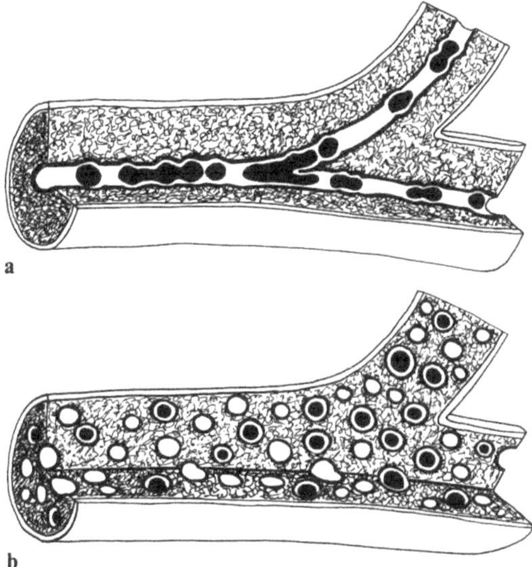

Fig. 4.50 a, b. Schematic drawings showing the location of the microcalcifications in the main histologic types of ductal carcinoma. **a** In comedocarcinoma the calcifications form at the center of the involved duct. **b** In cribriform carcinoma the psammomatous calcifications form in the cavities of the spongy tumor tissue

sponge") are filled with an albuminous, eosinophilic, and PAS-positive secretion. "Changes in the viscosity in this 'stagnant pool' create conditions favorable for the precipitation of calcium salts, and in this way the sievelike lumina can become filled in varying degrees with rounded calculi, creating the picture of a cribriform, psammomatous carcinoma" (BÄSSLER 1978). Thus, the calcifications form *within the cavities* of the spongy mass (Figs. 4.50b, 4.80b, c, and 4.86d). No difference exists between the psammoma bodies of cribriform carcinoma and those of microcystic or sclerosing adenosis or milk of calcium cysts (HOLLAND 1984; HOLLAND et al. 1984, personal communication) (Figs. 4.38c and 4.80b, c).

The foregoing types of ductal carcinoma rarely occur in isolation. The larger the carcinoma and the greater the number of histologic sections examined, the more variegated the pattern of coexisting solid, minute papillary, and cribriform structures.

Paget's disease is not discussed here as a separate entity because it represents a ductal carcinoma that has invaded the epidermis of the nipple. Its radiographic features are identical to those of intraductal carcinoma.

d) Solitary Papilloma or Papillomatosis That Has Undergone Malignant Transformation

This condition is relatively uncommon. According to HAAGENSEN (1971) the potential for malignant transformation is highest with multiple papilloma and papillomatosis, which should constitute a separate entity with its own prognosis. Calcifications rarely occur in areas of papillomatosis, regardless of whether it has undergone malignant change.

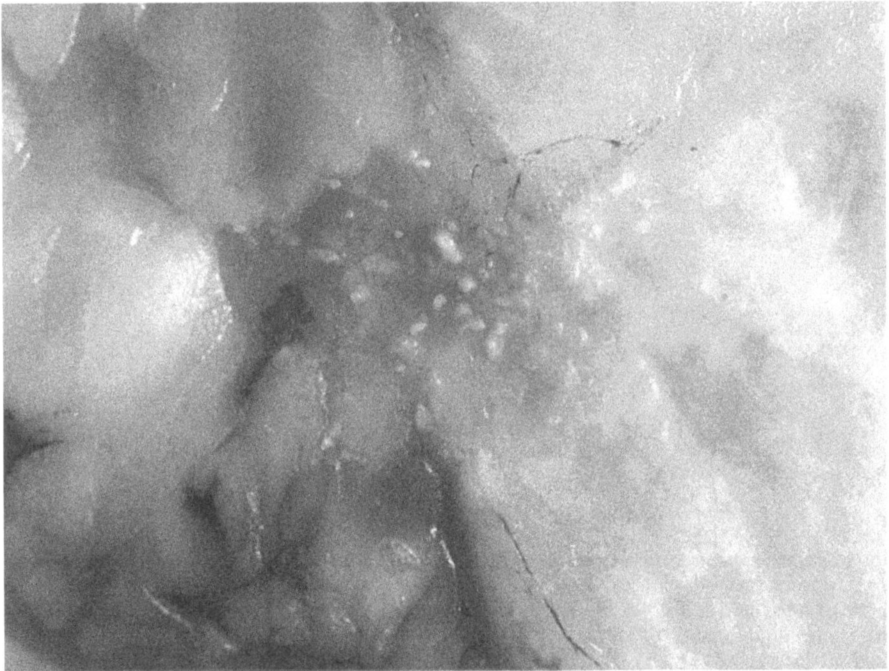

Fig. 4.51. The cut surface of a comedocarcinoma. Calcifications mixed with necrotic debris can be expressed like a comedo from the cut ducts (Professor LENNARTZ, Düsseldorf)

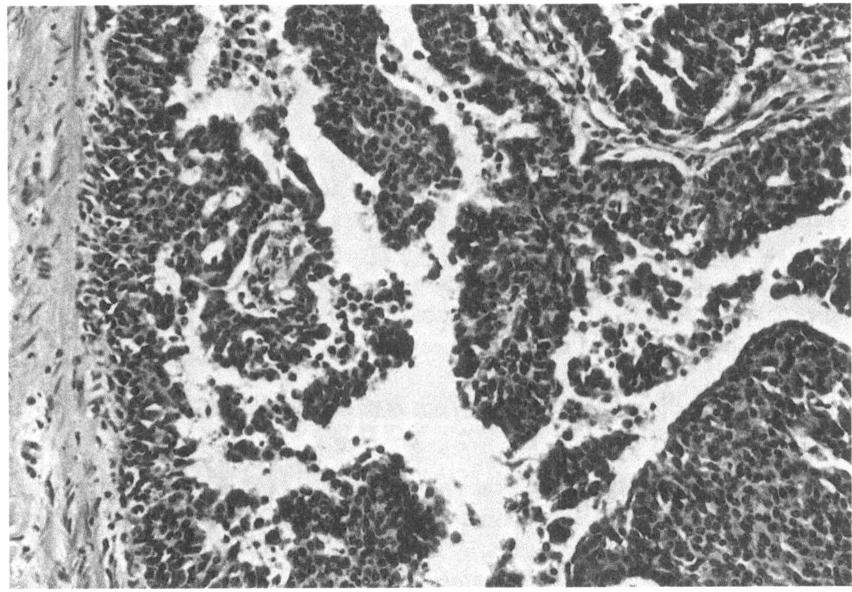

a

Fig. 4.52 a

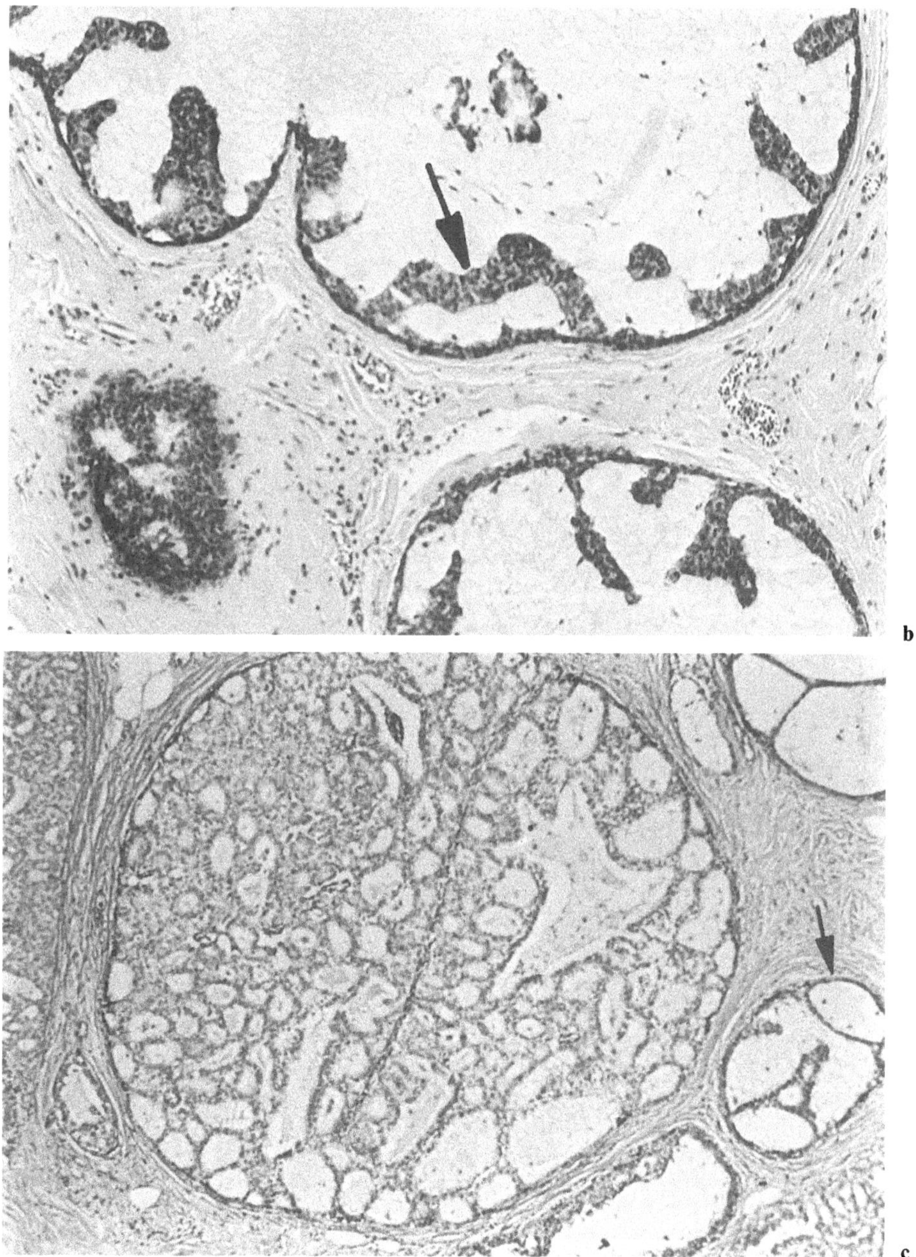

Fig. 4.52 a–c. Photomicrographs of histologic sections. **a** Intraductal papillary carcinoma with characteristic branching of the atypical cell masses (Professor CITOLER, Cologne) (150 ×). **b** Intraductal short papillary carcinoma. At the center, two papillary processes have fused together to form a lacuna – the precursor of a cribriform structure (Dr. HOLLAND, Nijmegen) (150 ×). **c** Intraductal, predominantly cribriform carcinoma forming numerous cavities that appear sievelike in cross section. The cavities contain secretions with minute, rounded calcifications. The *arrow* marks papillary structures that show the beginning of a cribriform pattern (Professor CITOLER, Cologne) (90 ×)

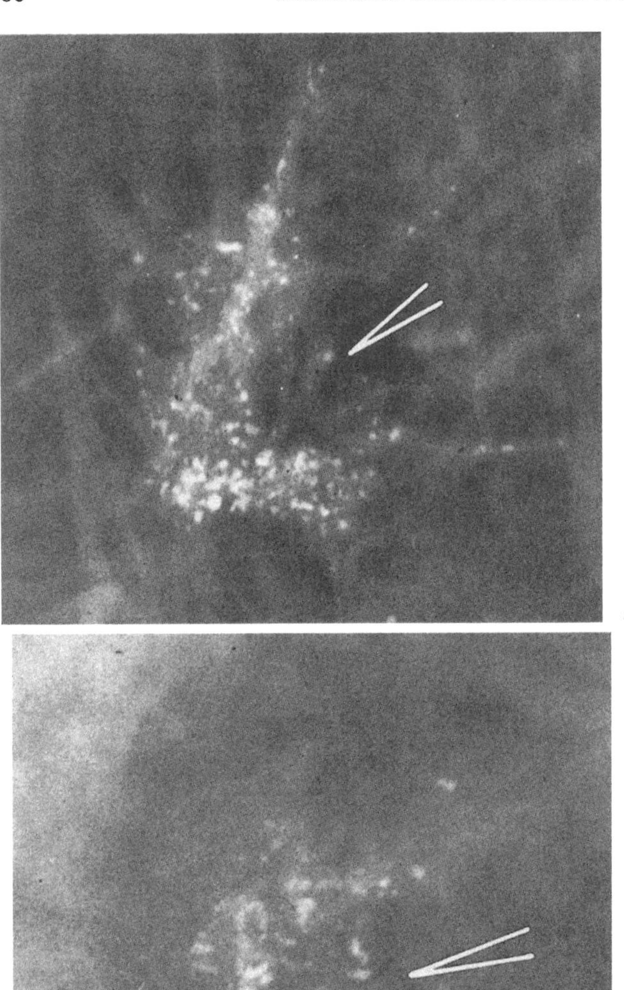

Fig. 4.53. a Detail of mammogram (4×): triangular cluster of numerous punctate, linear, comma-shaped, and several v-shaped microcalcifications. The apex of the triangle points toward the nipple, and the cluster is notched posteriorly *(arrow)* ("swallowtail sign") in this predominantly comedotype ductal carcinoma. **b** Similar pattern (3×) in a different comedocarcinoma. Again the cluster is triangular and notched posteriorly *(arrow)*; branched (v- and w-shaped) calcifications are more numerous

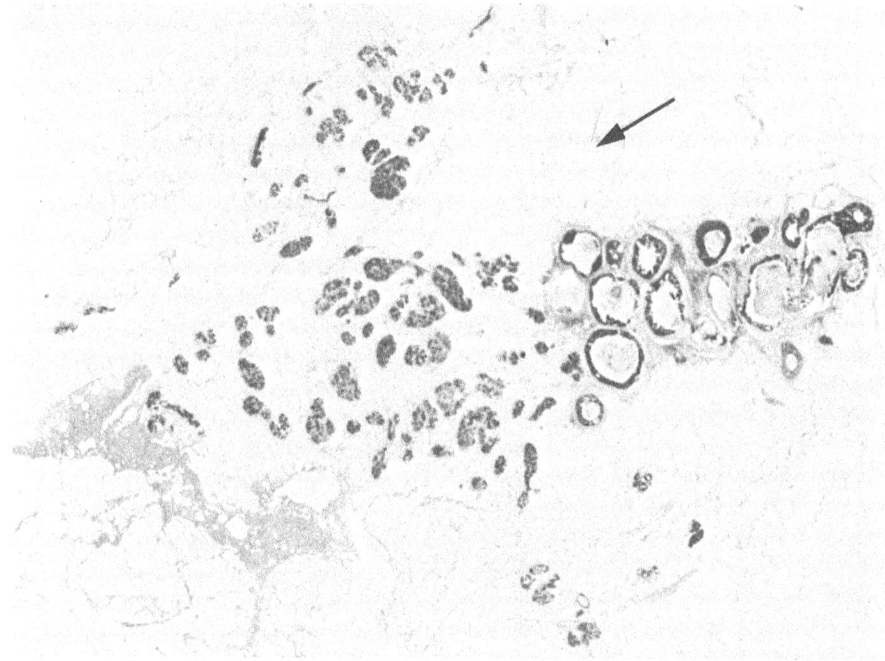

Fig. 4.53. c The histologic section of **b** (approx. 6 ×) shows that both the triangular shape and the swallowtail sign *(arrow)* can be appreciated on the histologic level (Professor CITOLER, Cologne) (approx. 25 ×)

Radiography of Intraductal Comedocarcinoma and Papillary or Cribriform Carcinoma

In a series of 501 histologically confirmed breast carcinomas at the Gummersbach Radiology Institute intraductal microcalcifications were demonstrated radiographically in only 181 (36%); of these, 74 cases (14.7%) were detected on the basis of microcalcifications alone.

In the analysis of microcalcifications, there are three diagnostic features that can be objectively evaluated with accuracy. These are:
1) The shape of the microcalcification *cluster*
2) The shapes of individual microcalcifications
3) The number of microcalcifications

A fourth feature – the intensity of the calcifications on the radiographic image – is not useful in practice, because it would require microdensitometry. Also, the intensity of the calcifications depends both on the radiographic technique (exposure, film, developing temperature) and on the scattering properties of the breast (fatty involution? dense glandular parenchyma?). Expressions such as "calcium dense," "moderately intense," "faint," etc. are too subjective to be of much value.

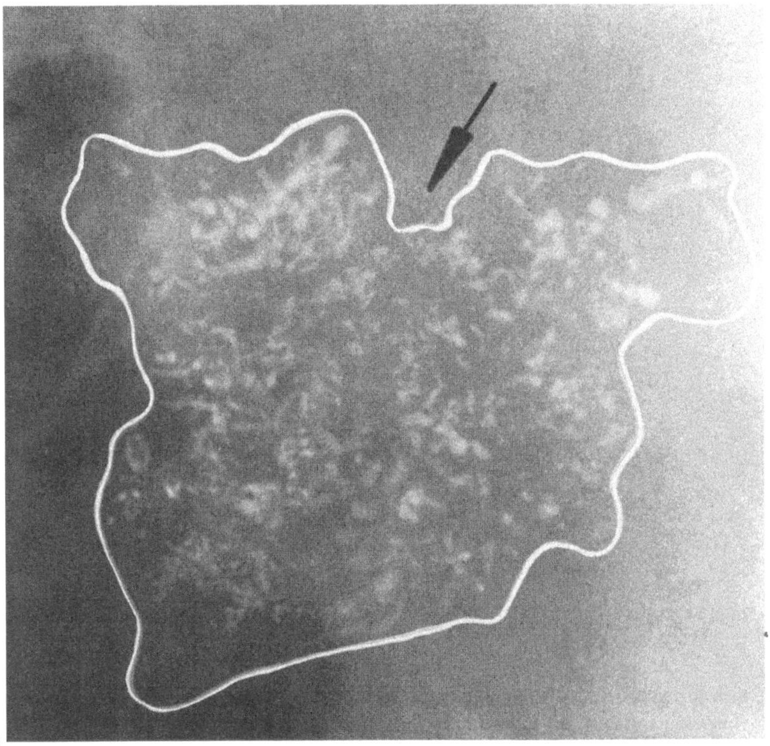

a

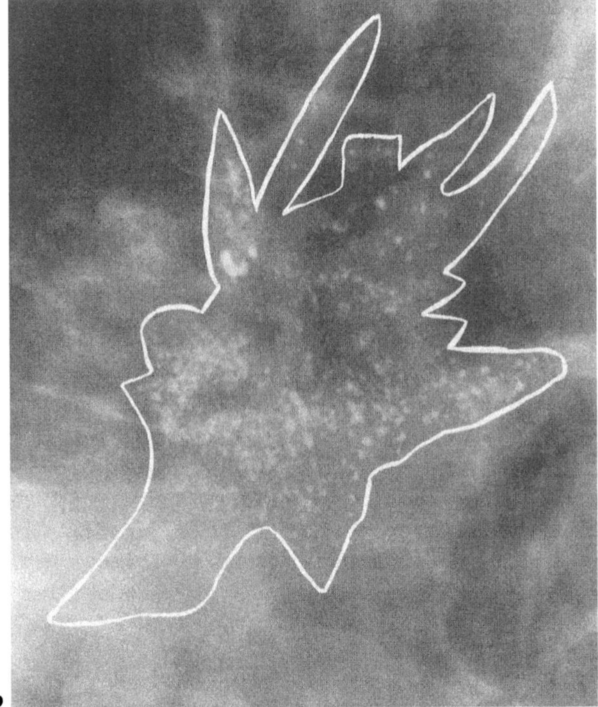

b

Fig. 4.54 a, b

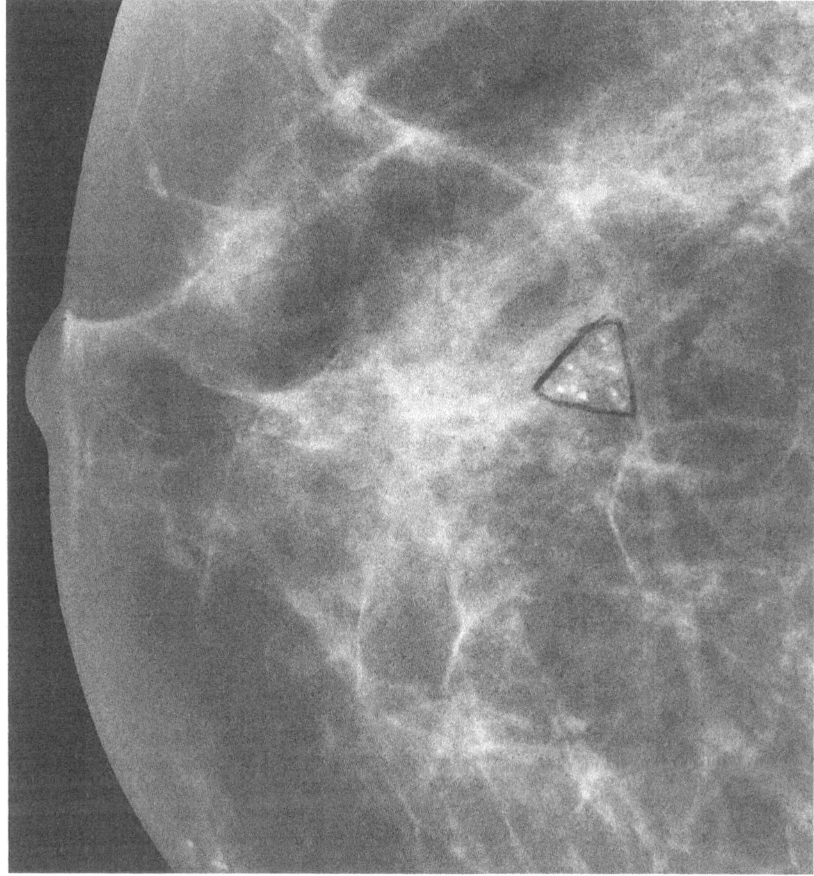

Fig. 4.55. Detail of mammogram (1.5 ×) showing a triangular cluster of 11 predominantly punctate microcalcifications (one Y-shaped and one V-shaped) in a small comedocarcinoma. Note: the smaller the comedocarcinoma, the less polymorphous it is. However, the triangular shape helps to differentiate this lesion from a small, calcifying fibroadenoma

◁ **Fig. 4.54. a** Triangular cluster of predominantly linear and branched microcalcifications in comedo-carcinoma (approx. 5 ×). The "lateral processes" are short, and the *arrow* marks the swallowtail sign (Dr. HENDRIKS, Nijmegen). **b** Another triangular cluster of punctate, linear, and a few branched microcalcifications. The lateral processes are more conspicuous than in **a**, and there are multiple posterior notches creating a stellate pattern (4.5 ×). Histology: mixed comedo- and cribri-form carcinoma

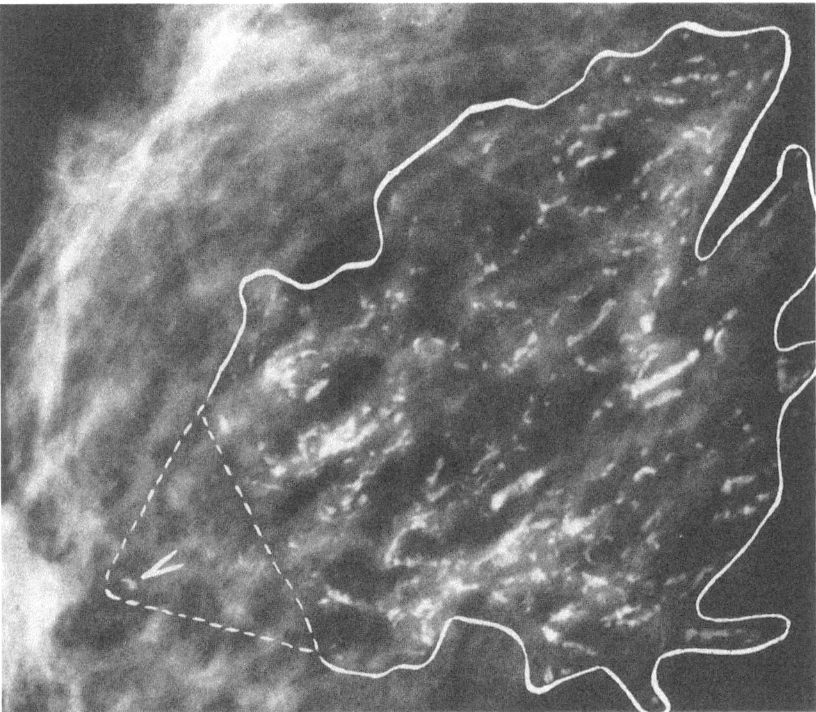

Fig. 4.56. Mammogram (slightly magnified) showing a very large cluster of predominantly linear and branched (V, Y) microcalcifications in an extensive comedocarcinoma. The cluster shape may be described as triangular or trapezoidal, depending on whether the solitary calcification near the nipple *(arrow)* is included. The neoplasm appears to involve an entire mammary lobe. Note: the larger the comedocarcinoma, the more polymorphous it is. Close analysis of the cluster contour shows wavy processes and posterior notching (Professor HOEFFKEN, Cologne)

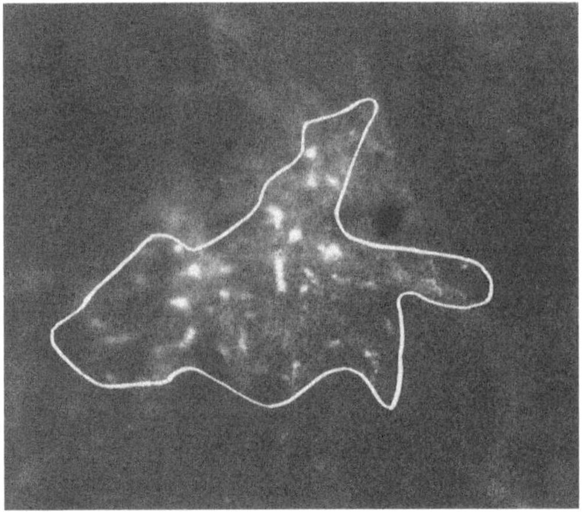
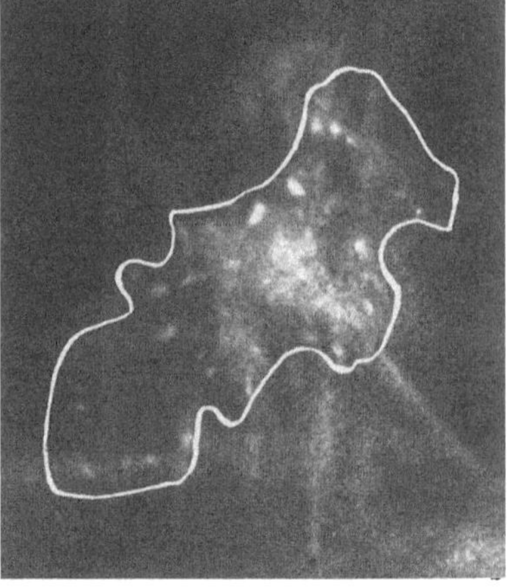

Fig. 4.58 a, b. Change of cluster shape with mammographic plane. **a** The lateral view shows a triangular cluster of somewhat polymorphous but predominantly linear microcalcifications with a posterior notch (swallowtail sign). **b** The same cluster on the craniocaudad view appears rectangular with a tapered end (3 ×). Histology: comedocarcinoma

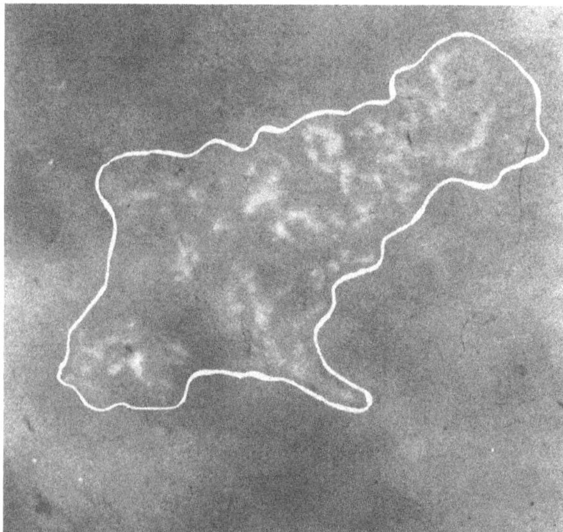

a

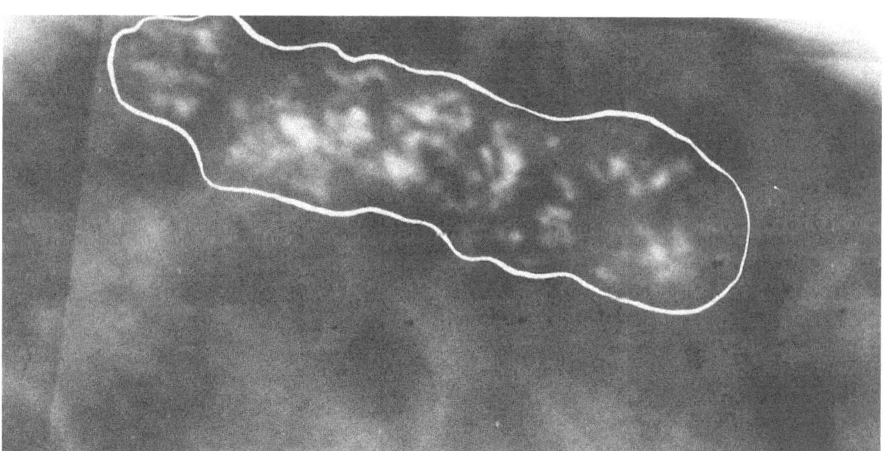

b

Fig. 4.57 a, b. Change of cluster shape with mammographic plane. **a** The craniocaudad view shows a rhomboid (kite-shaped) cluster of polymorphous microcalcifications in comedocarcinoma. **b** The same cluster appears rectangular on the lateral view (approx. 3 ×)

The Shape of the Microcalcification Clusters

The shape of a microcalcification cluster is best analyzed by drawing a line around its periphery two on mammographic planes (a sharp pencil is better for this than a wax marker). A magnifying lens should be used to make sure all peripheral calcifications are outlined. Rough estimation of the cluster shape with the unaided eye can be misleading!

One of the following cluster shapes is demonstrable on at least one radiographic plane in 97% of breast carcinomas:

1) Triangular or trapezoidal (Figs. 4.53–4.56, 4.58 a, 4.62 a, 4.69, 4.70 a).
2) Square or rectangular, possibly with a tapered end (Figs. 4.57, 4.58 b, 4.70 b).
3) Bottle- or club-shaped (Figs. 4.59, 4.92 c).
4) Propeller- or butterfly-shaped (Figs. 4.60, 4.61 a, b, 4.65 b, 4.70 b).

Calcifications Within the Lobular and Ductal System of the Breast

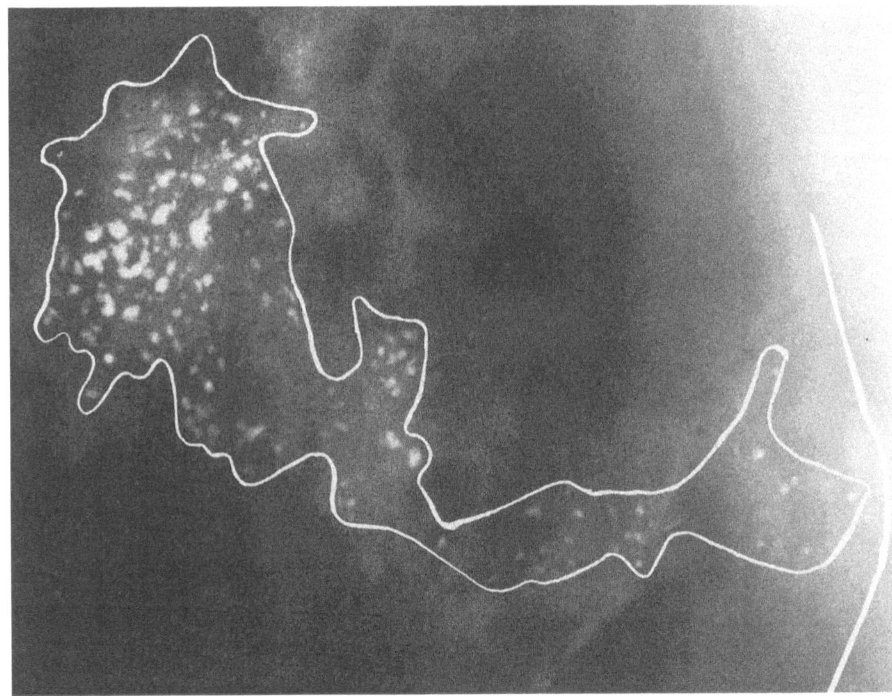

a

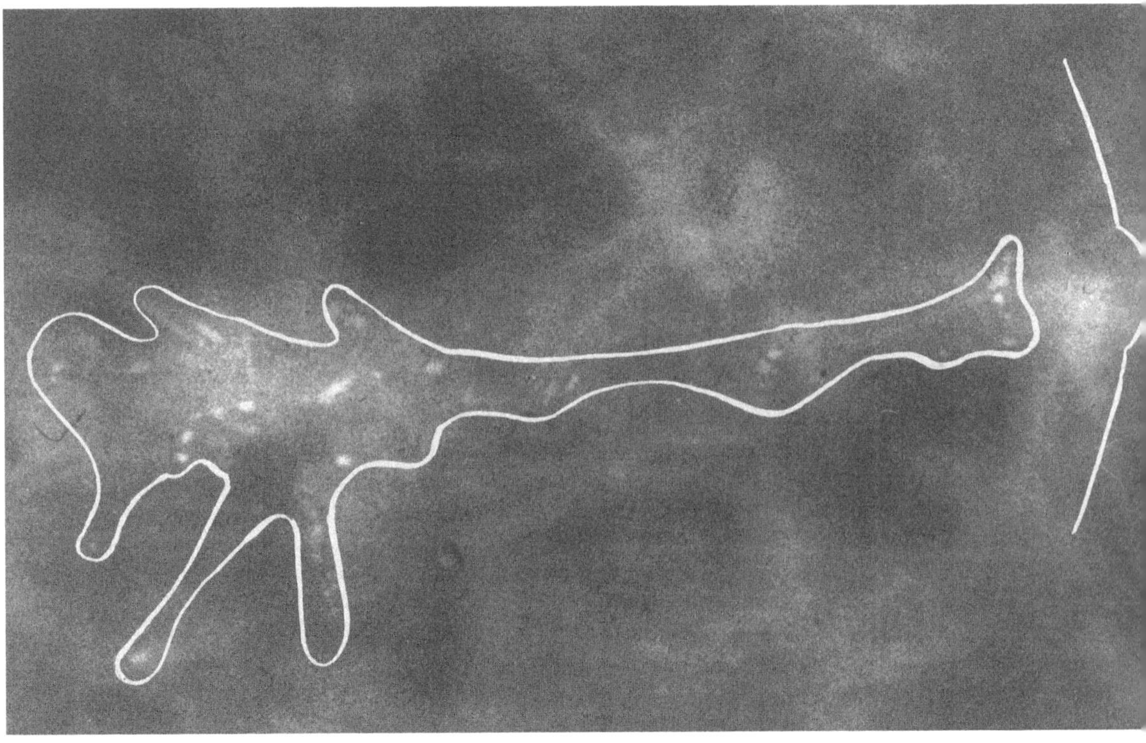

b

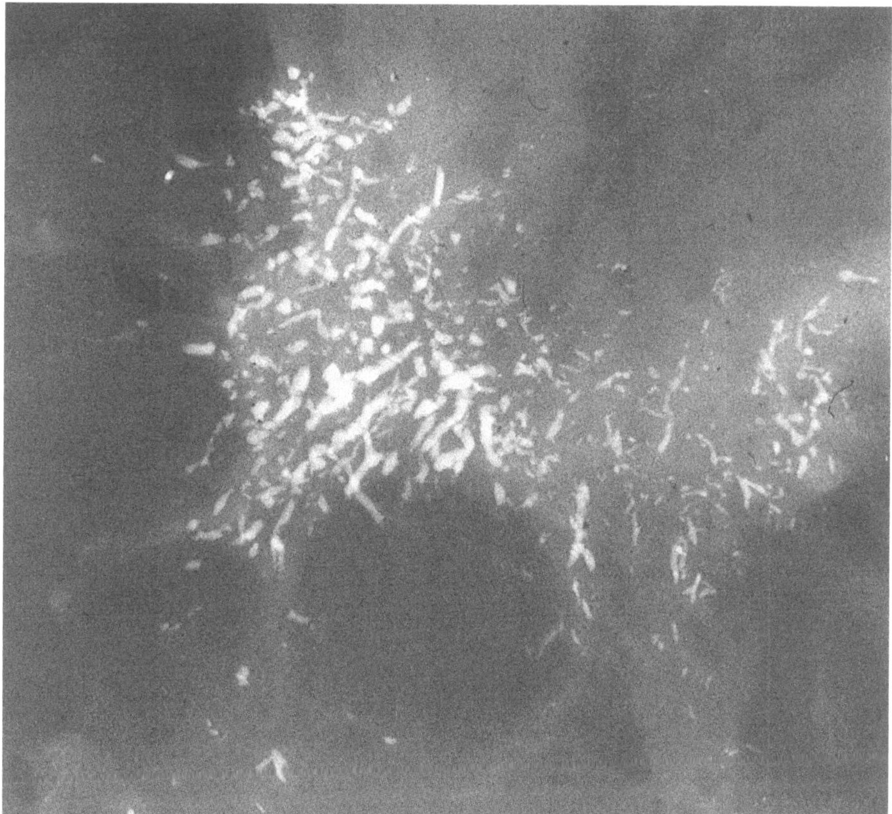

Fig. 4.60. Detail of mammogram (5 ×) showing a propeller- or butterfly-shaped cluster of polymorphous but predominantly branched microcalcifications in a histologically confirmed comedocarcinoma

◁ **Fig. 4.59 a, b.** Details of lateral mammograms (4.5 ×). **a** Club-shaped cluster of polymorphous punctate, linear, comma-shaped, and branched (Y-shaped) microcalcifications. Actually this is a triangular cluster that is elongated by a process extending toward the nipple, signifying involvement of an entire lobe and associated main duct by comedocarcinoma (Dr. LENDVAI, Porz). **b** Another club-shaped cluster of faint microcalcifications in an extensive comedocarcinoma. The number of calcifications (about 30) is remarkably small in relation to the cluster size, and apparently the tumor has little calcification tendency

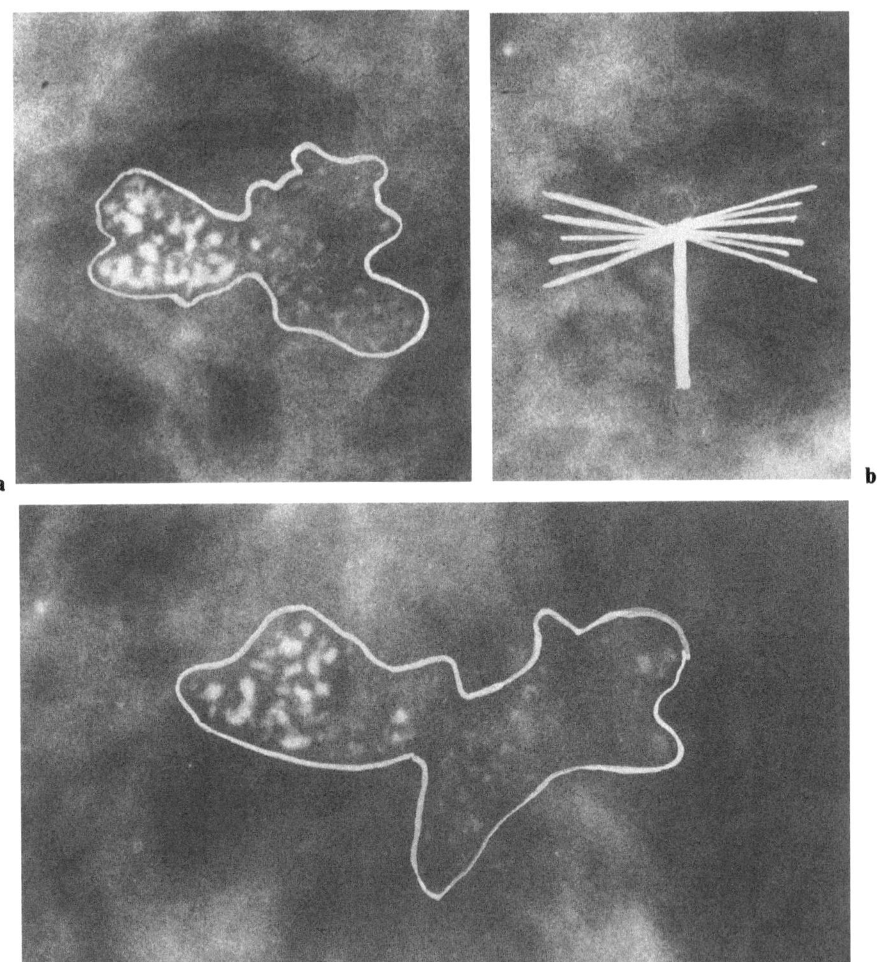

Fig. 4.61 a-c. Details of mammograms (4.5 ×) and schematic diagram (**b**). The cluster appears propeller-shaped on both the craniocaudad (**a**) and lateral (**c**) views. Almost all the microcalcifications are V- or Y-shaped. Histology: comedocarcinoma. In this case the propeller configuration is not a projection effect (cf. Figs. 4.68, 4.75 c, 4.76) but results from the tumor involvement of two opposed, triangular subsegments (**b**). This is confirmed by the swallowtail notches at both ends of the propeller (**a**). On the lateral view the propeller appears somewhat elongated (projection effect), and the notches are less pronounced (**c**). The microcalcifications are much more intense (older?) in one subsegment than the other

5) Rhomboid or kite-shaped (Figs. 4.57 a, 4.62 b).
6) Linear or branched (Figs. 4.63, 4.64).

In a morphologic analysis of 153 microcalcification clusters of malignant etiology (LANYI 1982 a), *no rounded or oval clusters were found,* and only 3% of the "malignant" clusters examined could not be assigned to any of the types listed above (Fig. 4.65 a). Experience teaches that the assessment of cluster shape can be difficult or even impossible in very small clusters. The longitudinal axes of cluster types 1, 3,

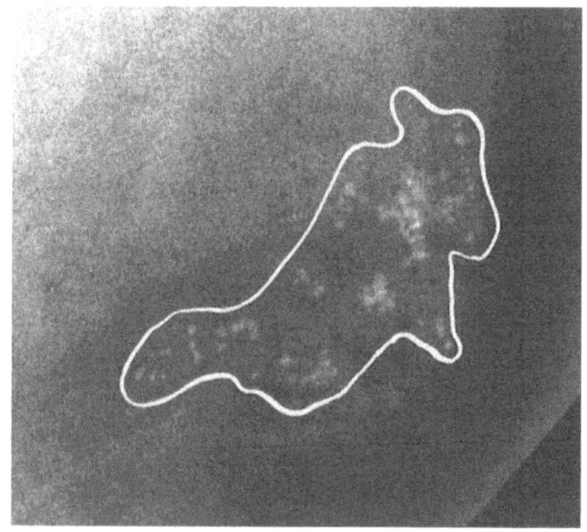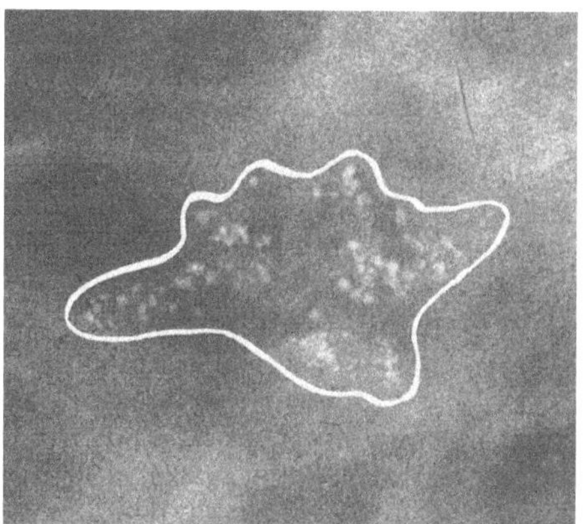

Fig. 4.62 a, b. Change of cluster shape with mammographic plane in an intraductal and intralobular carcinoma. **a** Lateral view: triangular cluster of microcalcifications with minimal polymorphism (most are punctate, a few comma-shaped). **b** Craniocaudad view: the cluster has a rhomboid (kite) shape

5, and 6 are always directed toward the nipple or the sagittal axis of the breast; this is not always the case with the other configurations. Figure 4.66 shows the percentage distribution of the different malignant cluster shapes found in one series.

Figure 4.67 shows the distribution of cluster shapes by mammographic plane. Analysis of the combination of different cluster shapes on two planes (Fig. 4.68) shows that the triangular or trapezoidal shape was evident on both planes in over 50% of cases (Fig. 4.69). In another 32% a triangular or trapezoidal cluster was found on one plane even when a different shape was present on the second plane (the "triangular principle") (Figs. 4.58, 4.62, 4.70, 4.92 b, c). Figure 4.71 shows the frequency of occurrence of the triangular or trapezoidal shape as a function of cluster size. The larger the cluster, the greater its tendency to assume a triangular or trapezoidal configuration.

On closer analysis of the clusters, it was determined that more than 30% exhibit wavy contours (Fig. 4.56). This feature is particularly characteristic of larger clusters. Clusters smaller than 100 mm^2 seldom have wavy contours (Fig. 4.69 a, b).

The baseline of triangular clusters, which usually faces the chest wall, often contains a notch that gives the cluster a "swallowtail" appearance (Figs. 4.53, 4.54, 4.56, 4.58 a, 4.61). Sometimes multiple posterior notches are present (Fig. 4.56). This phenomenon, too, is uncommon in clusters less than 100 mm^2 in size (as in Fig. 4.69).

Figure 4.72 shows the frequency of cluster shapes in breasts with intraductal carcinoma. The clusters were outlined on transparent sheets, brought to an approximately uniform size with an episcope, and projected onto one another such that the axes of the individual figures coincided. As the core of the superimposed contour lines indicates, the most common configuration on both planes is the triangle. The similarity between the malignant contours and the physiologic contours of the mammary ducts (Fig. 4.5) is unmistakeable.

The "triangular principle," the wavy contours, and the "swallowtail sign" can all be traced back to the intraductal location of the microcalcifications. Another sign of

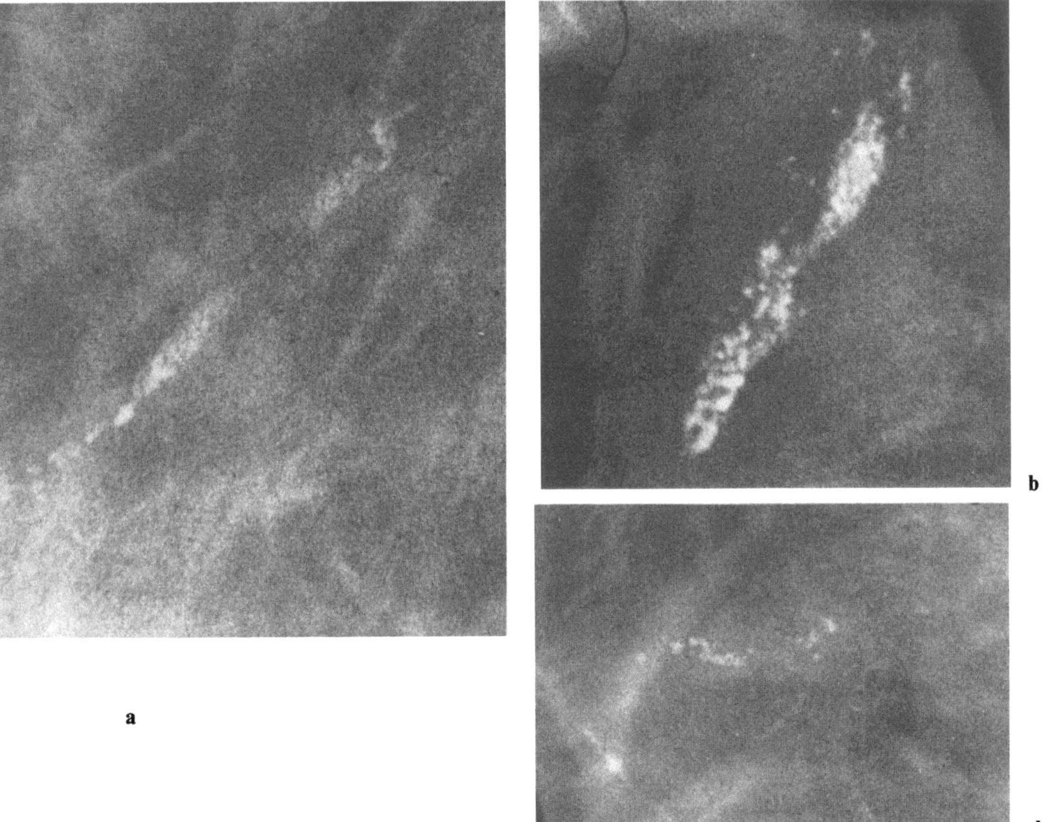

Fig. 4.63. a Detail of mammogram (6 ×) showing a milk duct completely filled with microcalcifications. The scaly ("snakeskin") appearance of the calcifications makes it impossible to analyze individual calcification shapes. **b** Detail from specimen radiograph (8 ×). Again we see a snakeskin pattern in a duct segment filled with microcalcifications (Dr. HENDRIKS, Catholic University, Nijmegen). **c** Detail of lateral mammogram (Professor HOEFFKEN, Cologne), slightly magnified. Here the microcalcifications fill an entire duct system, creating an image resembling a galactogram! Histology: all three cases are comedocarcinoma. **d** Detail of mammogram (2 ×) showing a linear (flat triangular) cluster of about 15 microcalcifications, 10 of which are grouped densely enough to create a snakeskin pattern. Comedocarcinoma. **e** The corresponding histologic section clearly shows the involved duct, which is filled with carcinoma cells and microcalcifications (approx. 40 ×) (Professor CITOLER, Cologne)

an intraductal localization is the presence of insular, microcalcification-free areas within larger clusters. These areas represent *inter*ductal, interstitial connective and fatty tissue devoid of microcalcifications (Figs. 4.73, 4.92 b). To test the validity of the triangular principle and to study the manner in which cluster shapes change with the direction of the X-ray beam, a three-dimensional model was constructed from a representative case (LANYI and CITOLER 1981) (Fig. 4.74).

The scale model of the carcinoma was mounted on an apparatus that could be rotated about two mutually perpendicular axes. The projected shapes of the model

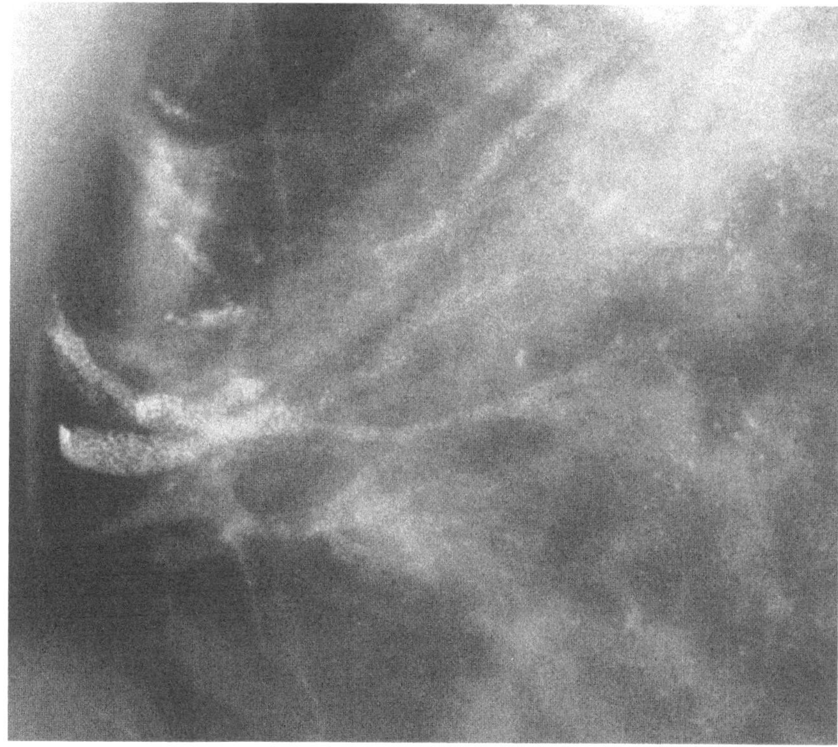

c

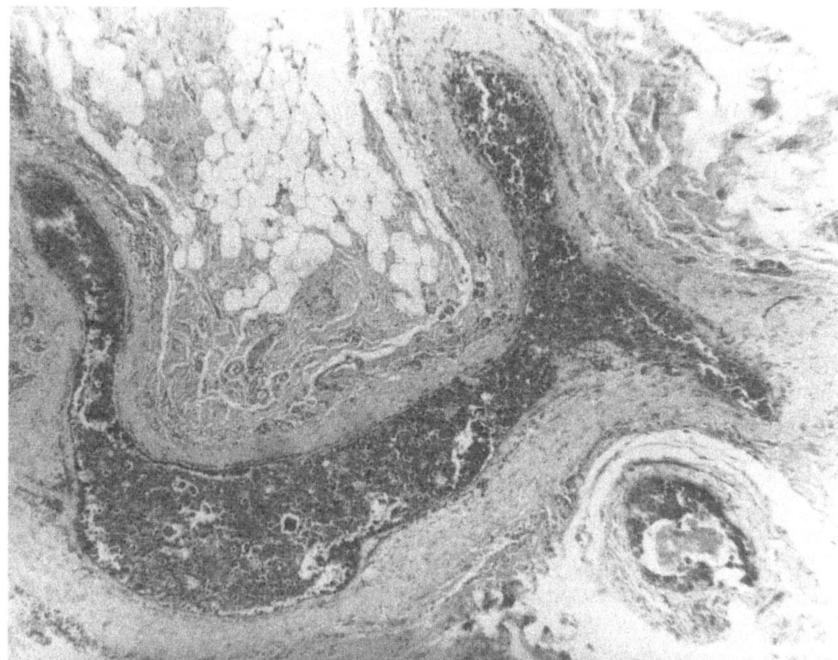

e

Fig. 4.63 c, e

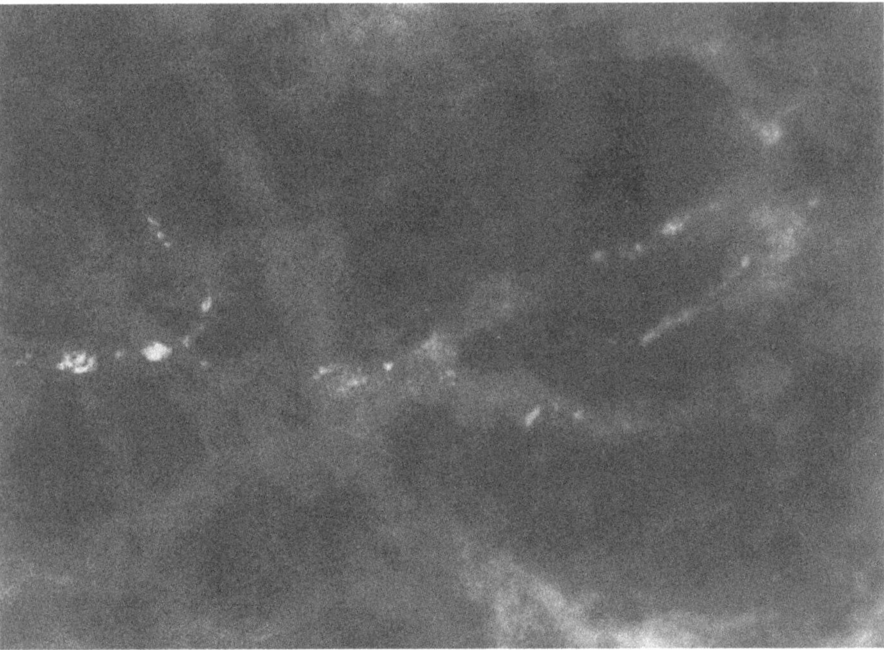

Fig. 4.64. Detail of mammogram (5 ×): branched cluster of punctate and linear microcalcifications in a histologically confirmed comedocarcinoma

was studied by tilting one axis and rotating the other in stages through equal angles in space, while using a strong light source to project the contour of the model onto a screen. To reduce subjective error we rotated the model 90° and repeated the experiment, making a total of 605 separate observations. This experiment made it possible to study shape changes relating both to the location of the mammary ducts involved by carcinoma and to the direction of the X-ray beam. The cluster configurations most often seen empirically were easily reproduced by manipulation of the model (Fig. 4.75). Comparison of the purely empirical data in Fig. 4.66 with the experimental data in Fig. 4.76 leads to the discovery of amazing similarities:

a) There is hardly any difference between the rates of occurrence of the triangular/ trapezoidal configurations (65% vs 73.6%).

b) The rates of occurrence of the diamond-shaped configurations are almost identical (5.5% vs 6.0%).

c) The total rates of occurrence of the square and bottle-shaped configurations, at 17.5% and 18%, are virtually identical.

This remarkable similarity between empirical and experimental data cannot be coincidental; it is highly probable that a true principle is involved.

The occurrence of *nontriangular* configurations depends not only on projection-dependent changes in the shape of the pyramid-shaped ducts (and thus of the carcinoma) but also on other anatomic factors (Fig. 4.61) and the degree to which the particular duct segment is filled with calcifications.

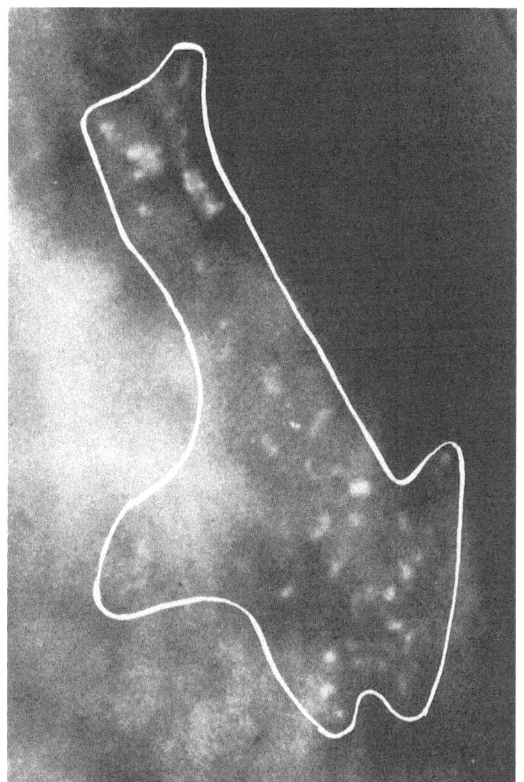

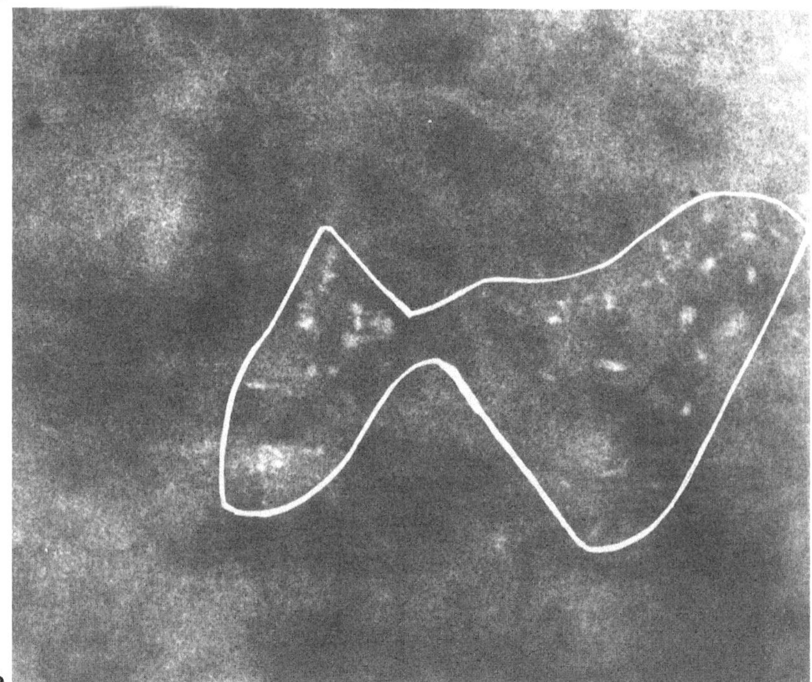

Fig. 4.65a, b. Details of mammograms (5 ×). **a** Lateral view: faint cluster of polymorphous microcalcifications. The cluster shape is difficult to evaluate (bottle-shaped? triangular?). **b** Craniocaudad view of the same area: the cluster is propeller- or butterfly-shaped

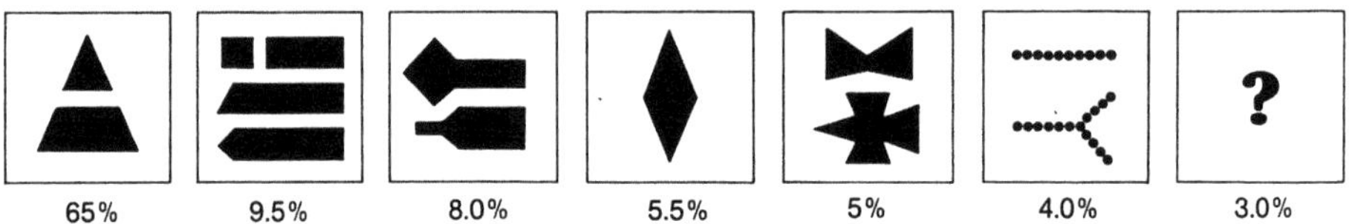

| 65% | 9.5% | 8.0% | 5.5% | 5% | 4.0% | 3.0% |

Fig. 4.66. Frequency of occurrence of different microcalcification cluster shapes in breast malignancies (total of 153 clusters on 290 mammograms: 137 clusters on two views, 16 on one view)

	▲	▦	◄	◆	✖	⤙	?
(craniocaudad)	88 +3	13	9	6	9 +1	6	6
(lateral)	88 +9	14	13 +2	9 +1	4	5	4

Fig. 4.67. Distribution of cluster shapes by mammographic plane, based on 137 clusters on two views and 16 clusters on one view; 91 triangular or trapezoidal clusters were observed on the craniocaudad films, and 97 on the lateral films. The remaining 50 or 52 clusters manifested any of five other well-defined cluster shapes, or were irregularly shaped (symbolized by ?)

	▲	▦	◄	✖	◆	⤙	?
▲	71						
▦	11	4					
◄	7	2	3				
✖	5	4	0	0			
◆	6	2	0	1	3		
⤙	1	0	0	0	0	5	
?	4	0	1	1	0	0	2

Fig. 4.68. Simultaneous occurrence of the different cluster shapes on the craniocaudad and lateral projections, based on an analysis of 137 clusters. Of these, 71 clusters appeared triangular or trapezoidal on both views, and another 34 clusters exhibited that shape on at least one view (including four clusters that were amorphous on the second view!)

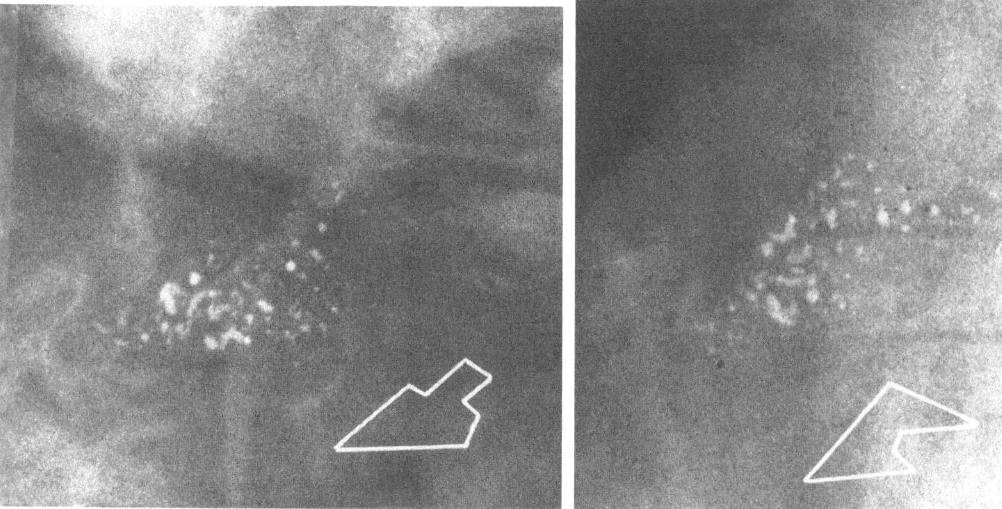

Fig. 4.69 a, b. Details of mammograms (3 ×). **a** Craniocaudad view: triangular cluster of polymorphous (punctate, linear, comma-shaped, branched) microcalcifications with a shallow posterior notch. **b** Lateral view of the same cluster: again the cluster is triangular, but the posterior notch is absent. A fine, knoblike "process" is visible on both views. Histology: comedocarcinoma

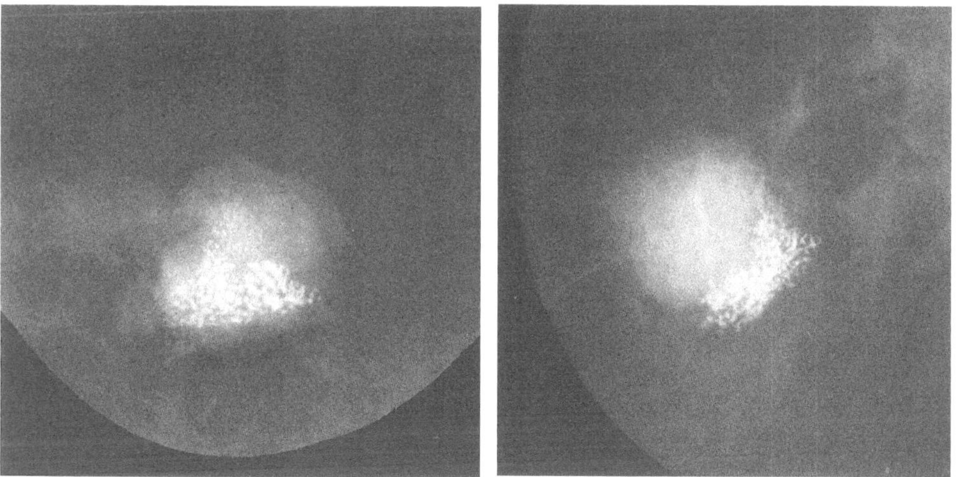

Fig. 4.70 a, b. Details of mammograms (original size). **a** Craniocaudad view: a dense, triangular cluster of polymorphous microcalcifications, all very intense, are projected onto a round shadow with partly smooth and partly ill-defined margins. A small notch is visible on one side of the cluster. **b** Lateral view: The cluster is rectangular (or slightly propeller-shaped?) (Advanced Medical Training University, Budapest). Histology: medullary carcinoma and comedocarcinoma

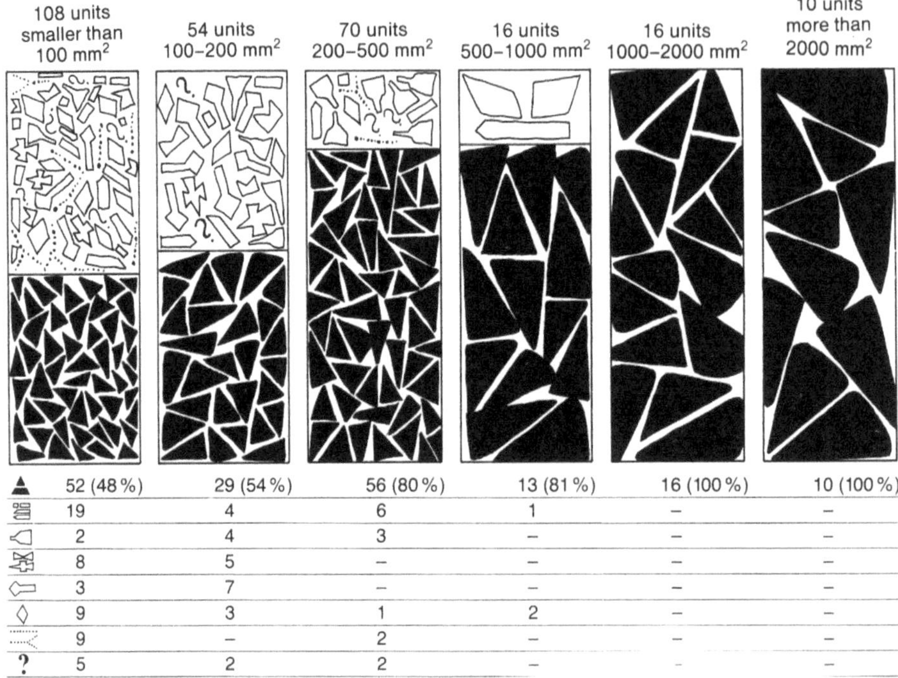

	108 units smaller than 100 mm²	54 units 100–200 mm²	70 units 200–500 mm²	16 units 500–1000 mm²	16 units 1000–2000 mm²	10 units more than 2000 mm²
▲	52 (48 %)	29 (54 %)	56 (80 %)	13 (81 %)	16 (100 %)	10 (100 %)
(stacked)	19	4	6	1	–	–
(trapezoid)	2	4	3	–	–	–
(bowtie)	8	5	–	–	–	–
(pentagon)	3	7	–	–	–	–
◇	9	3	1	2	–	–
(dotted)	9	–	2	–	–	–
?	5	2	2	–	–	–

Fig. 4.71. Graphic representation of the relationship between cluster size and shape: while only about half the clusters in the first three columns (i. e., clusters smaller than 500 mm²) have triangular shapes, the great majority of clusters 500–1000 mm² in size are triangular, and all the clusters larger than 1000 mm² are triangular or trapezoidal

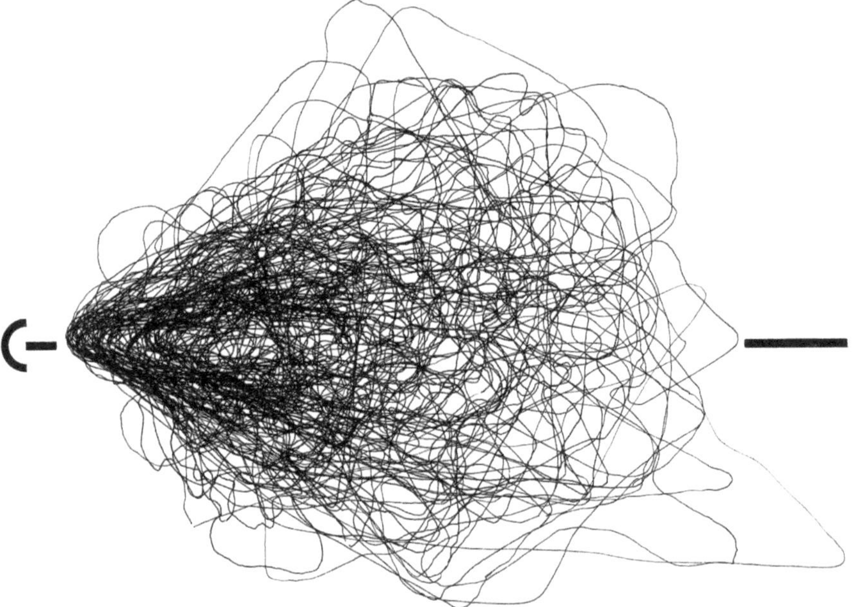

Fig. 4.72. Superimposed contour lines (lateral projection) of 153 microcalcification clusters of malignant etiology. The "core" of the tracings confirms that the most frequent cluster shape is triangular

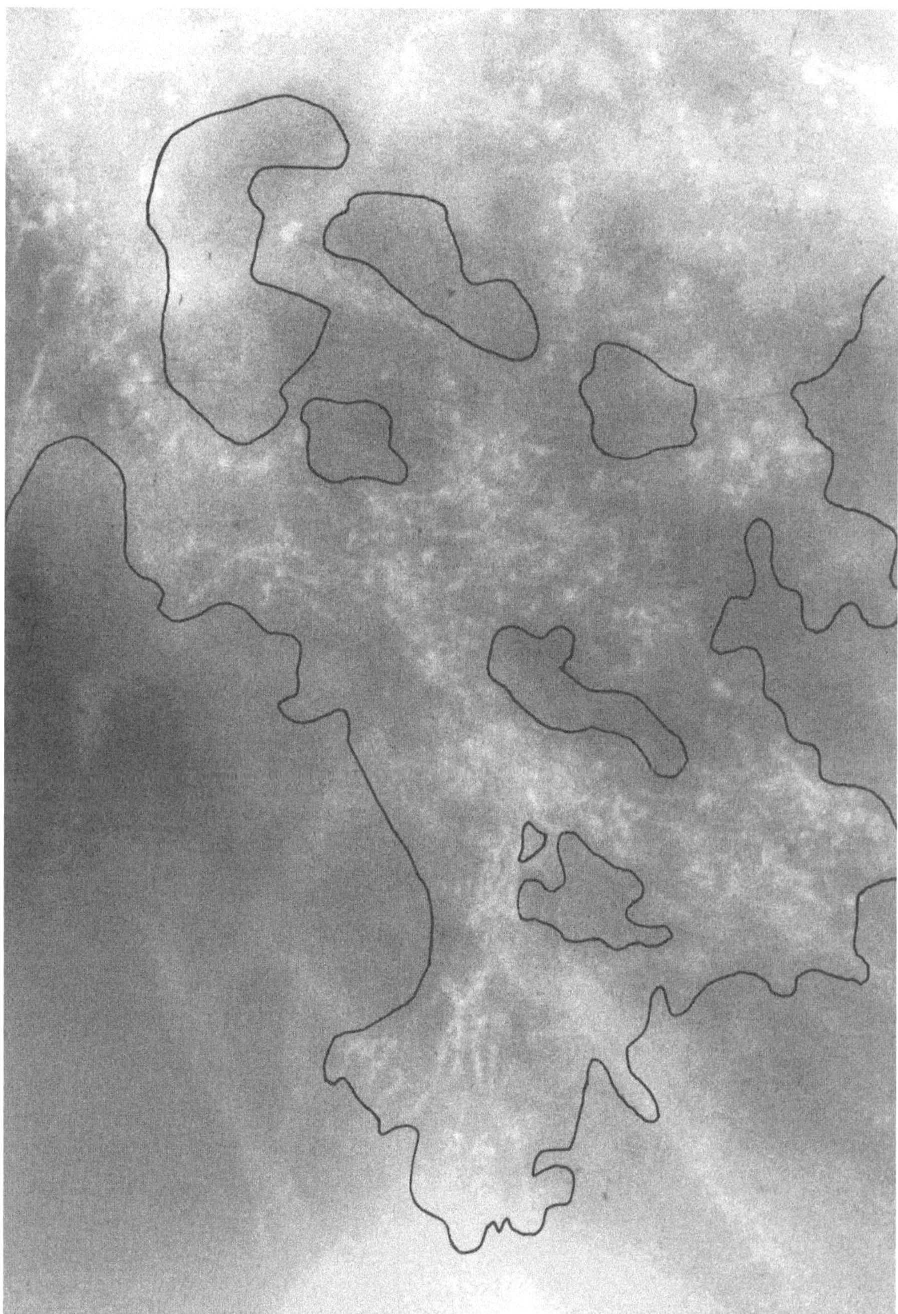

Fig. 4.73. Detail of mammogram from the periphery of an extensive microcalcification cluster in comedocarcinoma (5 ×). The calcifications are numerous, polymorphous, and uniformly faint. The processes extending from the cluster represent the ends of the mammary ducts. The cluster contains insular zones devoid of microcalcifications; these represent interductal, interstitial connective tissue (fat)

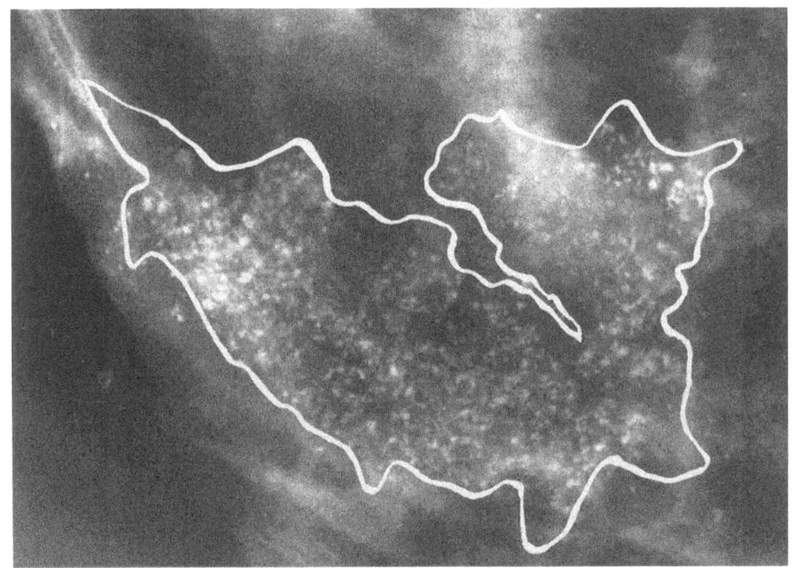
a

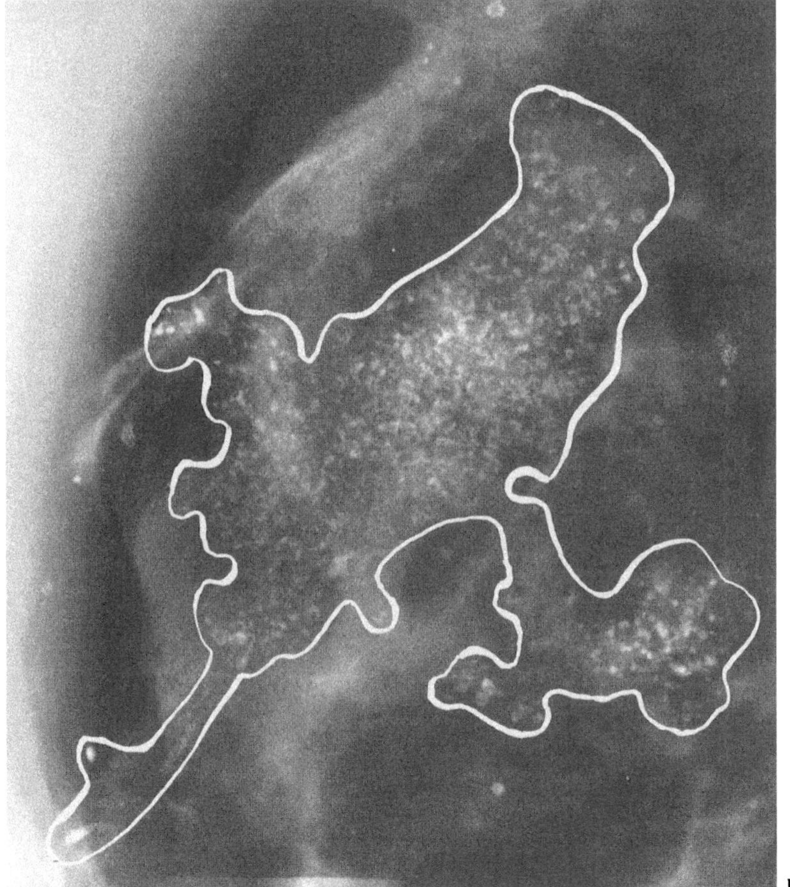
b

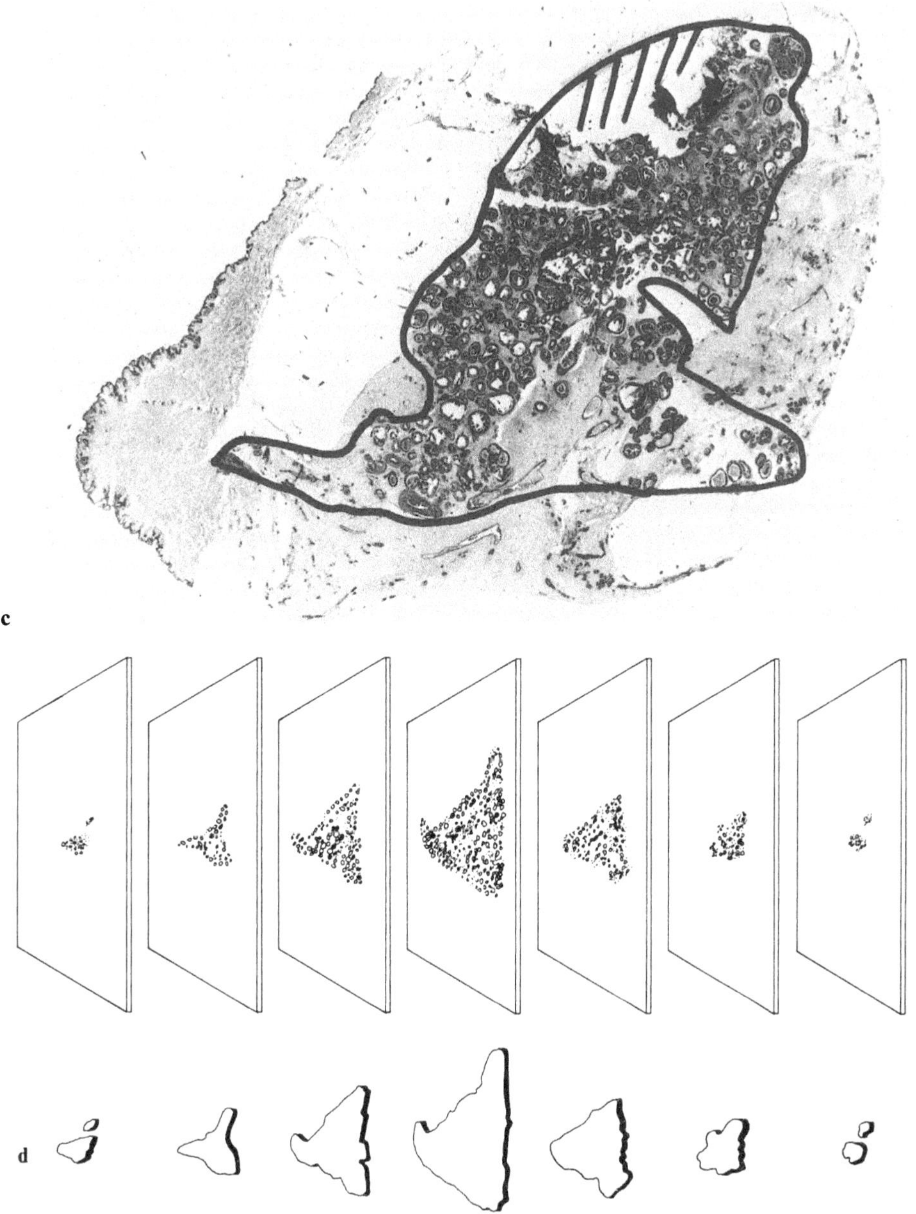

c

d

Fig. 4.74a-d Legend on p. 106

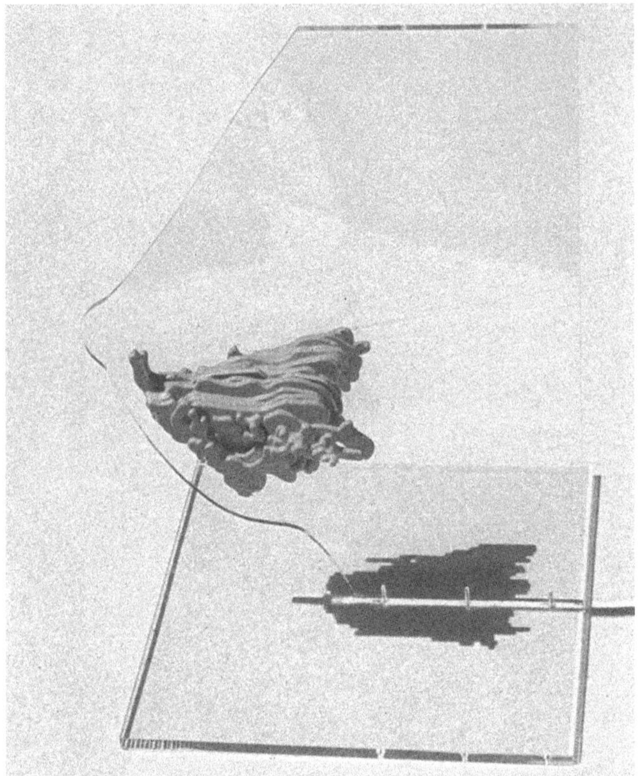

Fig. 4.74e

Fig. 4.74. a Lateral view: triangular cluster of innumerable, polymorphous microcalcifications. **b** Craniocaudad view: triangular (club-shaped?) cluster. The cluster contours are wavy and show small processes. Note the swallowtail sign on the craniocaudad view. The snoutlike anterior process pointing toward the nipple signifies involvement of the main duct and lactiferous sinus. Calcified sebaceous glands are visible outside the lesion. **c** Extensive, predominantly intraductal (comedo) carcinoma with areas of central necrosis and calcifications. The missing tissue piece *(hatched)* was taken for frozen section. The carcinoma, measuring 3.5 × 2 × 2 cm in size, was cut longitudinally into three blocks of roughly equal size, and 11 serial sections approx. 600–800 μm apart were prepared from each block. **d** Diagrams showing how the model of the carcinoma was made. *Top row:* the tissue sections were projected onto wooden boards 5 mm thick at a magnification of 4 ×, and the contours of the area involved by carcinoma were traced onto the board. *Bottom row:* the outlined shapes (33 in all) were cut from the boards and assembled in proper sequence. **e** The finished model

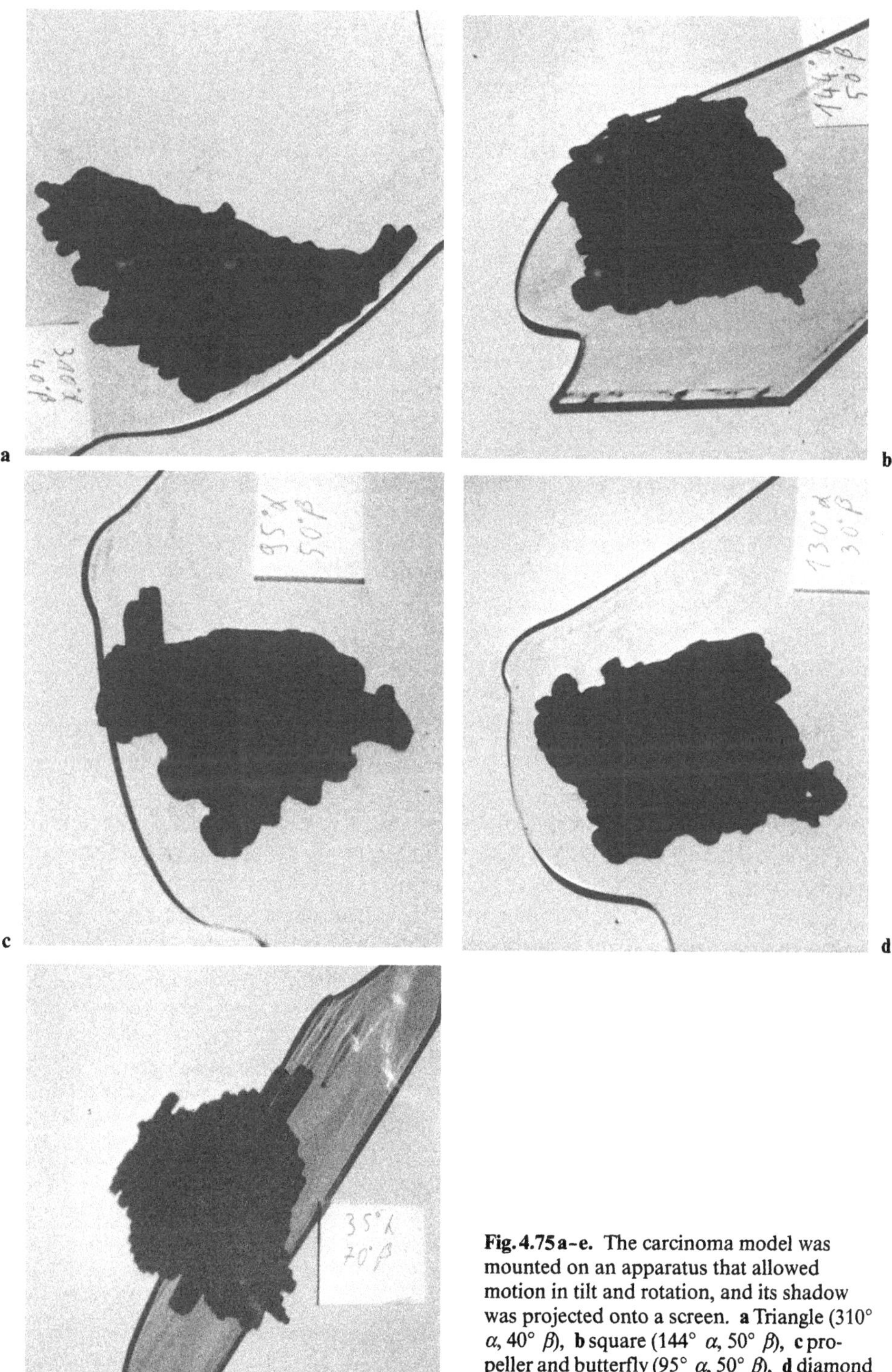

Fig. 4.75 a–e. The carcinoma model was mounted on an apparatus that allowed motion in tilt and rotation, and its shadow was projected onto a screen. **a** Triangle (310° α, 40° β), **b** square (144° α, 50° β), **c** propeller and butterfly (95° α, 50° β), **d** diamond (130° α, 30° β), **e** bottle/club (35° α, 70° β)

	▲	⬛	◀	◆	⨝	?	Total
Number of observations	445	102	7	36	10	5	605
%	73.6	16.8	1.2	6	1.6	0.8	100

Fig. 4.76. Frequency of occurrence of the different projected shapes observed experimentally (compare with Fig. 4.66)

The Shapes of Individual Microcalcifications

The shapes of the individual microcalcifications should be analyzed with at least a $4\times$ magnifying lens, and each calcification should be carefully examined.

To perform this analysis, we made high-quality contact copies from the original mammogram, selected a field measuring 6×6 cm, and projected it onto a drawing board, enlarged 20 times. This enabled us to trace the individual microcalcifications onto a sheet of paper. Overlapping or poorly defined microcalcifications were disregarded. Microcalcifications of like shapes were drawn with the same color to facilitate counting (Fig. 4.77). Four well-defined calcification shapes occur with different frequencies in breast carcinoma. They are:
1) Punctate calcifications of variable size
2) Bean- or comma-shaped calcifications
3) Wavy (wormlike) or linear calcifications of variable length
4) Branched calcifications resembling the last letters of the alphabet (V, W, X, Y, Z)

Microcalcifications that do not fit these categories may be found, but they are uncommon.

The analysis of 7028 individual microcalcifications in 121 intraductal carcinomas (Fig. 4.78) based on earlier studies (LANYI 1977b, 1983) yielded the following results.

Monomorphism of the punctate microcalcifications is very rare (5 cases = 4%) and is most apt to occur in short papillary/cribriform carcinomas (Fig. 4.79). Only one tiny comedocarcinoma in our material exhibited this feature (Fig. 4.63a). If the number of microcalcifications exceeds 15, only polymorphous microcalcifications can be demonstrated in ductal carcinomas ("principle of polymorphism").

Analysis of calcification shapes as a function of number shows the following relationships, which hold true with few exceptions. The smaller the microcalcification cluster, the greater the tendency of punctate calcifications to predominate. As the number of calcifications increases, the punctate forms tend to become less prevalent, regardless of the histologic type of the carcinoma (Fig. 4.78d). The ratio of punctate to nonpunctate calcifications for *all* the cases studied is 51:49.

Of the 121 cases investigated (Table 4.7), 10 were not further specified histologically. In the remaining 111 cases that were specified, the following relationship exists between histology and number of microcalcifications. An average of 66 microcalcifications were found in each of the 60 comedocarcinomas. The ratio of punctate to nonpunctate calcifications is 43:57, signifying a greater polymorphism within the cluster (Fig. 4.78a).

Table 4.7. Histologic diagnoses for 121 ductal carcinomas that were biopsied on the basis of microcalcifications alone, without a visible tumor shadow

Comedocarcinoma	60
Fine papillary/cribriform carcinoma	11
Mixed forms (comedo and cribriform)	40
Ductal carcinoma (further differentiation was not possible retrospectively)	10
Total:	121

An average of 42 microcalcifications were found in the 11 short papillary-cribriform carcinomas. The ratio of punctate to nonpunctate calcifications, 73:27, is markedly higher than in the other cases. The punctate shape obviously predominates in this histologic type of ductal carcinoma (Fig. 4.78 b). A similar phenomenon was seen in the 40 "mixed carcinomas" (comedo, short papillary, and cribriform growths coexisting in the same lesion) (Fig. 4.78 c). Although the histologic diagnoses for these mixed carcinomas show some variation (e.g., predominantly comedo combined with papillary, comedo-papillary-cribriform, papillary-cribriform combined with comedo), it is nevertheless clear that all these cases involve a mixed form. The ratio of punctate to other configurations is 55:45 in these lesions and thus is similar to the 51.2:48.8 established for *all* forms of ductal carcinoma (Fig. 4.78 d).

When the number of microcalcifications and ratio of punctate to nonpunctate calcifications are known, one sometimes can deduce the particular histologic pattern that is present (Figs. 4.80, 4.81, 4.86). This "quasi-histologic" diagnosis is made possible by the distinctive structural features of the comedo and short papillary-cribriform carcinomas, i.e., the different calcification shapes that are associated with these growths.

In comedocarcinomas the calcifications occur at the center of the duct lumina (Fig. 4.50 and 4.82). The linear or wormlike calcifications are probably derived from compressed punctate and bean-shaped calcifications. If the calcifications occur in branching ducts, a "V" or "Y" shape will form at bifurcations, a "W" shape at trifurcations, or an "X" or "Z" shape when the branches are cut by the beam in an orthograde direction.

In the short papillary-cribriform carcinomas, on the other hand, the psammoma bodies do not occur centrally, but are irregularly disposed in the cavities of the spongy cancer tissue, probably floating in calcific secretion, as in microcystic adenosis and milk of calcium cysts (see p. 42) (Figs. 4.50 b and 4.83).

All these calcification shapes described for intraductal carcinoma can be demonstrated in the debris scraped from a comedocarcinoma (Fig. 4.84). The percentage distribution of the various calcification shapes varies according to the prevalence of the basic histologic types in each carcinoma. Apparently none of the types occurs in isolation, and all breast carcinomas appear to be mixed to some degree. Thus, a linear or branched calcification is occasionally seen even in the very smallest papillary-cribriform carcinomas with predominantly punctate microcalcifications (Fig. 4.85 a, b). Besides the shape of the cluster, this "minimal polymorphism" is the second hallmark of an intraductal localization. In contrast, the individual calcifications of comedocarcinomas show a very strong polymorphism (Fig. 4.85 c).

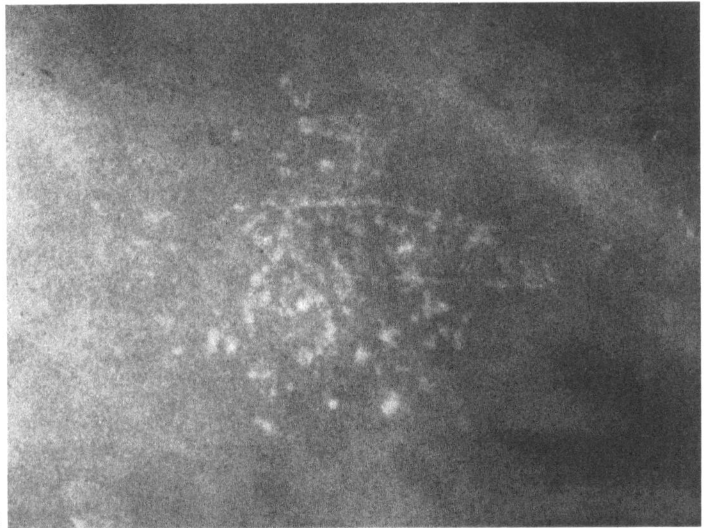

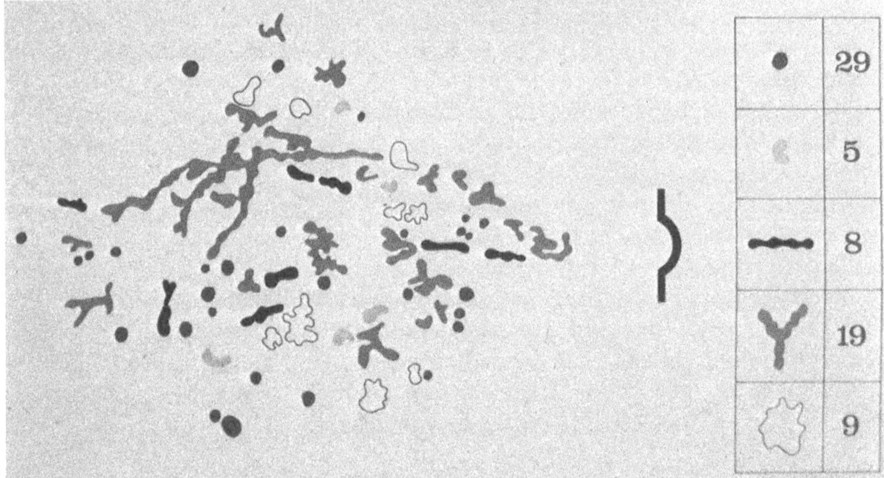

Fig. 4.77. a Diamond-shaped cluster of microcalcifications in a comedocarcinoma. **b** The cluster image was enlarged 20 times with a projector, and the individual microcalcifications were traced onto paper – punctate forms in red, comma-shaped in green, linear in black, and branched in blue (see p. 244). Amorphous calcifications were outlined but not colored. The nonpunctate shapes predominante by 41:29

Fig. 4.78a-d. Scatter diagrams for 111 ductal carcinomas given a specific histologic diagnosis. The object was to determine whether a correlation existed between histologic type (papillary, cribriform, comedo) and the ratio of punctate microcalcifications to other forms. Each case is represented by 1 *point* on the graph. **a** Comedocarcinomas, **b** papillary-cribriform carcinomas, **c** mixed carcinomas, **d** all cases (*open circles* represent cases not further specified). *Horizontal axis,* number of microcalcifications counted; *vertical axis,* percentage of punctate microcalcifications. On the basis of the U test (Mann and Whitney, quoted in Sachs 1978), the following statements may be made with a probability of error $d = 0.005$:

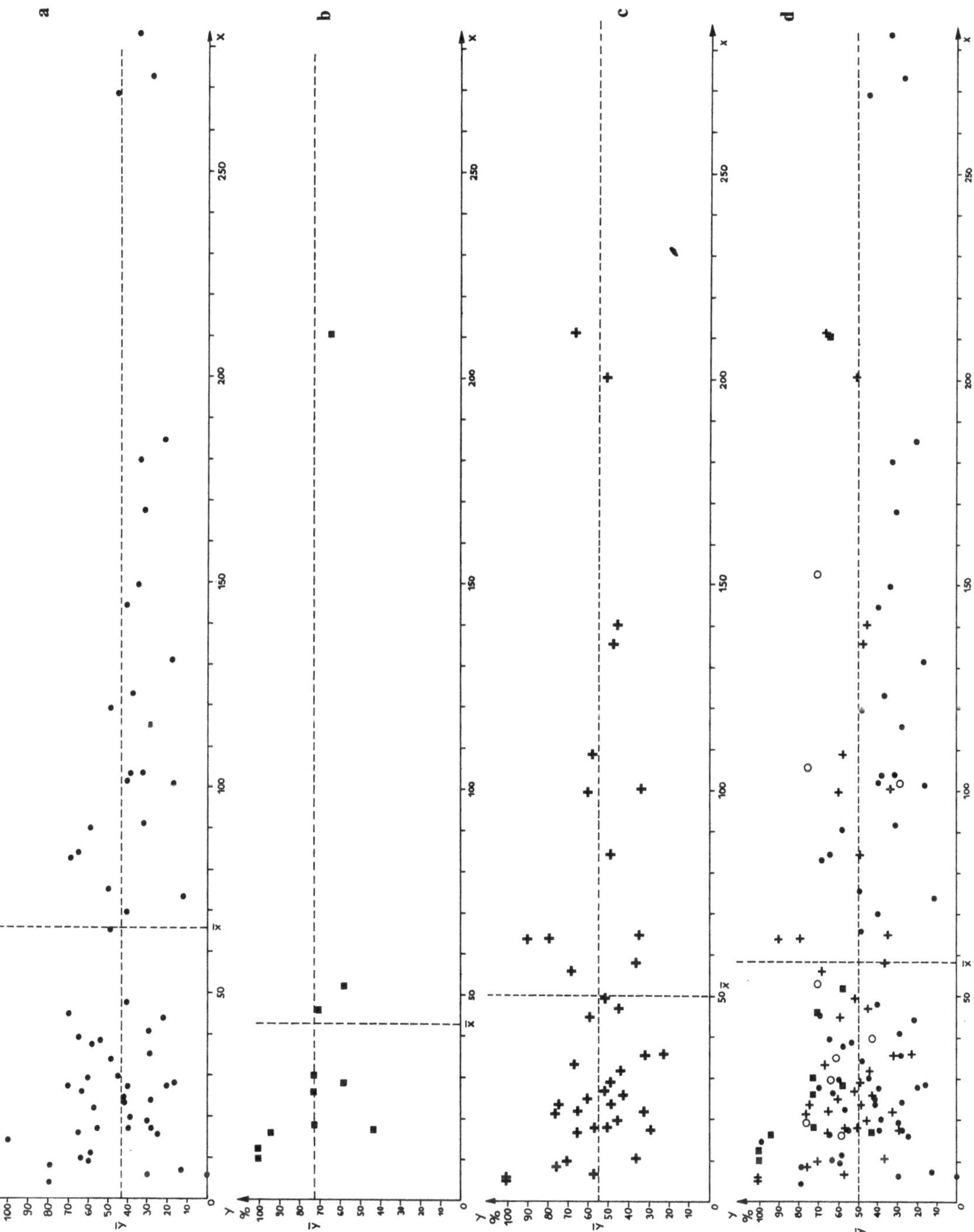

1) The percentage of punctate microcalcifications is significantly higher in the papillary-cribriform cases than in the comedo/papillary/cribriform cases overall ($\hat{z} = 2.77$) or in the comedo cases alone ($\hat{z} = 3.93$).

2) The percentage of punctate shapes is significantly higher in the comedo/papillary/cribriform cases overall than in the comedo cases ($\hat{z} = 3.05$) (P. SCHWANNENBERG, Technische Hochschule, Gummersbach)

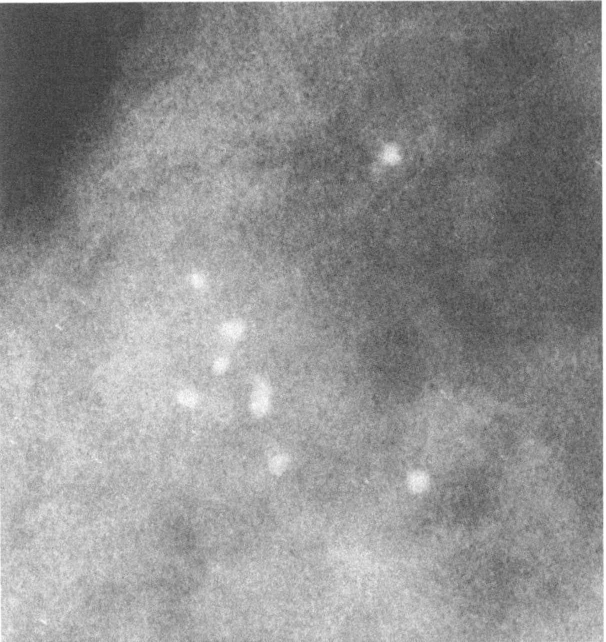

Fig.4.79. Detail of mammogram (4 ×): seven monomorphus, punctate microcalcifications forming a trapezoidal cluster in a small papillary-cribriform carcinoma

Fig.4.80. a Detail of lateral mammogram (4 ×): 13 punctate (1 linear?) microcalcifications in a pro- ▷ peller-shaped cluster, discovered on a routine mammogram (Drs.GÖRING and STOCKHAMMER, Braunschweig) and referred to the author for second opinion concerning the need for biopsy. Radiographic diagnosis based on the propeller shape of the cluster and minimal polymorphism: suspected papillary-cribriform carcinoma. **b** Histology (Professor CAESAR, Braunschweig): papillary carcinoma containing secretions and psammomatous calcifications (approx. 80 ×). **c** Cribriform carcinoma with intraluminal calcifications (approx. 40 ×)

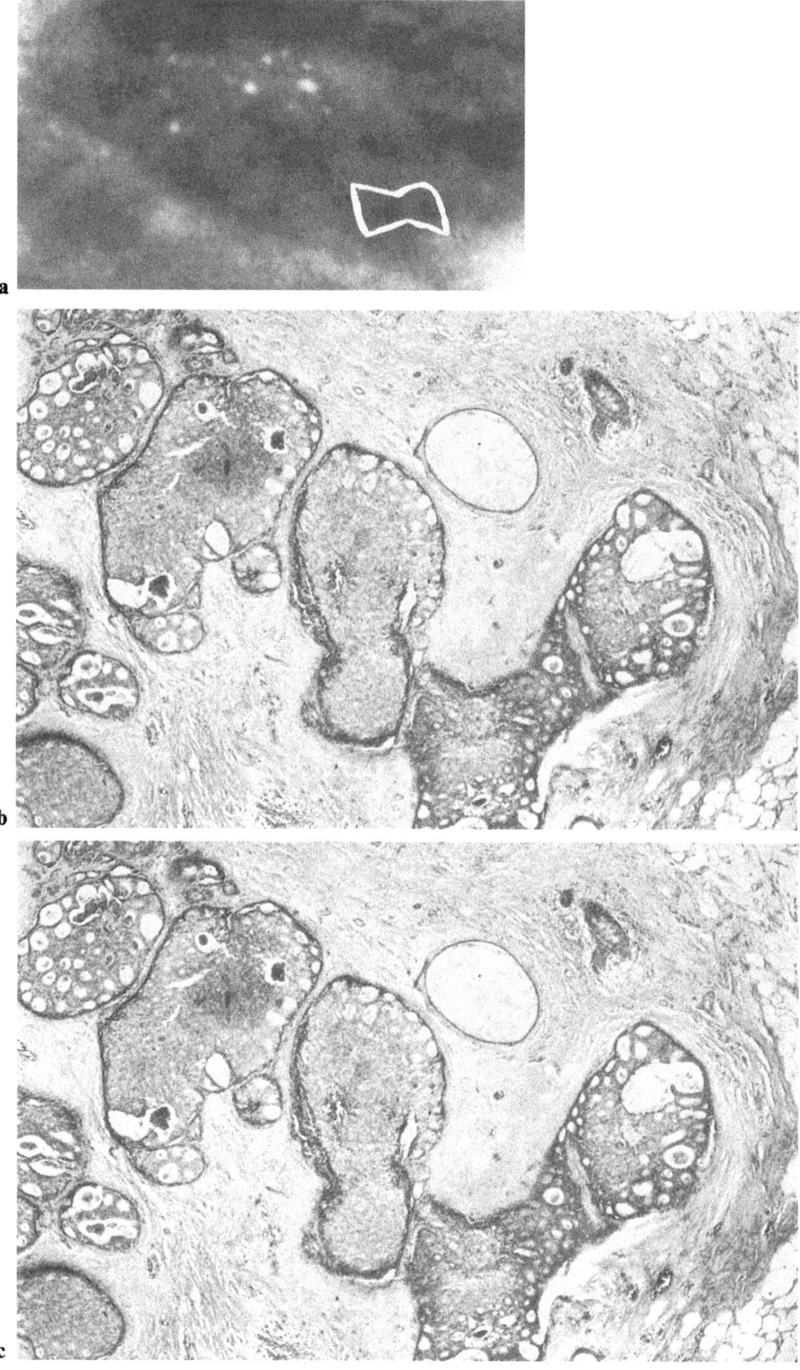

Fig. 4.80 a–c

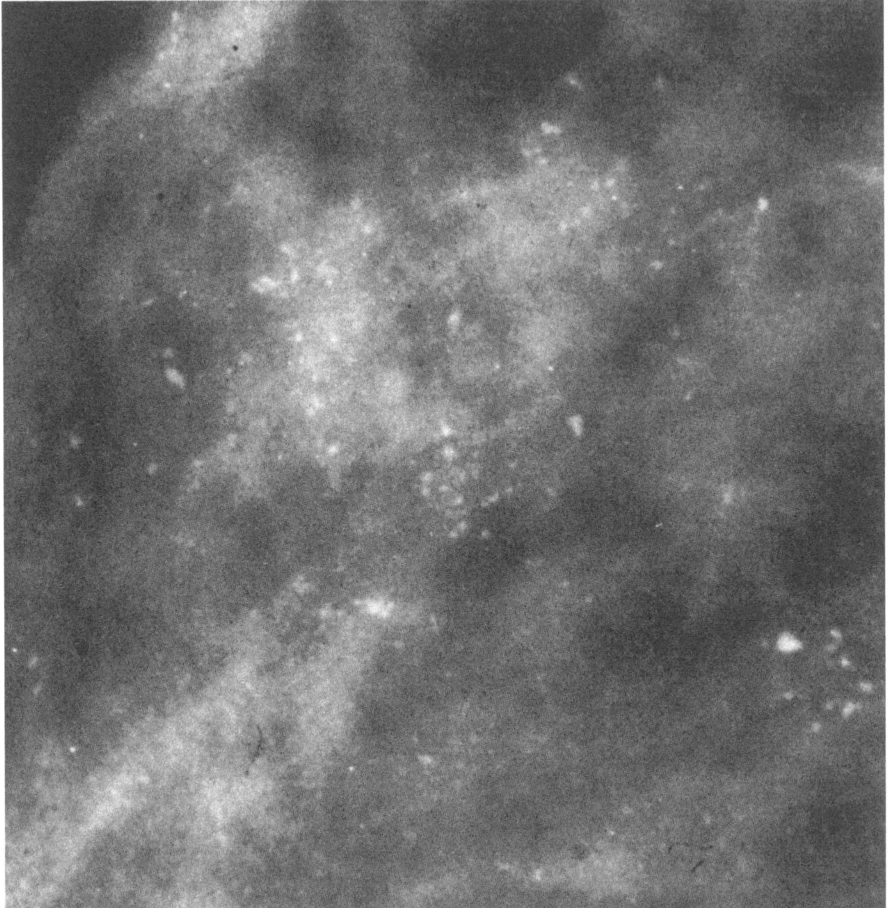

Fig. 4.81. Detail of lateral mammogram (4.5 ×) (case referred from Professor VAN DE WEYER, Trier). Question: do these lesions represent milk of calcium cysts? A relatively small number of linear, comma-shaped, and v-shaped microcalcifications are interspersed with numerous punctate calcifications. No teacup signs are visible. Radiographic diagnosis: predominantly papillary/cribriform, partly comedocarcinoma. This was confirmed histologically

Fig. 4.82. Detail of mammogram (5 ×) taken after galactography with iodized oil (lipiodol; per- ▷ formed elsewhere). The residual contrast medium shows the configurations typical of comedocarcinoma (linear, V-, Y-, and W-shaped); note also the triangular cluster shape with posterior notching (swallowtail sign). The punctate contrast residues probably represent small terminal cysts

Fig. 4.83 a, b. Model to explain the punctate microcalcifications of cribriform carcinoma. **a** The pores of a sponge were filled with contrast medium, and the model was radiographed. **b** The radiograph shows that the "microcalcifications" are mostly punctate, and that comma shapes appear when contrast medium fills two interconnecting pores

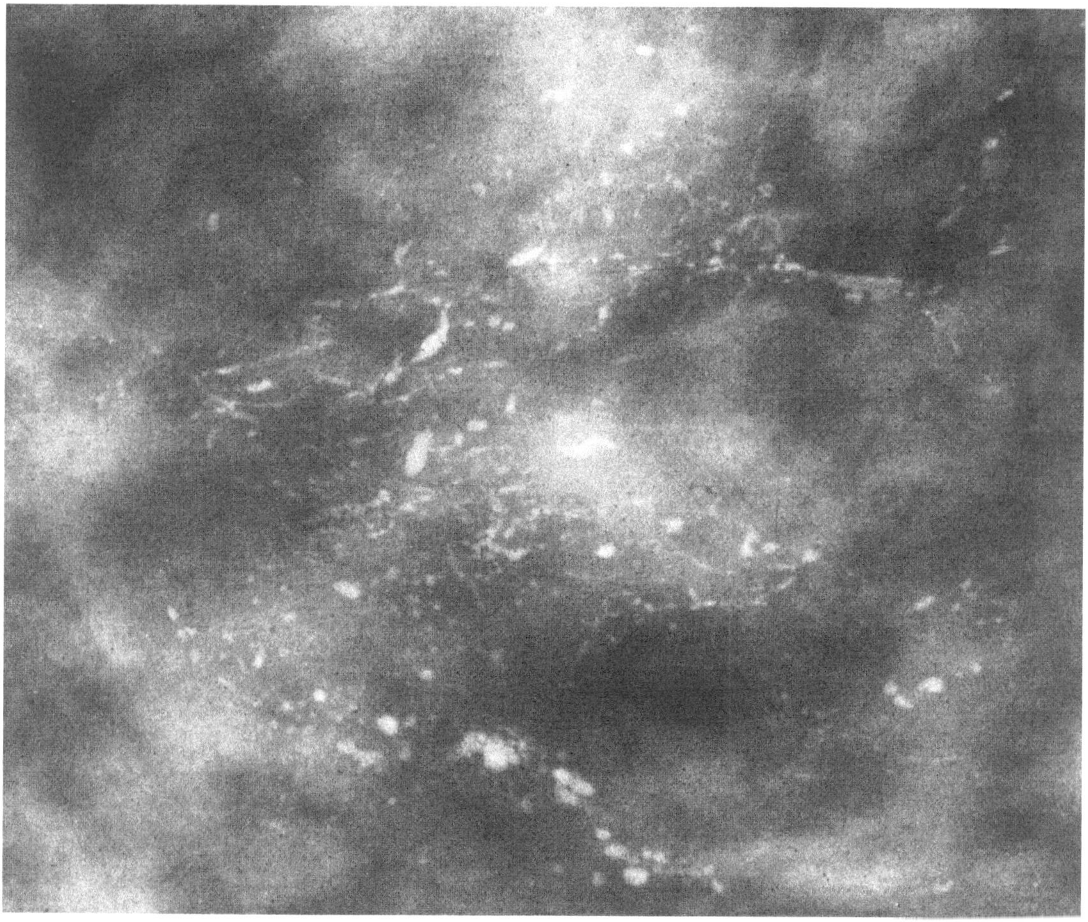

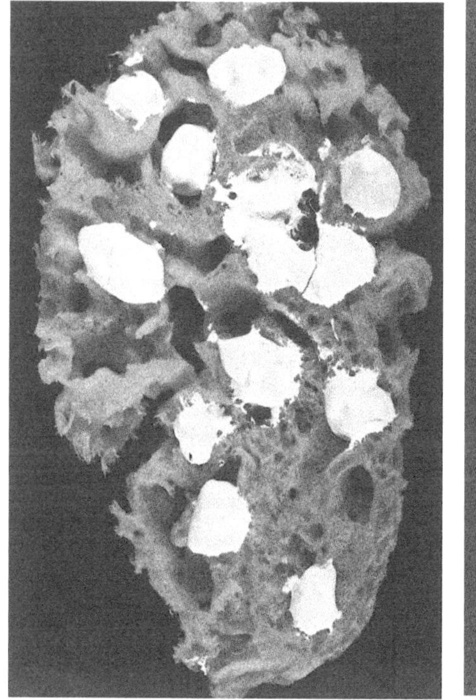
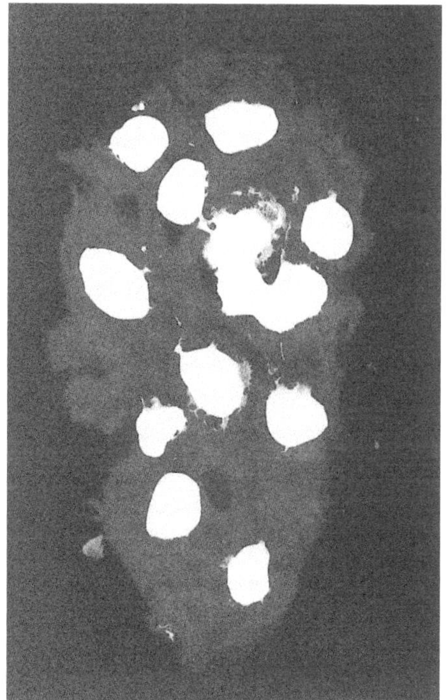

Fig. 4.82

Fig. 4.83 a, b

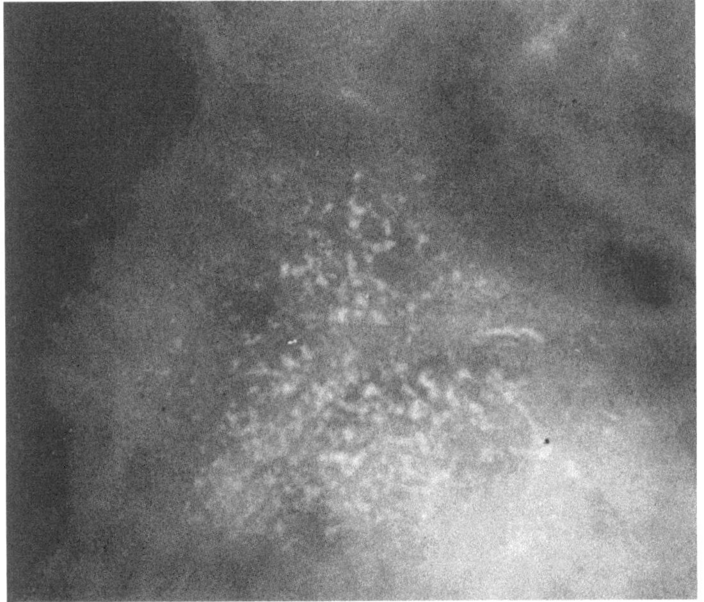

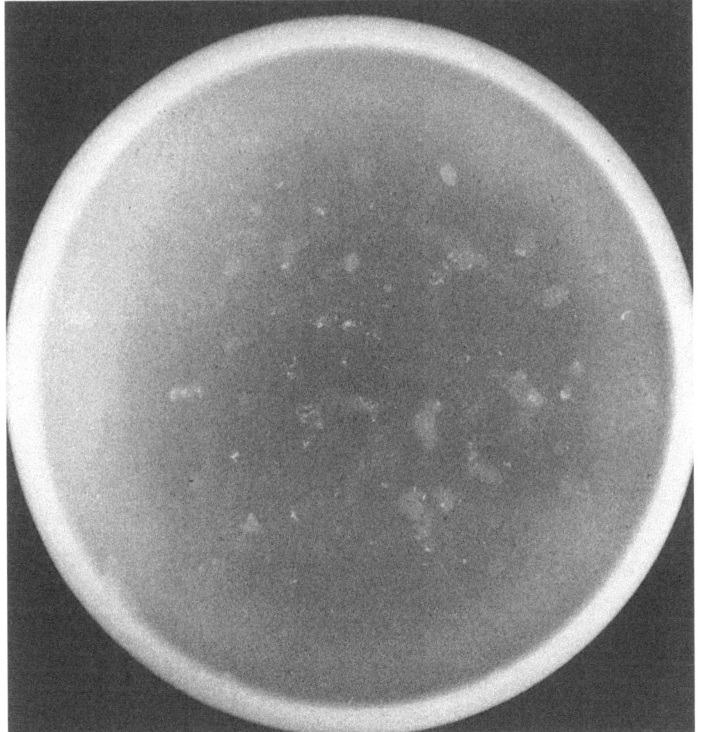

Fig. 4.84 a, b

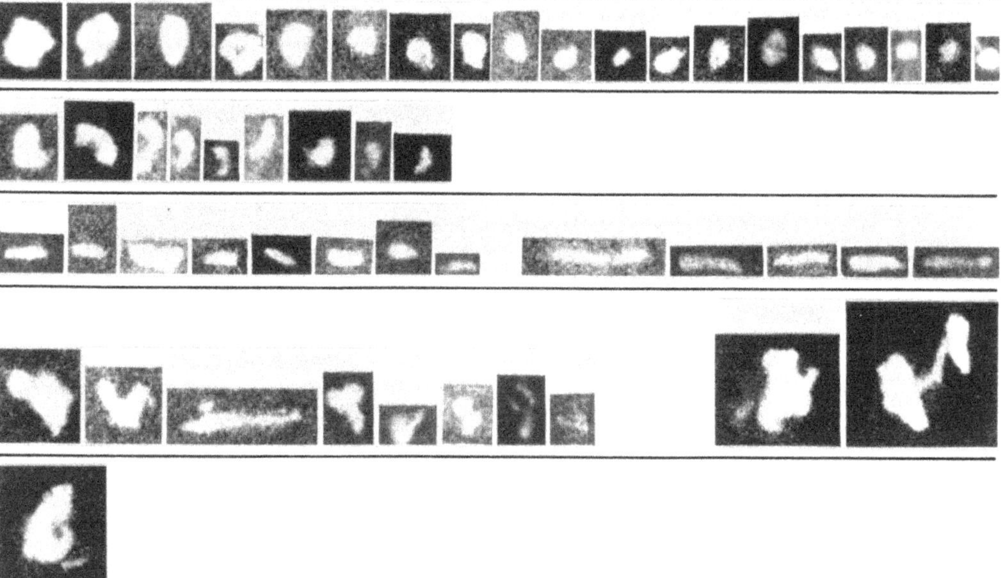

Fig. 4.84. a Detail of mammogram (4.5 ×): triangular cluster of polymorphous microcalcifications in a predominantly comedo-type ductal carcinoma. After the histologic diagnosis was made, the carcinoma was cut into thin slices, and the microcalcifications were scraped out. (**b**) These were radiographed, the radiograph was enlarged and printed on paper, and the individual microcalcifications were cut out. **c** Selections from over 100 microcalcifications. *First row,* punctate; *second row,* bean-shaped or comma-shaped; *third row,* linear; *fourth row,* branched. The last calcification could not be classified

As microcalcifications become more numerous, they tend to become more polymorphous. This suggests that even cases classified histologically as pure comedocarcinoma must contain a certain proportion of short papillary-cribriform structures (Fig. 4.86).

For most pathologists these distinctions are unimportant in making a diagnosis (carcinoma: yes/no? infiltration: yes/no?). But for the radiologist they are important because of their relevance to differential diagnosis. The fact that, statistically speaking, the monomorphism of the punctate microcalcifications increasingly gives way to polymorphism when the number of calcifications exceeds 15 aids the radiologist in the differential evaluation of cases where numerous *uniformly punctate* microcalcifications are found within a large area (Fig. 4.20) as opposed to cases where punctate figures coexist with polymorphism (Fig. 4.81).

The extent of the area occupied by microcalcifications does not necessarily correspond to the extent of the carcinoma. An intraductal carcinoma may be substantially larger than its radiographic substrate, yet it may remain clinically occult (Fig. 4.87). There is also no correlation between the extent of the calcifications and infiltrative growth. Thus, a microcalcification cluster less than 1 cm in size does not preclude an infiltrative carcinoma (Fig. 4.88), even if there are no radiographic signs

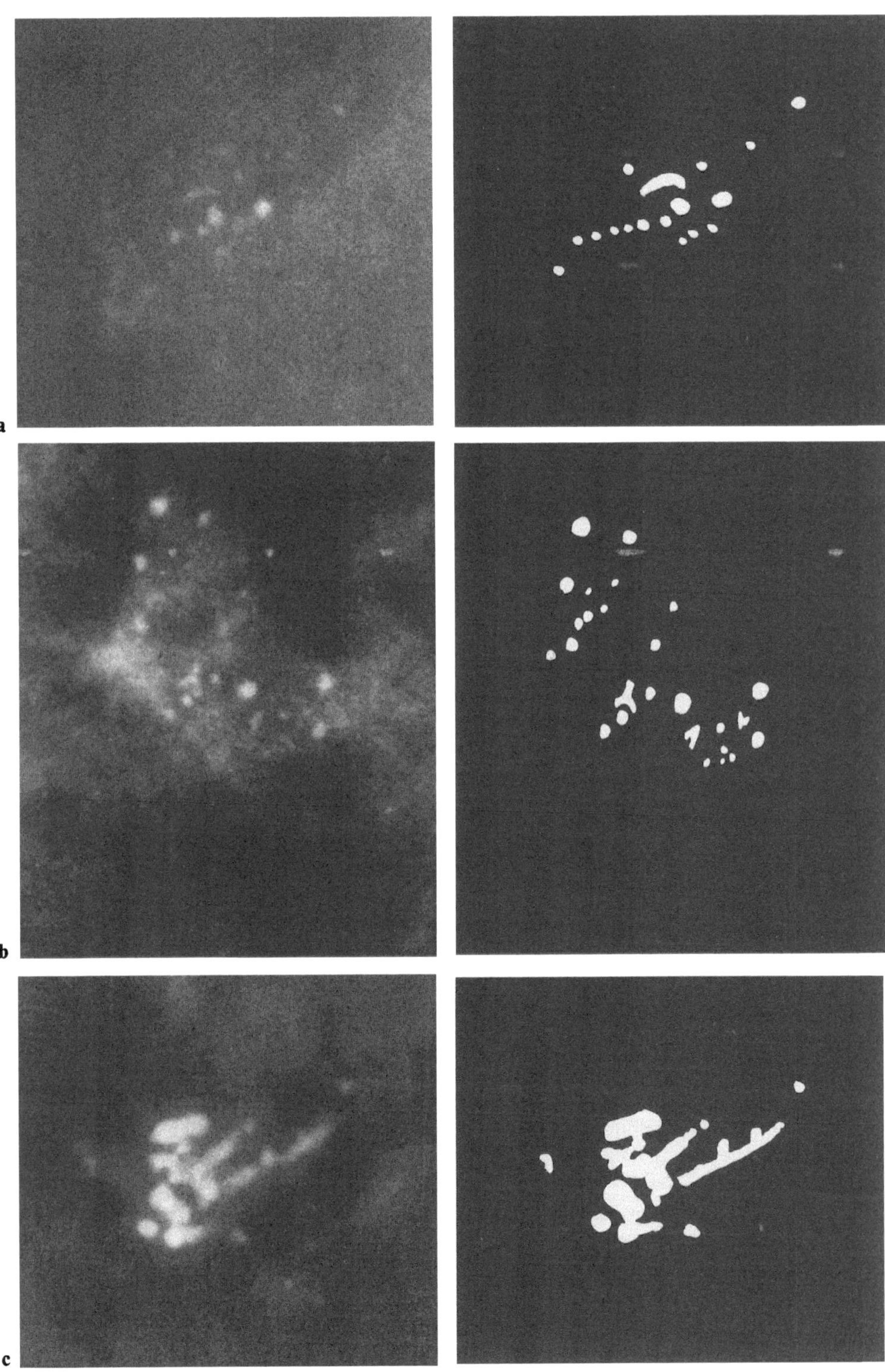

of infiltration. Conversely, the most careful histologic study of an extensive intraductal carcinoma on serial sections may fail to disclose infiltration anywhere around the lesion (Fig. 4.89). While pronounced infiltration may be found adjacent to a few microcalcifications (Fig. 4.90), infiltration may be minimal in an extensive intraductal carcinoma with numerous clustered calcifications (Fig. 4.91).

The proliferation of microcalcifications on follow-up mammograms of intraductal carcinoma was described as a diagnostic sign by MENGES et al. (1976). In our own material, we found only 3 such cases (4%) in 74 intraductal carcinomas detected on the basis of microcalcifications alone; in all 3 cases the increase in the number of microcalcifications prompted biopsy. The increase over a 3-year period is illustrated in Fig. 4.92a, b. One should be careful, however, not to ascribe too much differential diagnostic importance to a possible increase in the number of microcalcifications. The differential diagnosis of microcalcifications should be made during the initial examination if at all possible. An increase in their number is by no means pathognomonic for carcinoma and may occur, for example, in fibroadenoma (Figs. 5.11 and 5.12). A follow-up mammogram of a questionable microcalcification cluster after 6 weeks or 3 months is unlikely to be rewarding. If a diagnosis cannot be made on the initial examination of a patient with clustered microcalcifications, and if there are valid reasons for not performing biopsy (age, cardiac status, multiple prior biopsies, etc.), at least 6 months should elapse before the patient is reexamined. In our experience it is very unlikely that radiographically visible changes will develop prior to that time.

◁ **Fig. 4.85a–c.** Roughly equally sized ductal carcinomas of different histologic types. **a** Detail of mammogram (approx. 8 ×) and schematic diagram: minimal polymorphism in a papillary carcinoma (Dr. LeGAL, Curie Institute, Paris). Flat, diamond-shaped cluster of microcalcifications – 16 punctate and 1 linear. **b** Detail of mammogram and accompanying schematic diagram (approx. 5 ×). The cluster shape is difficult to evaluate (propeller?). The microcalcifications are mostly punctate, and three are y-shaped. Minimal polymorphism in a predominantly papillary-cribriform carcinoma with comedo elements. **c** Detail of mammogram and schematic diagram (approx. 5 ×). Triangular cluster of polymorphous microcalcifications in which linear shapes predominate. Histology: comedocarcinoma

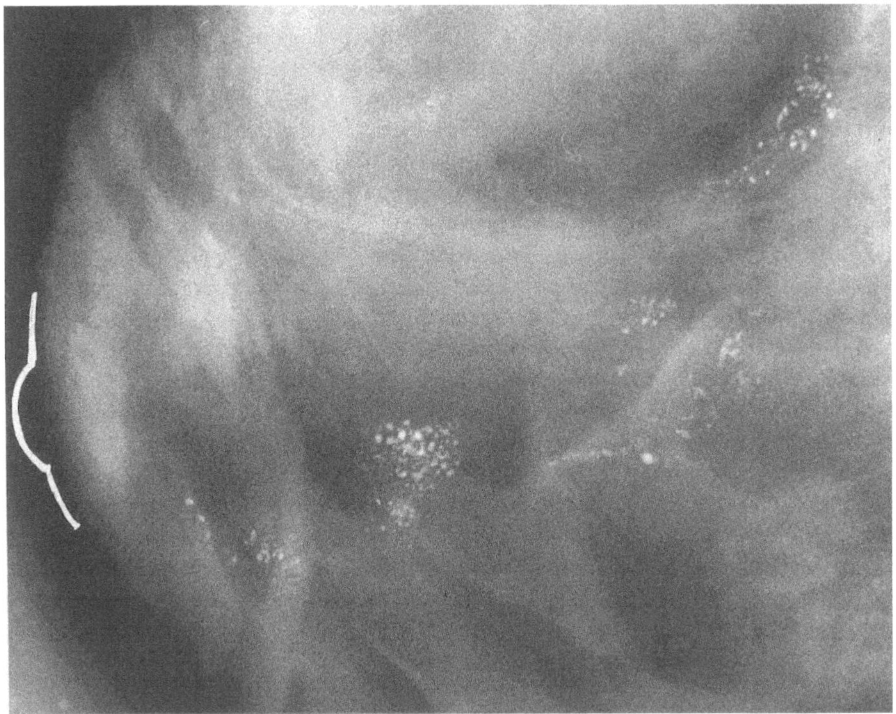

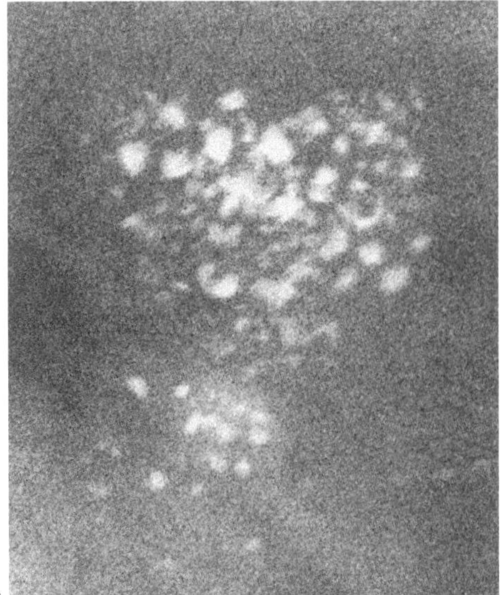

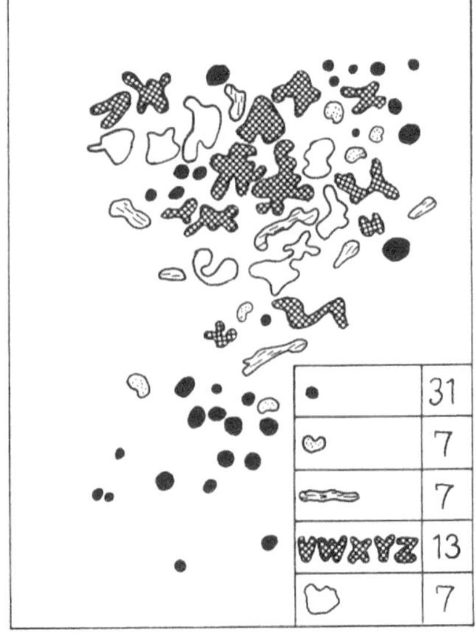

Fig. 4.86. a Detail of mammogram (slightly magnified): five triangular clusters of polymorphous microcalcifications. **b** Close-up view of one cluster (approx. 8 ×) and explanatory diagram. The calcifications are polymorphous, but about half are punctate. The original histologic diagnosis of comedocarcinoma was revised by the pathologist to "mixed comedo and cribriform"

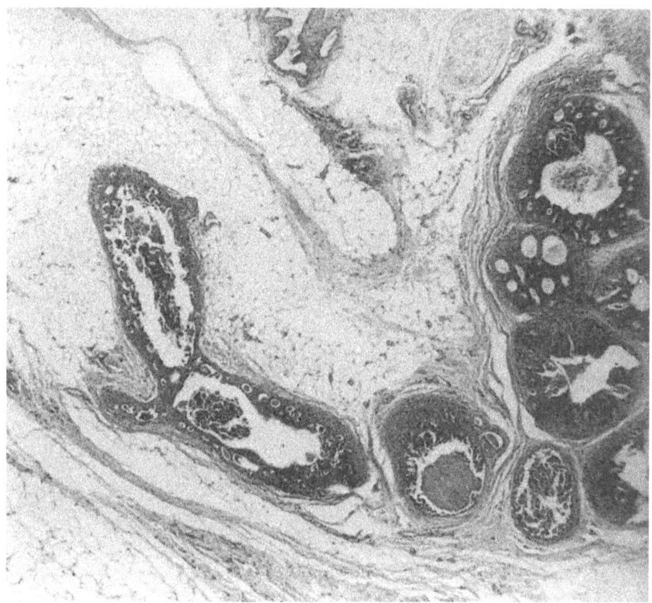

c

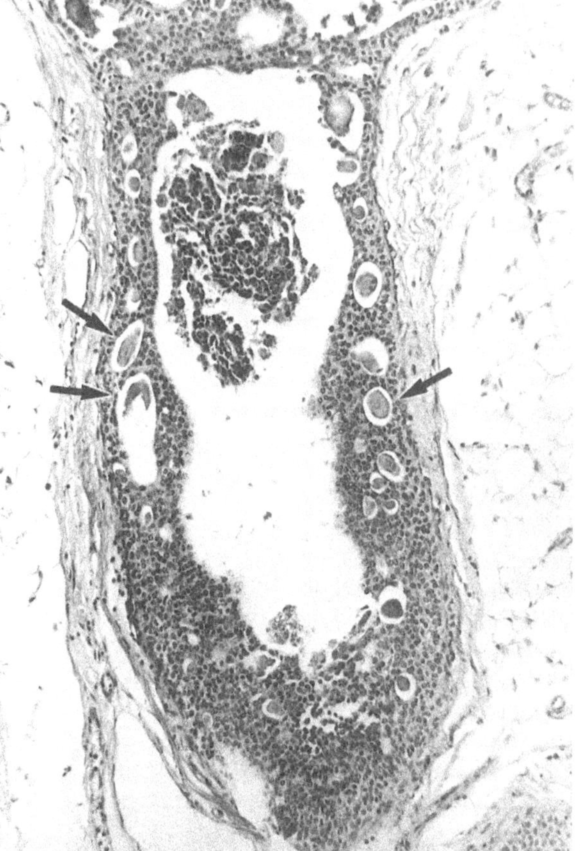

Fig. 4.86. c Histologic section from the same case (approx. 30×): carcinoma with partly solid and partly cribriform features. On the right we see obvious cribriform structures in the transversely sectioned ducts with rounded psammomatous calcifications. At the center is a longitudinally sectioned, y-shaped duct with central necrosis and calcifications.
d This is a more highly magnified view (approx. 100×) of the lower limb of the "Y" in c. Solid growths coexist with obvious cribriform structures, whose cavities contain microcalcifications of varying size. The largest of these *(arrows)* have an original size of 0.1–0.15 mm and hence are visible radiographically. (Professor CITOLER, Cologne)

d

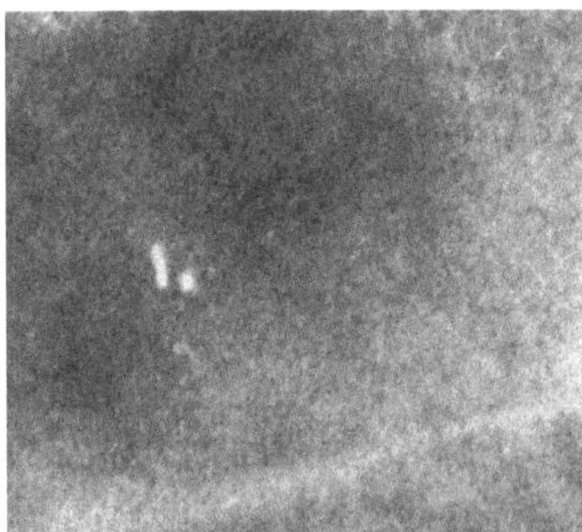

Fig. 4.87. Detail of mammogram: 4 mm triangular cluster of five microcalcifications, four punctate and one linear. No palpable tumor. Histology: 17 mm (!) comedocarcinoma with some papillary and cribriform elements

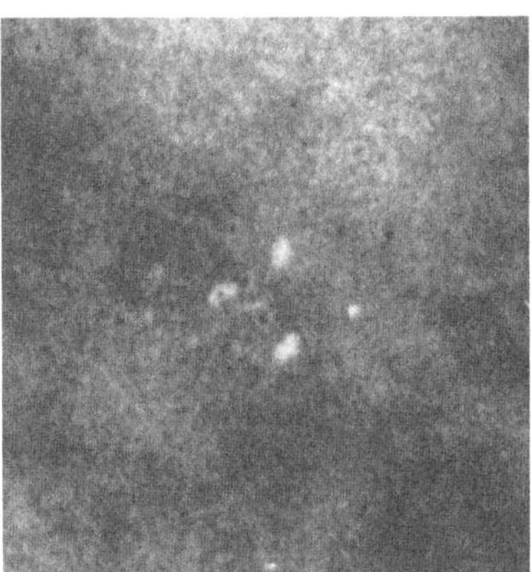 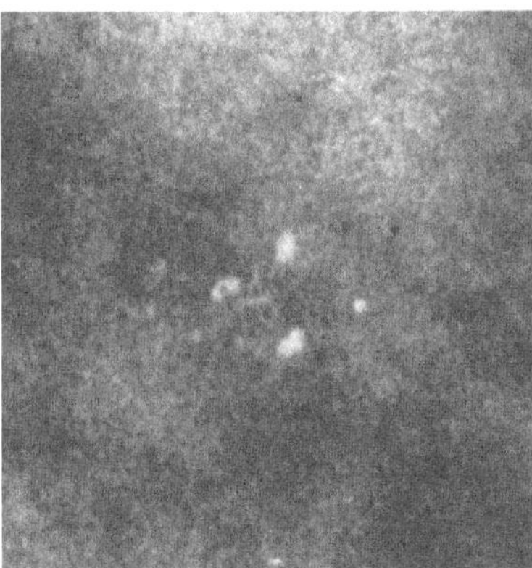

Fig. 4.88. Detail of mammogram (4×) and schematic diagram: tapered rectangular cluster of 10–12 microcalcifications showing a variety of shapes (punctate, comma-shaped, linear, y-shaped). Histology: 6-mm comedocarcinoma with early infiltration

The Number of Microcalcifications

Often the question is raised as to the minimum number of clustered microcalcifications beyond which one should suspect intraductal carcinoma. Answers such as "less than five not suspicious, from five to ten suspicious" are arbitrary and unsatisfactory. Even five microcalcifications may be suspicious under certain circumstances, e.g., with any degree of polymorphism (Fig. 4.87), with prior contralateral mastectomy, or if no microcalcifications were seen in the suspicious area 6 months previously. At the same time, it is not uncommon for 10–15 microcalcifications to occur in a focus of microcystic (blunt duct) adenosis, sclerosing adenosis, or fibroadenoma (Figs. 4.14, 4.23a, b, 5.11). Thus, the number of clustered microcalcifications is irrelevant for the differential diagnosis. Finally, there are intraductal carcinomas which, unfortunately, are devoid of calcifications or had not *yet* formed calcifications when the earlier mammogram was taken. These cases point out the limitations of the method.

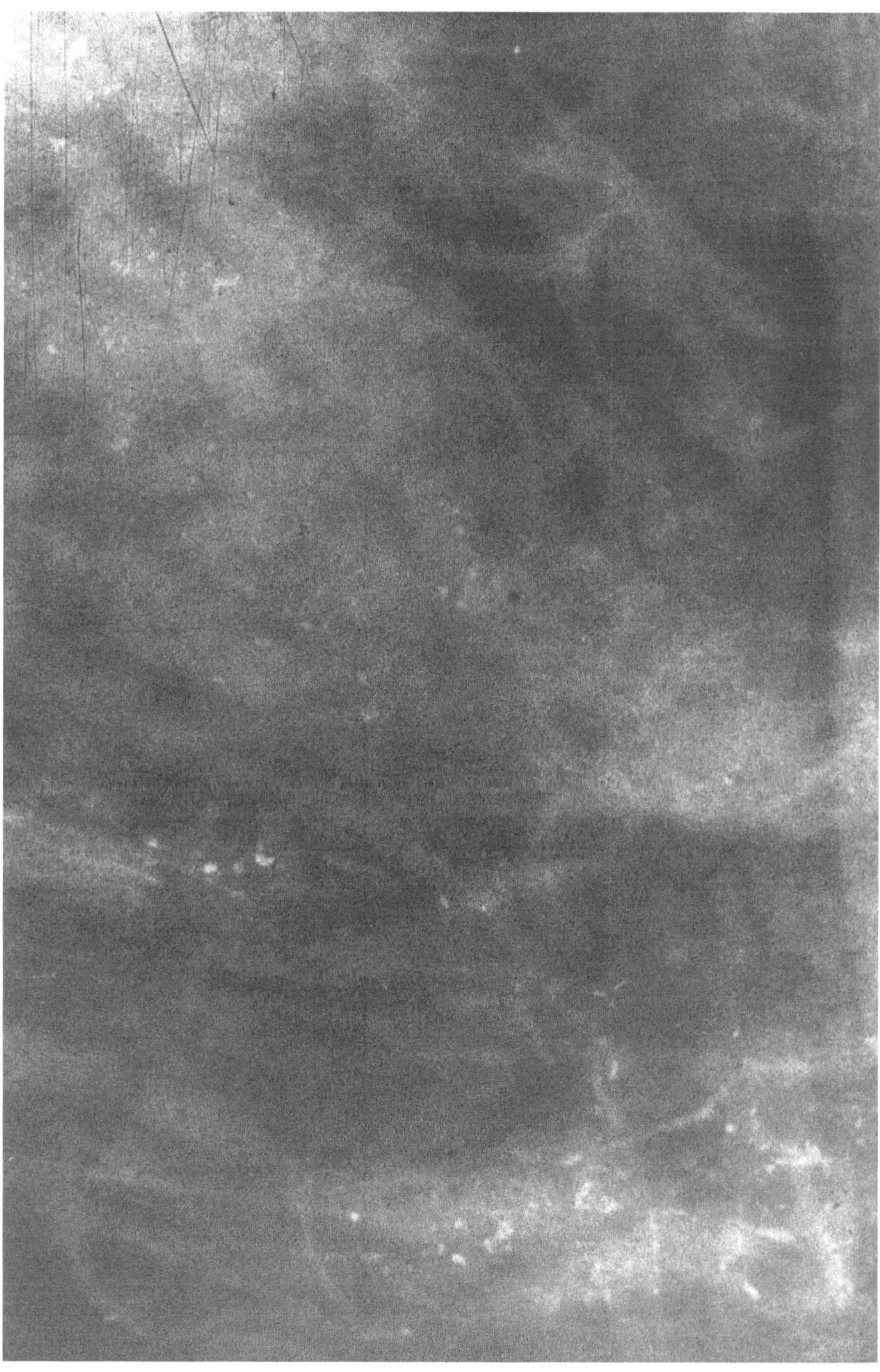

Fig. 4.89. Detail of mammogram (4×): innumerable faint, polymorphous microcalcifications occupying an entire quadrant of the breast. Their ductlike arrangement is most obvious in the lower right of the picture. Histology: extensive, noninfiltrating comedocarcinoma

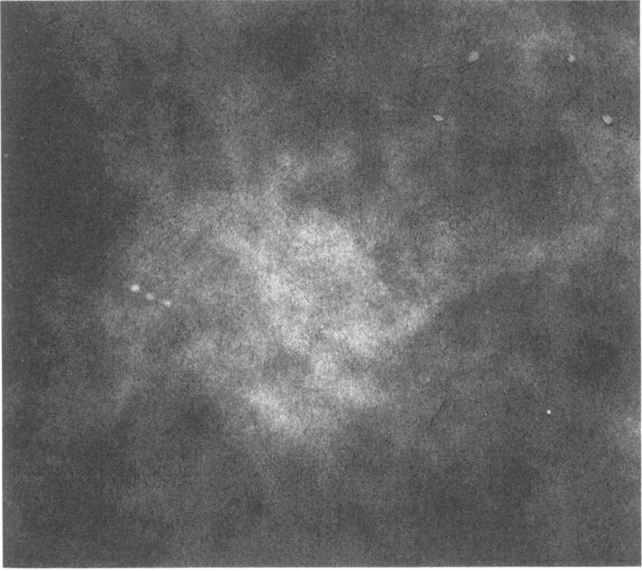

Fig. 4.90. Detail of mammogram (2 ×): three linearly arranged, punctate microcalcifications in an extensive, infiltrating malignancy

When intraductal carcinoma breaks through the basement membrane and infiltrates the periductal tissue, the organism responds either with fibrosis (scirrhus) or with liquefaction of the pathologic tissue (medullary or gelatinous carcinoma).

In our material malignant-type intraductal microcalcifications were demonstrated in 25% of the radiographically infiltrating carcinomas.

Following irradiation "malignant" microcalcifications may (a) remain unchanged, (b) become less distinct, or (c) disappear completely. However, the persistence of microcalcifications after radiation therapy implies nothing about the activity of the tumor (LIBSHITZ et al. 1977).

Microcalcifications in male breast carcinoma are extremely rare (ROSEN and NADEL 1966; ROCEK et al. 1968; TABÁR et al. 1972; PÉNTEK et al. 1975; BRYANT 1981) (Fig. 4.93).

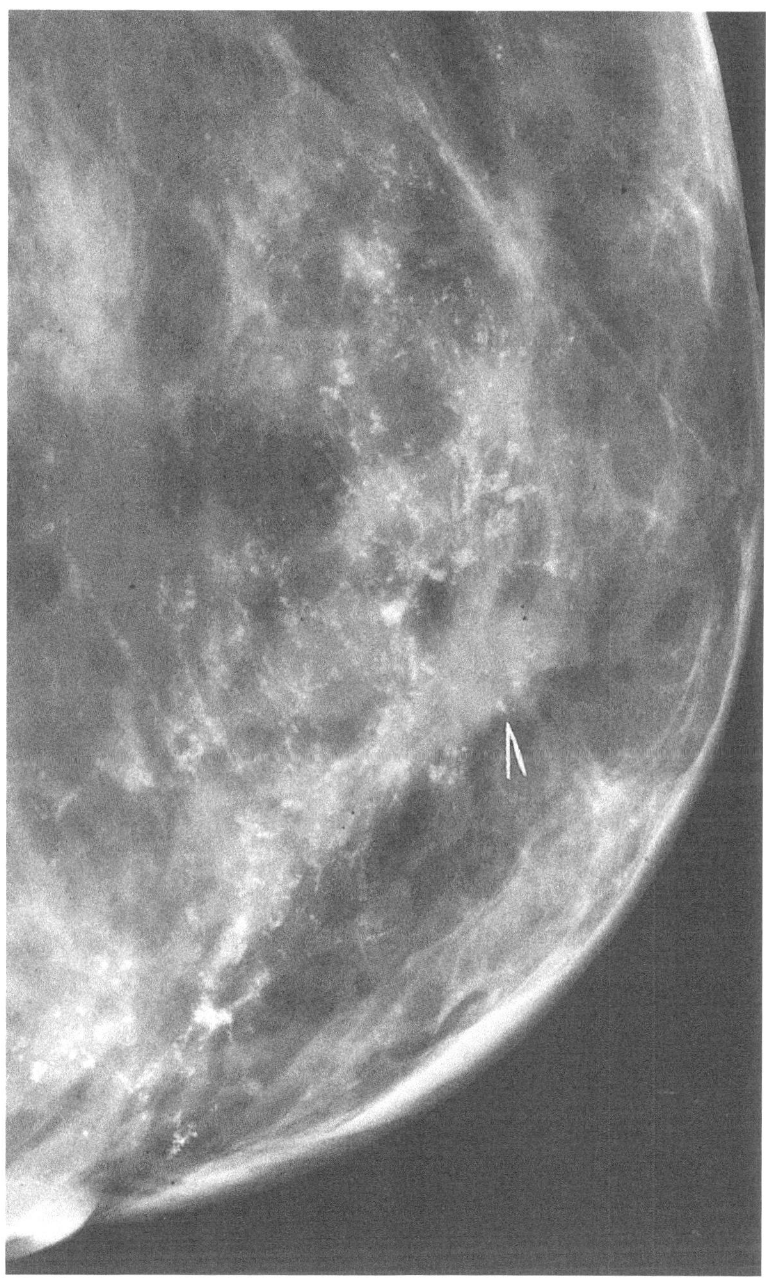

Fig. 4.91. Detail of mammogram (1.5 ×): extensive triangular cluster of polymorphous microcalcifications having all the radiographic features of comedocarcinoma (e. g., islets devoid of microcalcifications, swallowtail sign). Both mammography and histology showed only one area of frank infiltration *(arrow)*, but skin thickening from dermal lymphatic carcinomatosis is already apparent

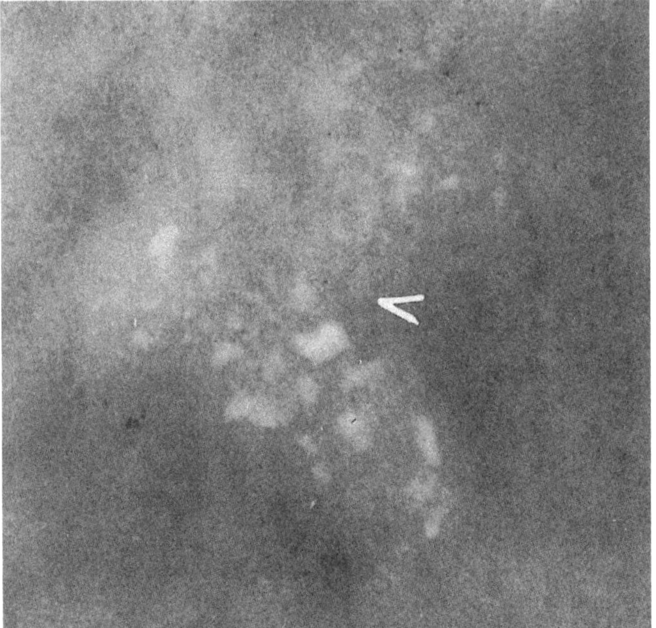

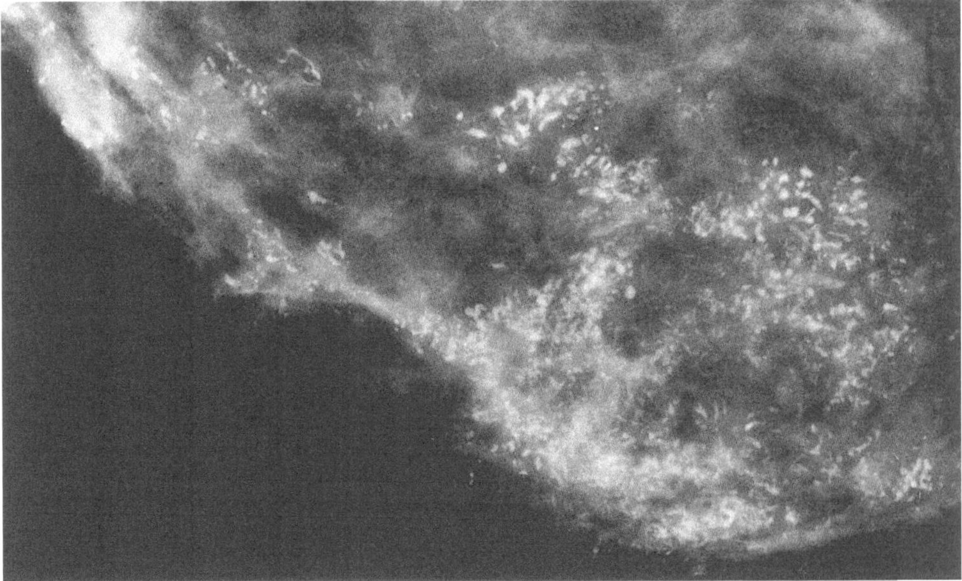

Fig.4.92a-c. Details of mammograms. a This craniocaudad view (5×) taken in 1975 (elsewhere) shows a triangular cluster of faint polymorphous microcalcifications. A posterior notch is present *(arrow)*. The significance of the lesion was not appreciated. b Craniocaudad view of the same breast in 1978 (slightly magnified): extensive, triangular cluster of polymorphous microcalcifications of equal intensity. The apex of the triangle is toward the nipple, the outer contours are wavy, and there are two posterior notches. The cluster contains insular areas devoid of microcalcifications. c Lateral view of the same breast in 1978 (slightly magnified). Here the cluster appears club-shaped; the process extending toward the nipple represents the main duct of the affected lobe. Histology: comedocarcinoma

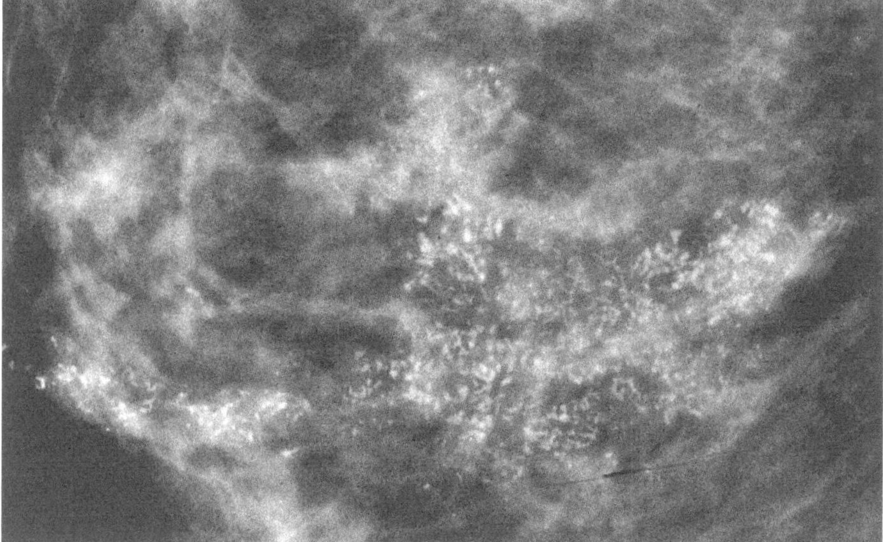

Fig. 4.92c

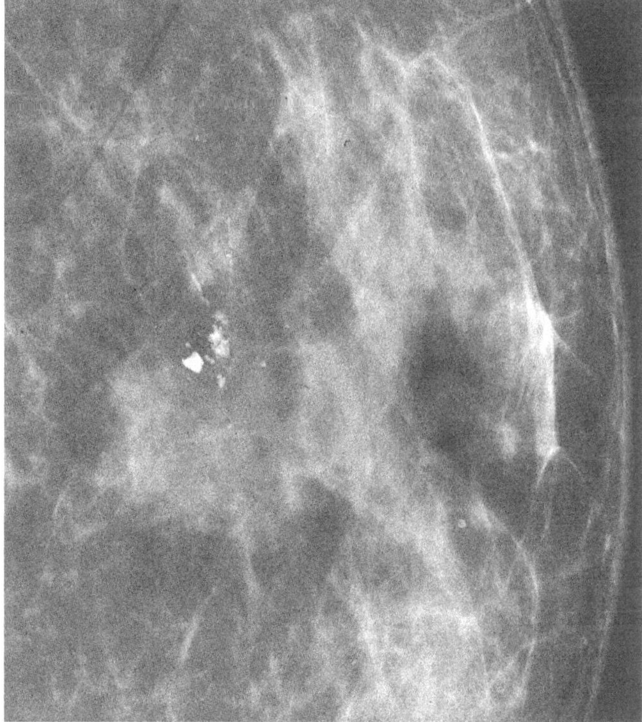

Fig. 4.93. Clustered microcalcifications in a histologically confirmed male breast carcinoma. Again we see a ductlike arrangement and polymorphism (Dr. PÉNTEK, Szekszárd, Hungary)

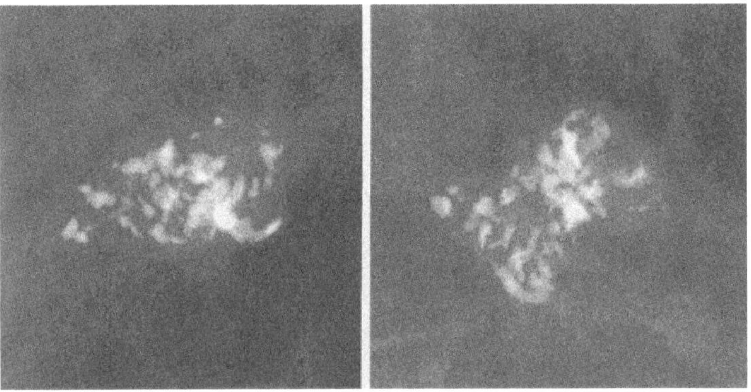

a
b

Fig. 4.94a, b. Details of mammograms (2 ×). **a** Triangular cluster of polymorphous calcifications, some very coarse, within a fine soft-tissue shadow. **b** Propeller-shaped cluster on a different plane. The soft-tissue shadow also has changed its shape. Histology: intraductal papillary carcinoma (papilloma which has undergone malignant transformation)

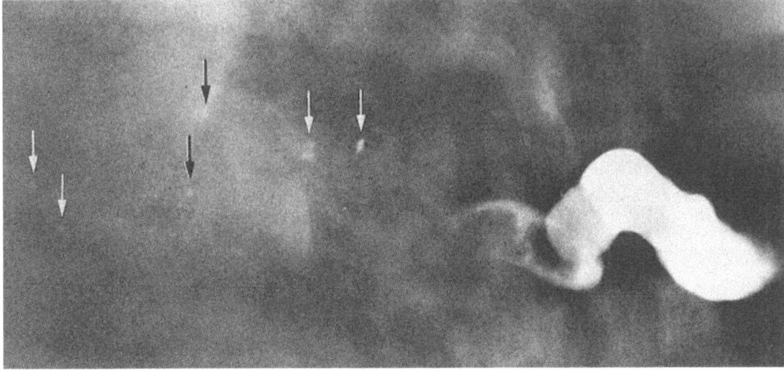

Fig. 4.95. Detail of galactogram (approx. 3 ×) showing an almost complete filling defect in the lactiferous sinus. Behind it are six or seven faint punctate microcalcifications *(arrows)* in the area of an extensive ductal papillary carcinoma

Radiography of Malignantly Transformed Solitary Papilloma and Papillomatosis

Papillomas that have undergone malignant change are detected primarly by galactography. The radiologist should diagnose the intraductal papilloma without attempting to classify it as malignant or benign. In the author's experience, malignant transformation takes place in 6% of papillomas thus diagnosed. Cancerous papillomas account for 1.4% of breast carcinomas in the material studied.

By analyzing the shapes of microcalcification clusters on mammograms, the author was able to detect an intraductal papillary carcinoma whose radiographic image (Fig. 4.94) corresponded to an ordinary intraductal carcinoma (cluster appeared triangular on one plane and propeller-shaped on the other). The shapes of the individual microcalcifications more closely resembled those of fibroadenoma.

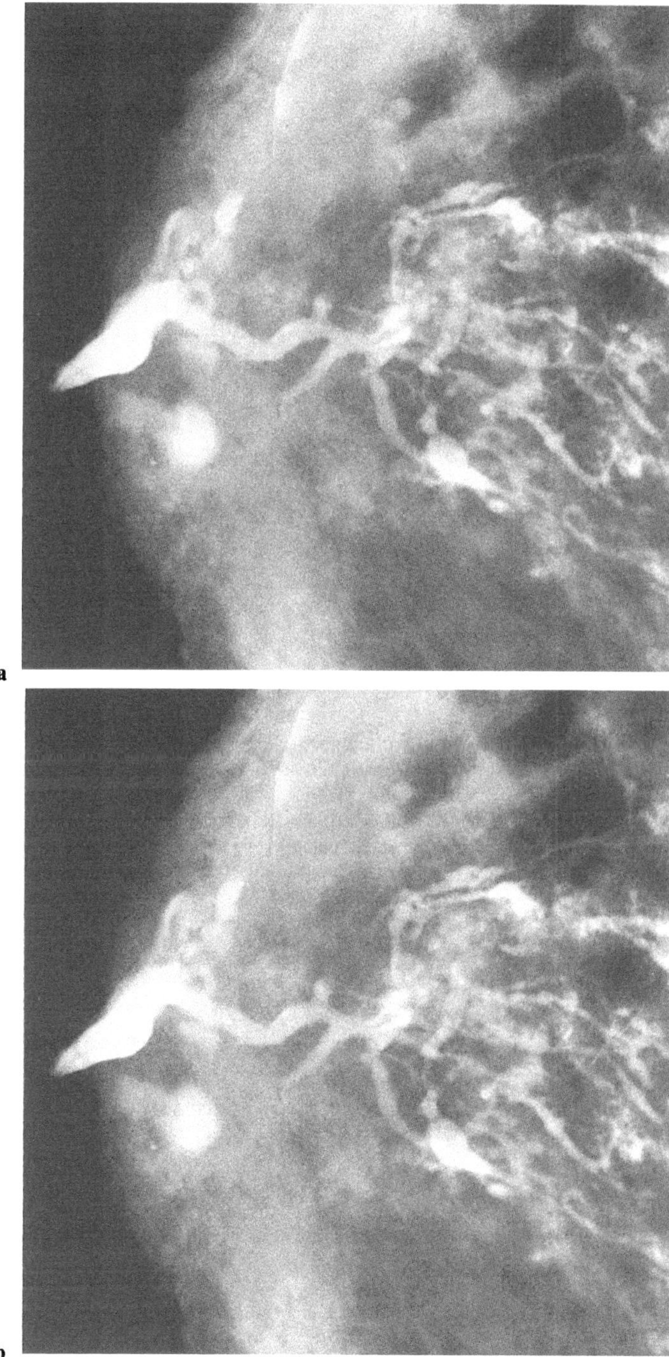

Fig. 4.96 a, b. Legend on p. 130

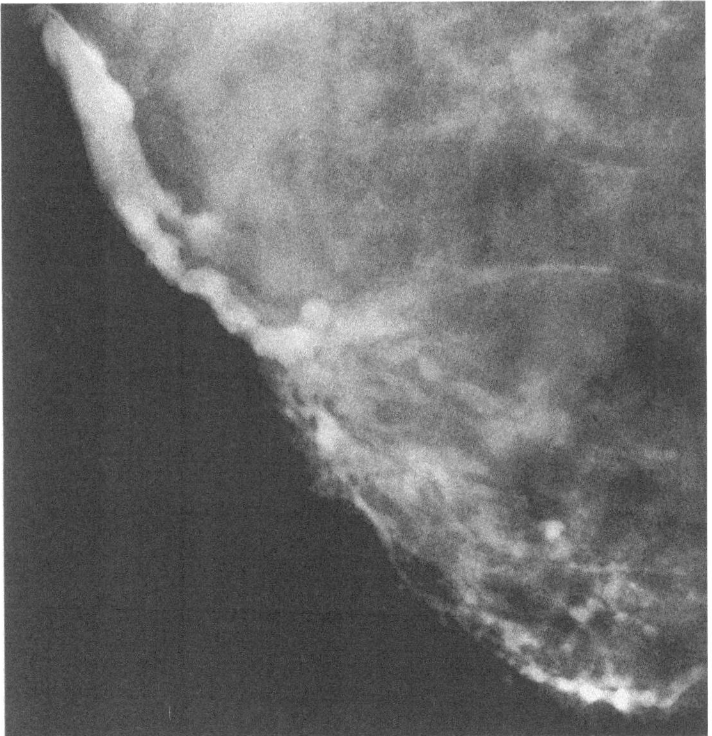

c

Fig. 4.96. a Detail of lateral mammogram (slightly magnified). The very fine, scattered, faint microcalcifications (some marked with *arrows*) are not characteristic of any pathologic, process! **b, c** Details of galactograms (same magnification as in **a**). **b** Lateral view shows an unusual forked shape of the main duct. The second order ducts show fine, circumscribed filling defects and variations of caliber, which are most clearly seen on the craniocaudad view (**c**). The localization of the obviously pathologic duct coincides exactly with that of the faint microcalcifications. Radiographic diagnosis: pathologic intraductal papillary process requiring histologic evaluation. Histology: papillary carcinoma

The microcalcifications of papillomatosis that has undergone malignant change are punctate and scattered sparsely over a lobe-shaped (trapezoidal?) area. They are not pathognomonic, and similar microcalcifications are seen in papillomatoses that are completely benign (Figs. 4.95 and 4.96).

Retained Secretions With or Without Epithelial Proliferation or Galactophoritis (Plasma Cell Mastitis)

Pathology

This section encompasses a range of fundamentally different processes whose only common clinical and pathologic feature is the secretory activity associated with duct ectasia ("secretory disease" of GERSHON-COHEN 1970). Pathologically, either these processes are the result of *intraductal epithelial proliferation* (papilloma, papillomatosis; solid, papillary, or cribriform epithelial proliferation in the setting of proliferative mastopathy with or without cellular atypia), or they are inflammatory in nature (e.g., galactophoritis and plasma cell mastitis). It is not unusual for proliferative and inflammatory processes to coexist.

Drops of secretion can be seen histologically in the lobules or small milk ducts at any age and in normal individuals. This latent secretion becomes clinically evident only when the material reaches the nipple through the major ducts.

The *fluid, milky-white, or yellowish secretion* contains protein with lipid cells, foam cells, and cellular debris. This type of secretion almost always produces a *bilateral* discharge from multiple ducts, either spontaneously or when pressure is applied. Possible causes include prolactin-secreting adenomas, suprasellar pituitary tumors, various drugs (e.g., psychotherapeutic agents), and contraceptives. This type of secretion has become more prevalent in recent years. It is not typical of carcinoma, and the author has seen only one case of a papillary carcinoma associated with a milky secretion.

The *serous, clear, watery, or amber-colored fluid secretion* contains few foam cells or duct epithelia, is mostly unilateral, and comes from a *single* duct. It occurs in cystic disease and duct papilloma or papillomatosis; it is rarely seen in papilloma or papillomatosis that has undergone malignant change.

The *greenish, grayish ("dirty") fluid secretion* of cystic disease contains an abundance of foam cells and cellular debris. It is always bilateral and occurs in multiple ducts.

Retained secretions that are yellowish, show increasing viscosity, and can be expressed from the duct like paste are symptomatic of galactophoritis (synonyms: comedomastitis, obliterative mastitis, plasma cell mastitis). Very often the ducts are palpable as closely spaced, pencil-thick, wormlike masses in the peri- or subareolar area (varicocele tumor of the breast, BLOODGOOD 1923). In the late stage, periductal fibrosis causes some degree of nipple retraction. The histologic picture of this abacterial inflammation is marked by a more or less pronounced lymphocytic or plasmacytic periductal infiltration (further details on the natural history of plasma cell mastitis are given in Sect. 6.1).

Blood-stained or bloody secretions contain foam cells with hemosiderosis and epithelial cells, erythrocytes, and possibly cells from a papilloma or malignant growth. Bloody secretions do not occur exclusively in benign or malignant papillary processes. It may occur in the absence of a galactographically visible cause, or it may occur in galactophoritis (plasma cell mastitis) after the retained material has eroded through the duct epithelium (GERSHON-COHEN et al. 1956).

Radiography

Retained secretions may calcify regardless of whether or not a visible discharge is present (INGLEBY and HERMEL 1956). The unclustered monomorphous, linear calcifications occur close to the nipple and usually are easily distinguished from an intraductal malignancy, unless branched calcifications are present (Fig. 4.97) or the number of microcalcifications increases. The simultaneous appearance of calcified secretions and microcalcifications in intraductal carcinoma is very unusual

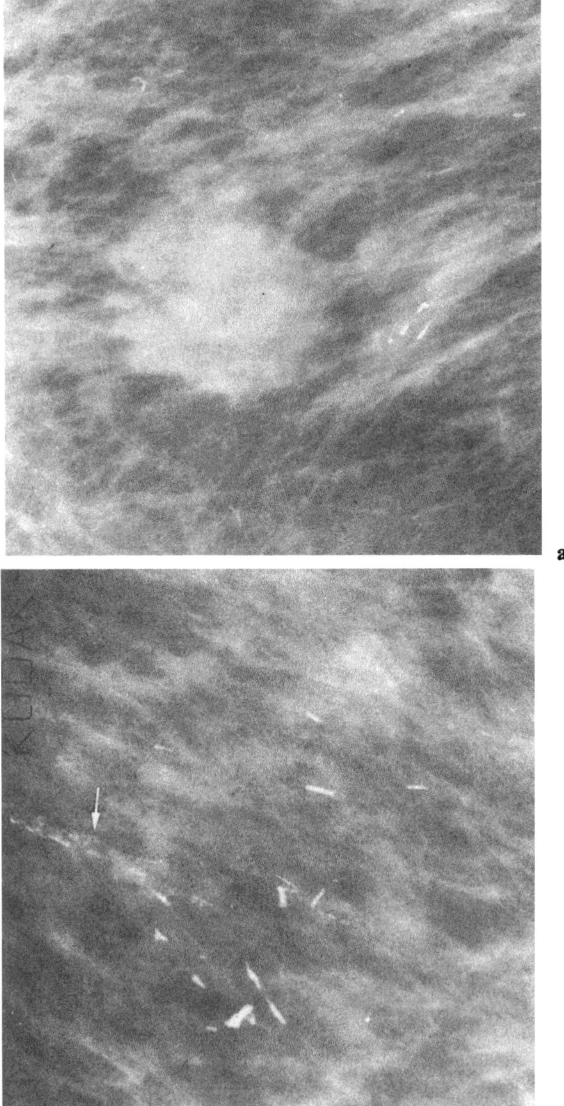

Fig. 4.97 a, b. Details of mammograms (bilateral, slightly magnified). **a** Right side: several linear microcalcifications are seen behind the round shadow, which is characteristic of solid or medullary carcinoma. **b** Left side: loose cluster of predominantly linear and some v-shaped calcifications, accompanied by vascular calcification *(arrow)*. Radiographic diagnosis: because carcinoma exists in the right breast, a biopsy of the left breast is prudent, although this is very likely plasma cell mastitis with calcified secretions. Histology: right side, carcinoma accompanied by calcified secretions; left side, calcified secretions and lymphoplasmocytic infiltration

(Fig. 4.98). It may be impossible to distinguish inspissated secretions from early carcinoma if the calcified secretions are clustered.

The clusters in such cases usually are triangular in shape (Figs. 4.99 and 4.100) or may change shape with the beam direction as in ductal carcinoma (see p. 91). If marked polymorphism is also present, a radiographic diagnosis of carcinoma is justified; a subsequent histologic diagnosis of plasma cell mastitis with inspissated secretions will then be a pleasant surprise (Fig. 4.101). False-positive diagnosis of this kind are rare but unavoidable, because "stony casts" in the form of microcalcifications will be seen regardless of whether the patient has a comedocarcinoma or comedomastitis. Obliterative comedomastitis can mimic an intraductal papilloma with calcifications (Fig. 4.102), and conversely, calcified secretions may be seen in association with intraductal papilloma and papillomatosis (Fig. 4.103). In the immediate vicinity of the "inspissated and calcified" secretion the pathologist may find either a completely normal epithelium or the entire scale from normal epithelium or epitheliosis, to precancerous changes such as epithelial proliferation and papillomatosis with or without atypia, to type 3 cystic disease[4] (Fig. 4.104). It should be noted, however, that
a) the dividing lines between these histologic diagnoses are indistinct,
b) routine histologic sections are not always representative, and
c) evaluation of the degree of proliferation is often subjective.

Thus, the benign epithelial processes found on the basis of clustered microcalcifications, whatever their degree of proliferation, do not prove the success of microcalcification diagnosis. Indeed, as we saw in Table 4.3, these processes are found more frequently in association with radiographic signs other than microcalcifications. Attempts by PATEROK et al. (1983) and others to augment the number of carcinomas found on the basis of microcalcifications with that of atypical epithelial proliferations only lead to confusion.

---

[4] See footnote 1 on p. 50.

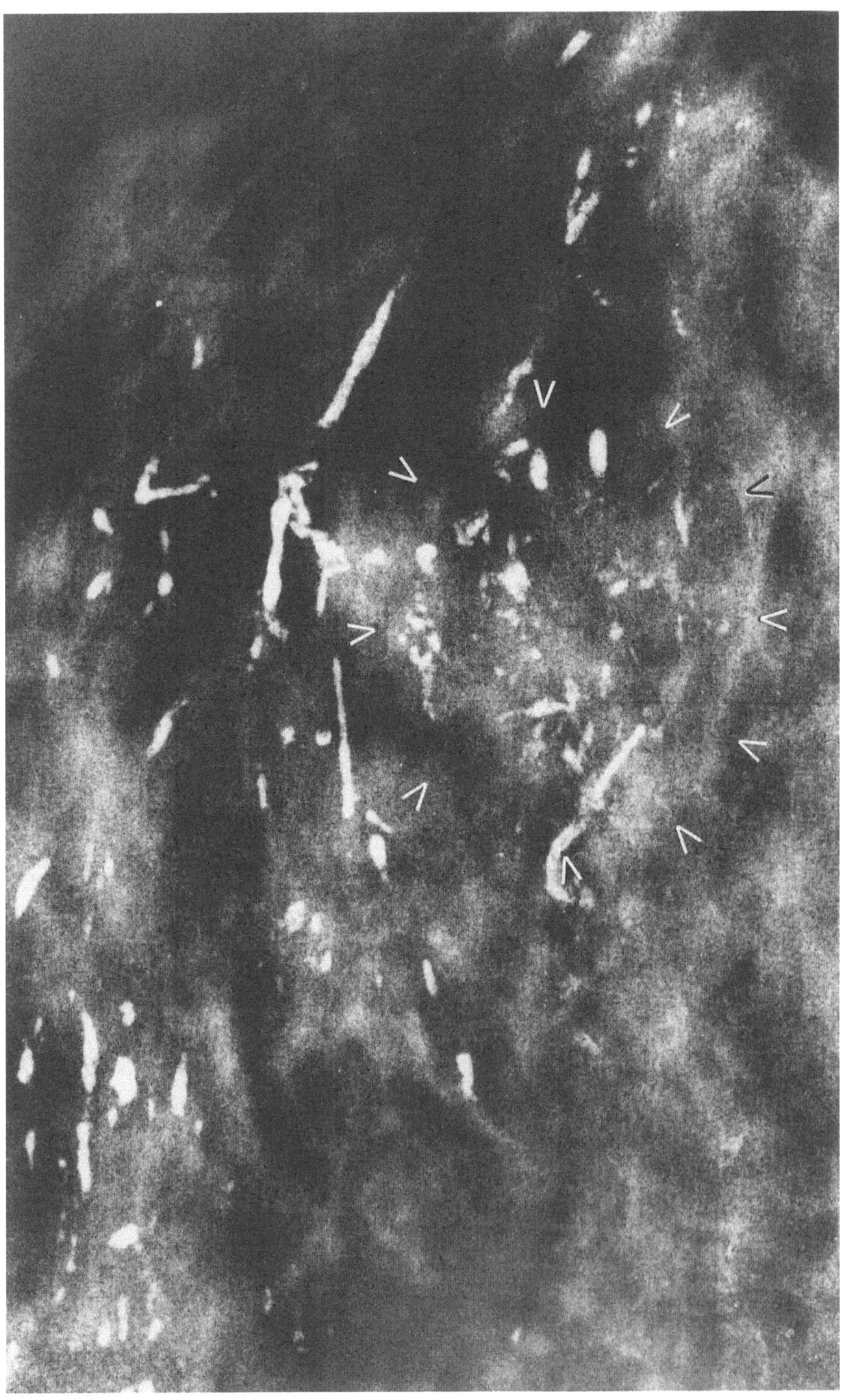

Fig. 4.98

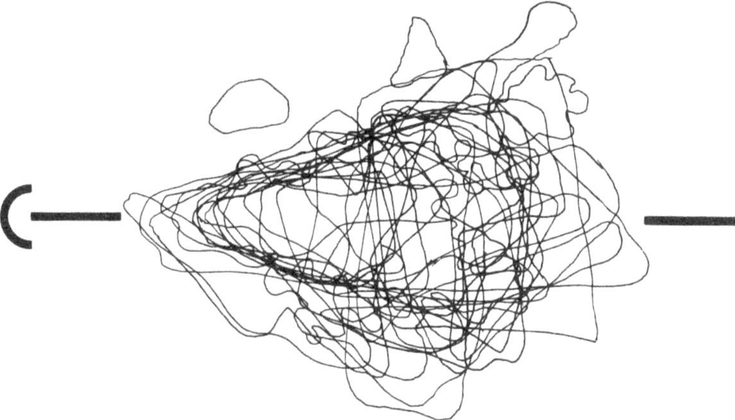

Fig. 4.99. Superimposed contour lines of 29 intraductal microcalcification clusters of benign etiology (retained secretions in comedomastitis or intraductal proliferation of varying degree). The triangular configuration is apparent

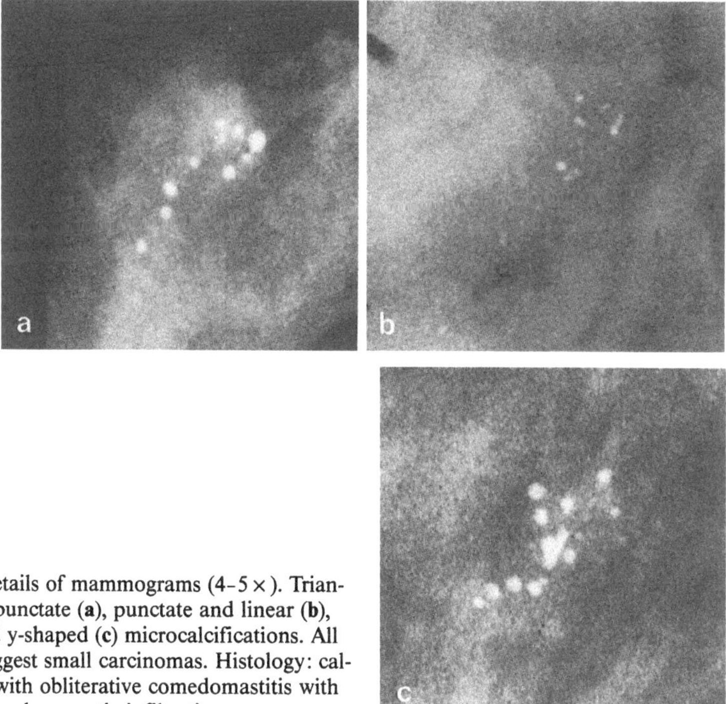

Fig. 4.100 a-c. Details of mammograms (4-5 ×). Triangular clusters of punctate (**a**), punctate and linear (**b**), and punctate and y-shaped (**c**) microcalcifications. All three patterns suggest small carcinomas. Histology: calcified secretions with obliterative comedomastitis with or without lymphoplasmocytic infiltration

◁ **Fig. 4.98.** Simultaneous manifestation of calcified secretions and microcalcifications in a ductal carcinoma (comedocarcinoma; *arrows*). The calcified secretions are considerably longer and thicker than the calcifications in the carcinoma (approx. 4 ×) (Professor KÜNZIG, Siegen). Histologically both lesions can be seen together (Professor CITOLER, Cologne)

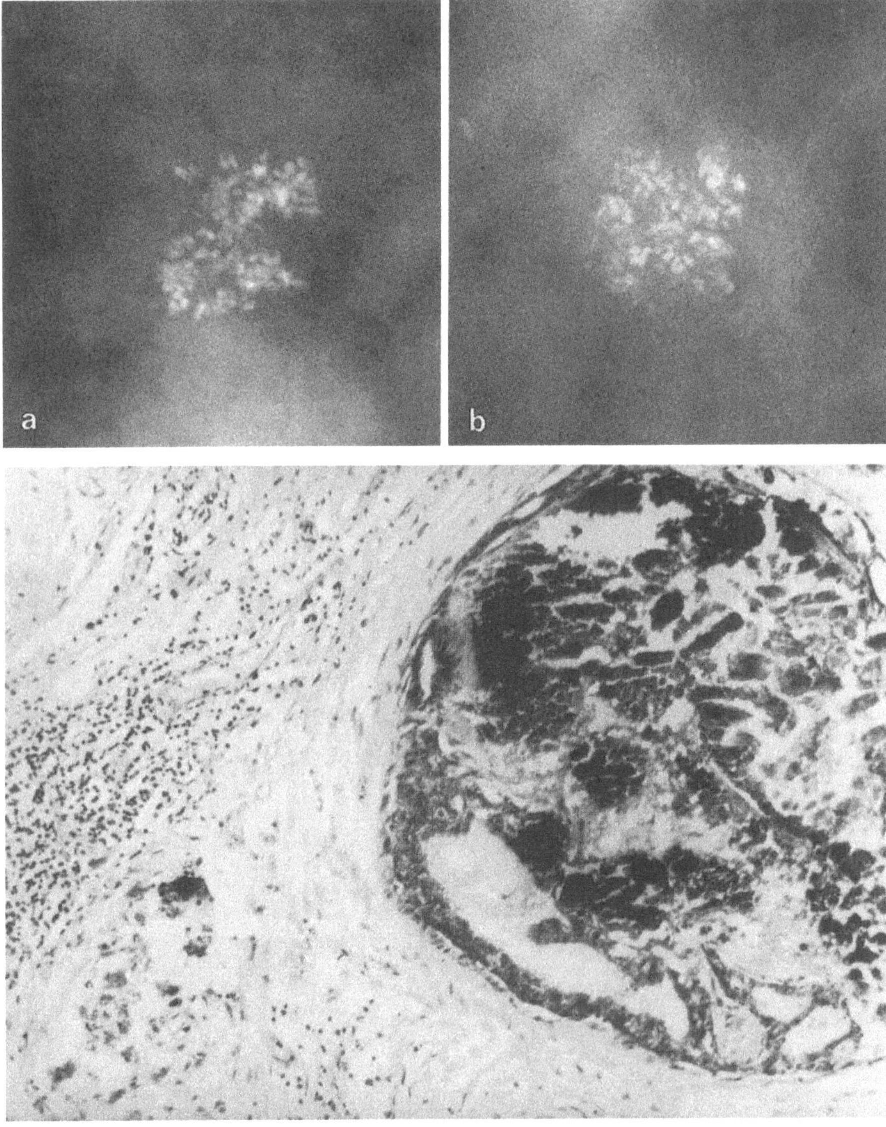

Fig. 4.101 a–c. Details of mammograms showing polymorphous (punctate, linear, comma-shaped, stelate) microcalcifications in a 9-mm cluster that appears propeller-shaped on the craniocaudad view (**a**) and square on the lateral view (**b**). Radiographic diagnosis: comedocarcinoma. Histology: chronic abacterial galactophoritis, plasma cell mastitis. **c** The histologic section (approx. 100 ×) shows marked intraductal calcification, periductal lymphoplasmocytic infiltration, and a circumscribed interstitial calcification (Professor CITOLER, Cologne)

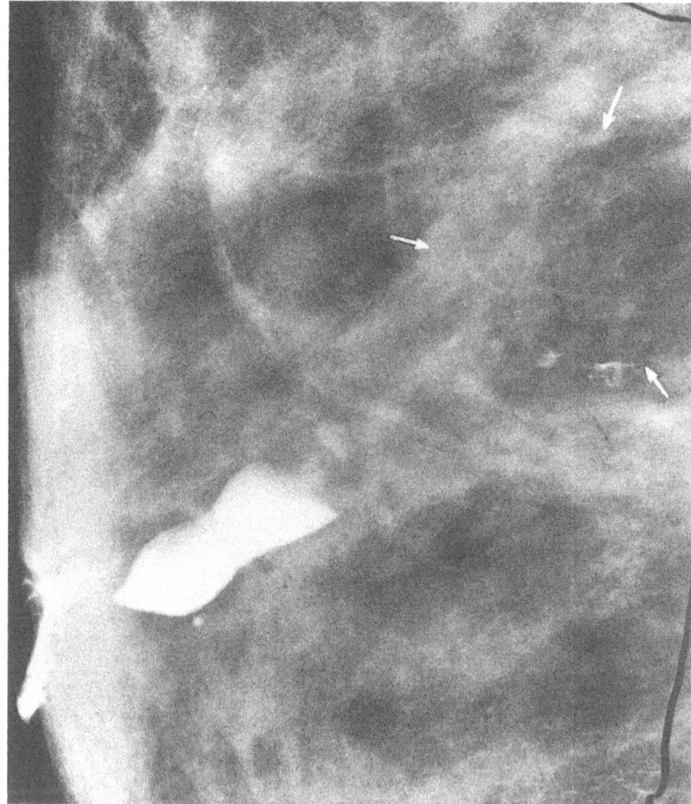

Fig.4.102. Detail of galactogram (approx. 3 ×) showing a filling defect in the lactiferous sinus. Behind it, near the chest wall, are punctate and amorphous microcalcifications (between *arrows*); the amorphous ones probably represent a circumscribed calcified arterial segment. Radiographic diagnosis: intraductal papilloma or papillomatosis, possibly with malignant transformation. Histology: obliterative mastitis

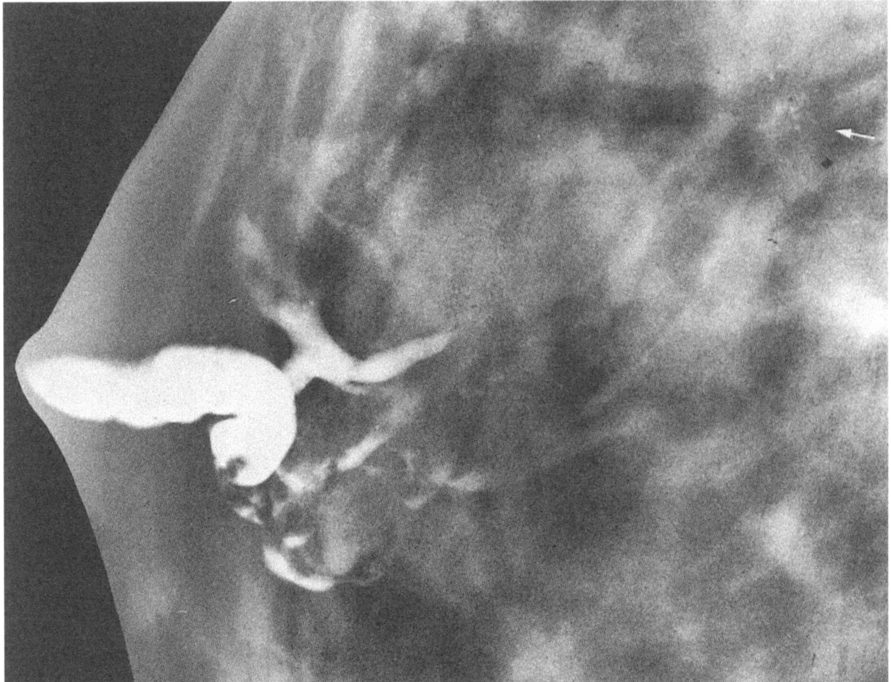

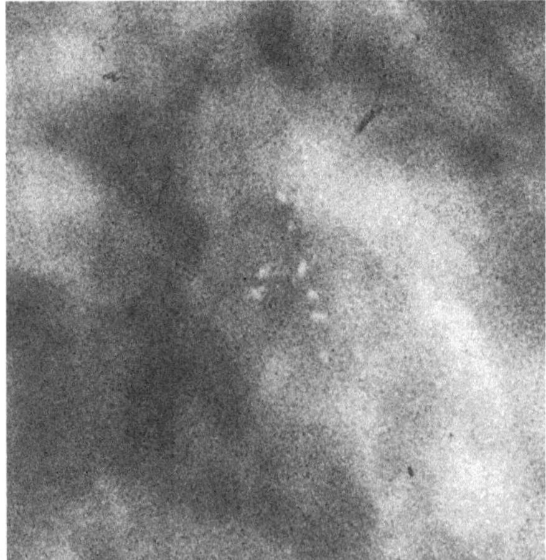

Fig. 4.103a, b. Details of galactogram.
a Multiple "duct amputations" and numerous filling defects in and behind the lactiferous sinus. The small triangular cluster of somewhat polymorphous microcalcifications *(arrow)* appears to belong to this duct system (2 ×). **b** 4 × magnification of the microcalcification clusters. Radiographic diagnosis: papillomatosis, possibly with malignant transformation. Histology: papillomas, papillomatosis; inspissated and apparently calcified secretions in the area containing the microcalcifications

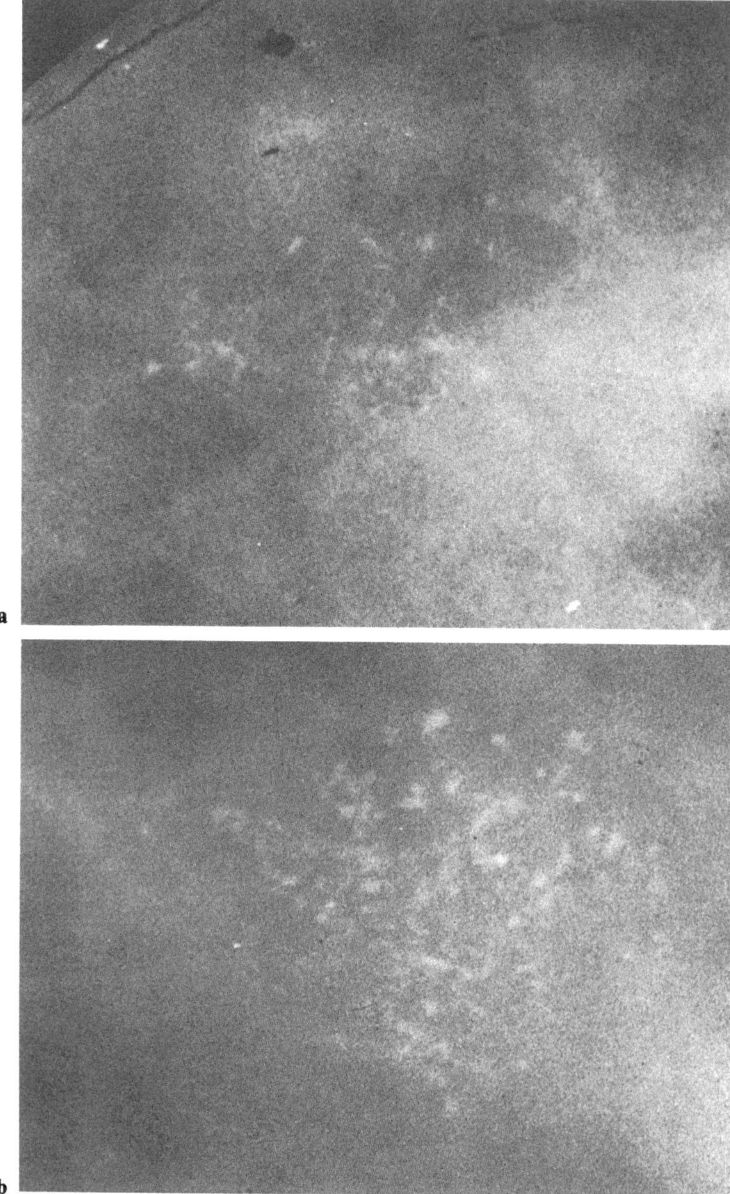

Fig. 4.104a, b. Details of mammograms. **a** Extensive, triangular, or rhomboidal cluster of faint, obviously polymorphous microcalcifications. Histology: multicentric papillomatosis with atypia (3×). **b** Picture similar to **a**: rhomboid cluster of very faint, definitely polymorphous (punctate, comma-shaped, linear, branched) microcalcifications in a histologically confirmed comedocarcinoma (4.5×)

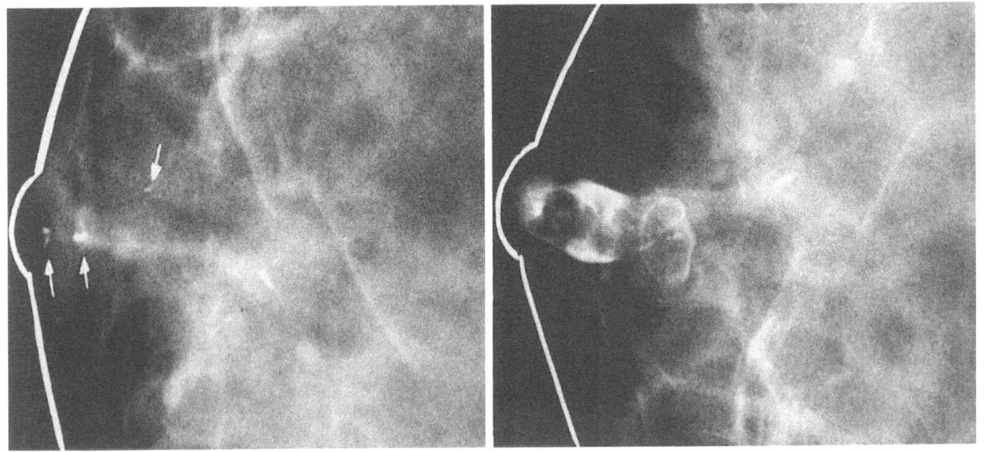

a   b

Fig. 4.105. a Detail of mammogram (3 ×): several punctate microcalcifications within the nipple *(arrows).* **b** Detail of galactogram (3 ×). The microcalcifications are located within an extensive nipple papilloma. Histology: sclerosed papilloma

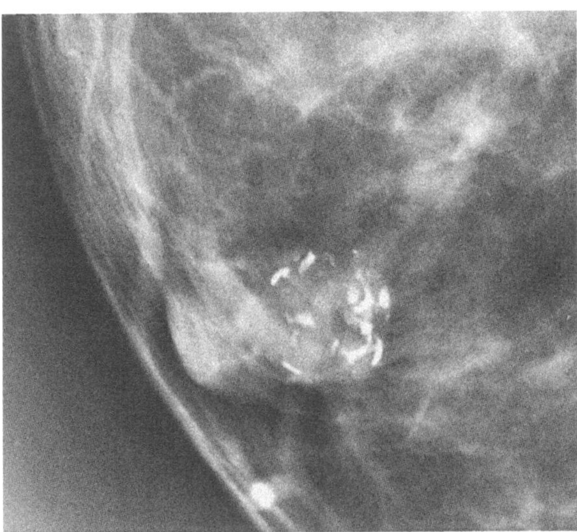

Fig. 4.106. Detail of mammogram (2 ×). A rounded feature with punctate, linear, and branched microcalcifications presents just behind the nipple (which was incorrectly placed). Pattern is suggestive of calcified fibroadenoma. Histology: hyalinized, calcified intraductal papilloma

Hyalinized, Sclerosed Intraductal Papilloma and Fibroadenoma

Pathology

This papilloma is characterized by a fine network of branched fibroepithelial proliferations. As the proportion of fibrous tissue increases relative to the epithelial component, the so-called sclerosed papilloma develops. It is nearly impossible to distinguish this type of papilloma from a histologically fibroadenoma.

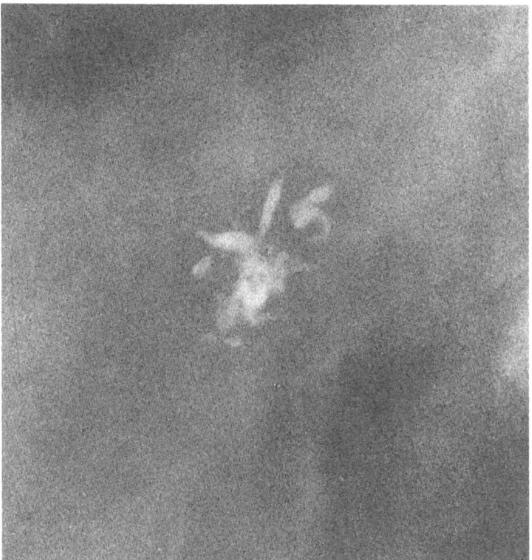

Fig. 4.107. Detail of mammogram (3 ×): ovoid cluster of polymorphous, irregularly shaped microcalcifications without a soft-tissue shadow. Intracystic hyalinized papilloma

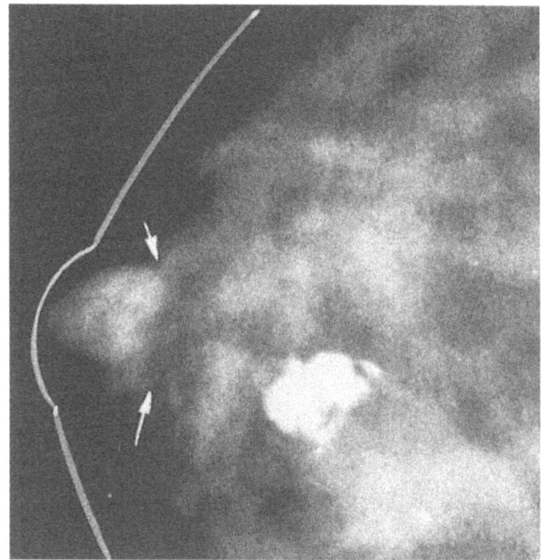

Fig. 4.108. Detail of galactogram (3 ×). The portion of the duct within the nipple is visualized by the contrast medium. Behind the site of complete blockage *(arrows)* is a large filling defect with large, flaky calcifications. Histology: calcified papilloma

Radiography

The microcalcifications of hyalinized, sclerosed intraductal papilloma typically occur within or beneath the nipple. They may be punctate (Fig. 4.105), polymorphous (Figs. 4.106 and 4.107), or flaky (Fig. 4.108), depending on the extent of the calcifying process. The flaky form is virtually indistinguishable from a liponecrotic microcyst. The cluster shape is usually round to ovoid. When secretion is present, galactography can be used to establish the intraductal location of the lesion and make a correct diagnosis.

Simultaneous Lobular and Ductal Calcifications

Calcifications occurring simultaneously in the lobular and ductal systems of both breasts can be found in primary (MARINESCU and DAMIAN 1984) and secondary hyperparathyroidism. This syndrome is known to be associated with the occurrence of calcifications in various soft tissues (arteries, cornea, conjunctiva, joint capsule, skin, lung, heart). SANG Y HAN and WITTEN (1977) reported on a case of secondary hyperparathyroidism in which extensive calcifications formed bilaterally *within the lobules and ducts.* Interestingly, the extent of the calcifications in this case decreased markedly following 20 months of dialysis. Similarly, extensive bilateral breast calcifications accompanied by arterial calcifications developed in a 42-year-old woman who had a disturbance of calcium phosphate parathormone metabolism secondary to renal failure. These changes are shown in Fig. 4.109.

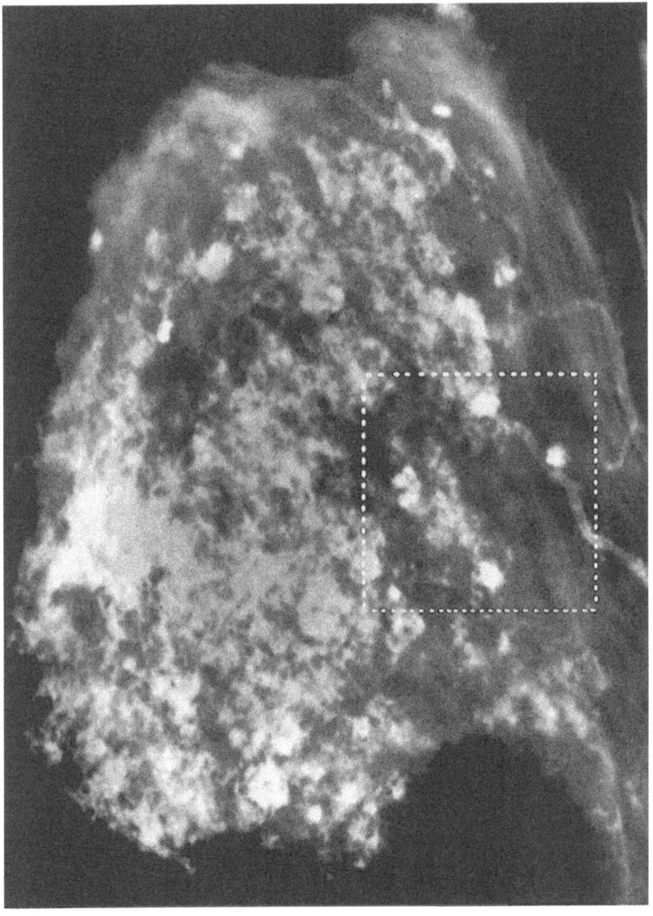

a

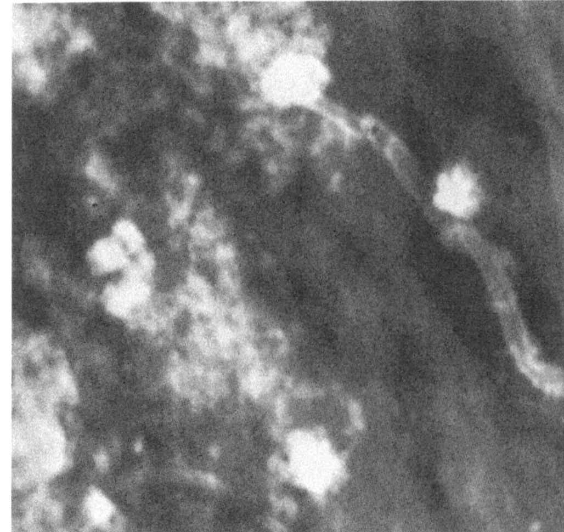

b

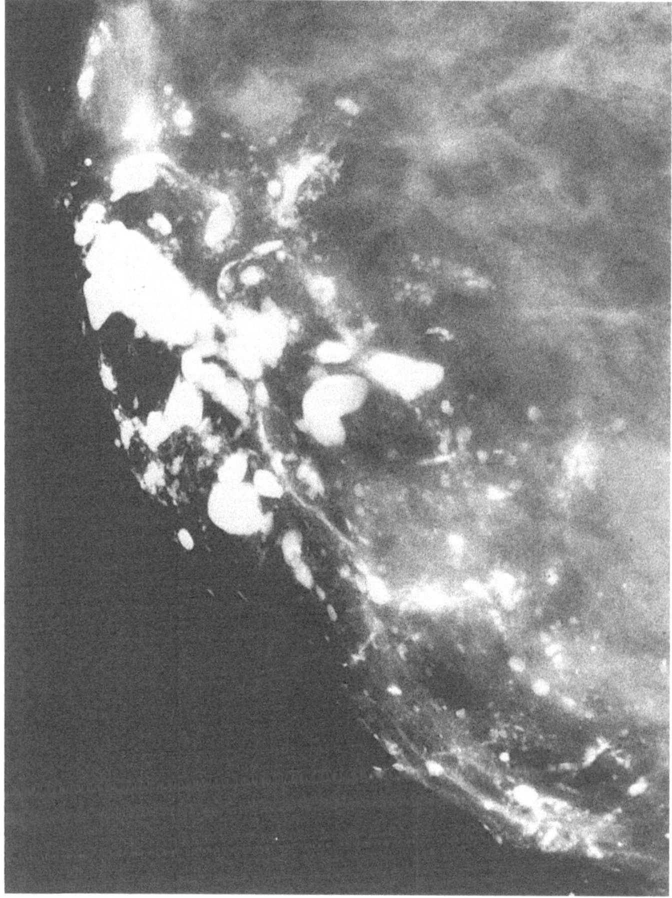

Fig. 4.110. Detail of mammogram. Galactography with iodized oil had been performed 5 years previously (elsewhere). Cysts of varying size and milk ducts are visualized. Some of the smaller cysts show a lobular arrangement with septation

An X-ray image after galactography with iodized oil (Lipiodol; Fig. 4.110) may be similar, however without interstitial or arterial calcifications. This technique is rarely used and only by a few radiologists. Differential diagnosis is not difficult because calcifications are bilateral in primary and secondary hyperparathyroidism, but unilateral in galactography with iodized oil.

◁ **Fig. 4.109. a** Mammogram (slightly reduced). Analysis of the scattered calcifications shows that some are definitely located in cystically dilated lobules, while others are intraductal. Some of the calcifications cannot be localized in the ductolobular system (interstitial calcifications?). Arterial calcification is also present. **b** This detail (3 ×) shows calcifications inside small lobular cysts; the intercystic septa are visible, and calcified ducts can be identified. Clinical diagnosis: renal failure, hyperparathyroidism with osteopathy (Professor STEGMANN, Düsseldorf)

5 Calcifications in Intra- and Pericanalicular Fibroadenomas

It is impossible to fit the calcifications of fibroadenoma into the framework of this book in a way that would satisfy both didactic and pathogenetic demands. As fibroadenoma arises from the connective tissue of the lobule, it should, from a pathogenetic standpoint, be included in a discussion of calcifications of lobular origin (Sect. 4.2). Yet as fibroadenoma contains ducts or ductlike spaces (canaliculi), it would be equally reasonable to place it in a discussion of calcifications of intraductal origin (Sect. 4.3). The only solution is to devote a separate chapter to the calcifications of this Janus-faced tumor.

Pathology

Fibroadenoma, the third most common disease of the female breast, is a mixed tumor composed of mesenchymal and epithelial elements. It usually is palpable clinically as a round-to-oval, smooth, elastic, easily movable nodule 1–2 cm in diameter. It may show transitory enlargement or tenderness in response to hormonal changes. Clinically occult fibroadenomas are frequently detected on mammograms.

Fibroadenoma develops from a confluence-prone hyperplasia of the connective tissue of the lobule (see p. 29) and, according to McDivitt et al. (1968), is indistinguishable in its early stage from the myoepithelial tumor of Hamperl (1939), i.e., from tumorlike sclerosing adenosis. The hormone-dependent swelling or proliferation of connective tissue envelops the acini (terminal duct) and compresses them into clefts. Pathologists call these cleftlike structures "canaliculi." If the hypertrophied, swollen, newly formed connective tissue grows into the lumina of these canaliculi and forms a pseudolining, the fibroadenoma is described as *intracanalicular.* If the neoplastic reticular and collagenous fibers do not invade the canaliculi, and these ductal structures remain intact (though still compressed to some degree), *pericanalicular* fibroadenoma is said to be present. Ductal structure in fibroadenoma can be analyzed easily by fibroadenogram (Wahlers et al. 1977; Sigfusson et al. 1982), as shown in Fig. 5.2b.

Thus, while the mesenchymal component is predominant in intracanalicular fibroadenoma, the glandular (adenous) component predominates in the pericanalicular type. Mixed forms are the rule, however. The lumina of the intact ducts or clefts are lined with epithelium that may form two rows of cells or may be atrophic due to external pressure from the fibrous tissue. The epithelium may show increased proliferation, especially in younger women, and it can even undergo malignant transformation, though this is very rare. Reports like that of Egger and Müller (1977) concerning a 20%–30% association between fibroadenoma and carcinoma are not consistent with personal experience. Cysts may form in intracanalicular fibroadenomas, and Bässler (1978) states that secretions may be observed in these cysts and in ectatic clefts in approximately one-fourth of tumors. In such cases calcium deposits may form from inspissated secretory residue or from cellular debris. The mesenchymal components of the fibroadenoma may also calcify as a result of regressive changes and hyalinosis. Calcifications can also form in fibroadenomas that have become infarcted and necrotic (necrobiotic calcification).

Radiography

The calcification shapes of fibroadenoma on mammograms are determined both by the *location* of the calcifications within the tumor and by the pathologic processes that are taking place. It is no longer possible to interpret these calcifications purely as sequelae of necrobiotic processes (Hoeffken and Lanyi 1973; Sickles 1986); it is necessary to differentiate between
1) calcified secretions in cysts or ductlike structures located within the fibroadenoma, and 2) calcifications in the hyalinized or necrotic stroma or in the capsulelike margin of the tumor.
While the latter types generally are easy to recognize, calcifications occurring in cysts and ductlike structures can raise serious problems of differential diagnosis, especially if they are very small and form a pattern resembling ductal carcinoma.

The following data will serve to illustrate these difficulties. A series of 297 cases biopsied for clustered microcalcifications at the Cologne University Women's Clinic included 18 histologically confirmed fibroadenomas. In a "blind experiment" the author, unaware of the histologic diagnoses, identified 11 of these cases as fibroadenomas and thus classified them as not requiring biopsy. In the remaining seven cases, however, the author was unable to make a definite diagnosis because neither the cluster shape nor the individual calcification shapes allowed for clear differentiation (Lanyi and Neufang 1984). Similar experience was made in a series of examinations conducted at the Nijmegen Catholic University in the Netherlands; of six fibroadenomas biopsied on the basis of microcalcifications, only three were identifiable as such on mammograms.

Analysis of Calcification Cluster Shapes in Fibroadenoma

The calcifications form rounded clusters in the overwhelming majority of cases. Very often they are surrounded by a distinct soft-tissue margin, or they are contained within a round soft-tissue shadow (Figs. 5.1 and 5.2). If the soft-tissue shadow is sharply marginated or if there is a fatty margin around the tumor shadow producing a "halo sign," it is easy to differentiate fibroadenoma from medullary carcinoma. This becomes difficult if the margins are not well defined, the "halo" is interrupted, or the soft-tissue shadow is absent (Fig. 5.3), or especially if the cluster is very small (Fig. 5.4) or presents a triangular shape (this was true in four of the seven cases in the Cologne series, and one of the three Nijmegen cases) (Figs. 5.3b, 5.5, 5.6).

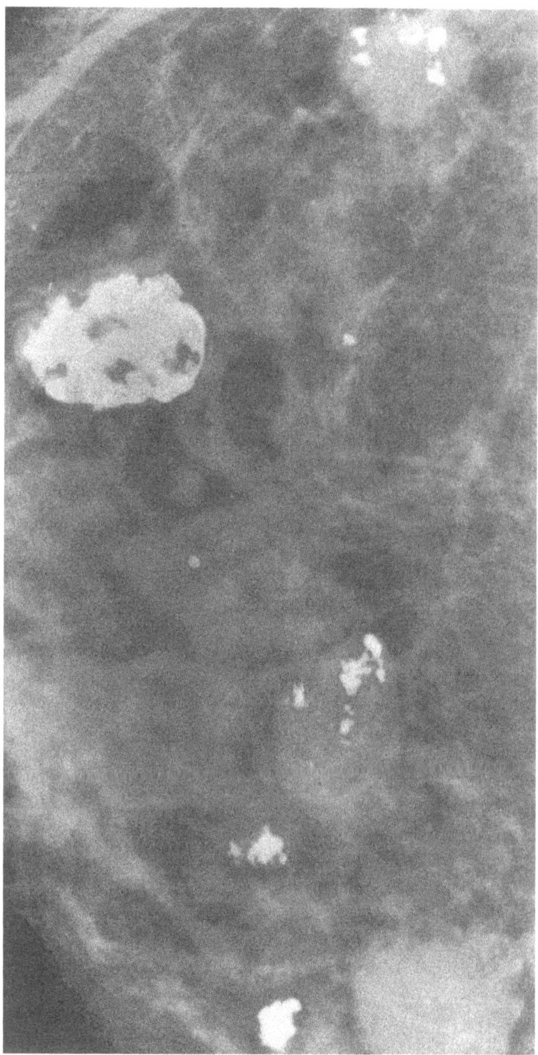

Fig. 5.1. Detail of mammogram (slightly magnified) showing multiple fibroadenomas. The lesion at lower right is devoid of calcifications. The fibroadenomas adjacent to it and at the upper right are completely or almost completely calcified; three others are partially calcified

Analysis of Microcalcification Shapes in Fibroadenoma

Cystic Calcifications. These form in the cysts of the predominantly intracanalicular fibroadenoma (Bässler 1978) and represent calcified secretions. They are rounded, and they may be finely punctate or large and densely clustered, possibly manifesting a uniform size. Septa are visible between the cysts, creating a morulalike pattern similar to that in microcystic adenosis (Fig. 5.7). Clustered, punctate microcalcifications can also form in the cystically dilated acini of predominantly pericanalicular fibroadenoma that are separated ("dissociated") by intervening connective tissue (Fig. 5.8).

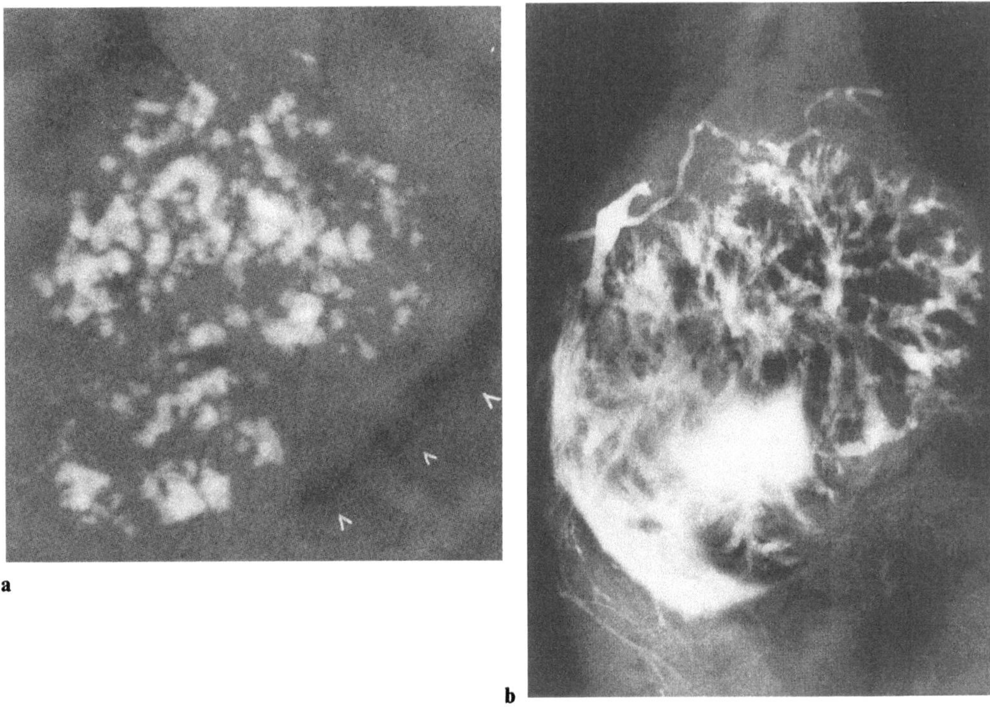

a

b

Fig. 5.2. a Detail of mammogram (approx. 3 ×): rounded cluster of polymorphous (punctate, linear, comma-shaped, v-shaped) microcalcifications within a faint soft-tissue shadow partly surrounded by a fatty margin *(arrows)*. Original size: 2 cm in diameter. The calcifications are larger than those ordinarily seen in carcinoma. **b** Fibroadenogram of another case shows the structure of the canaliculi within the fibroadenoma. The sample is almost identical to that of the calcifications shown in **a** (Dr. R. MÜLLER, Siegburg)

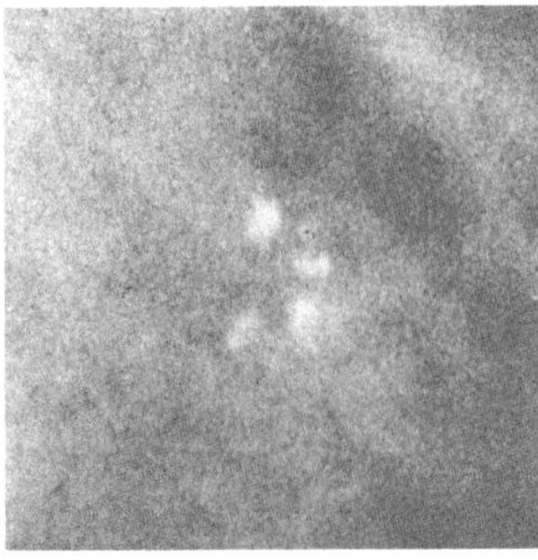

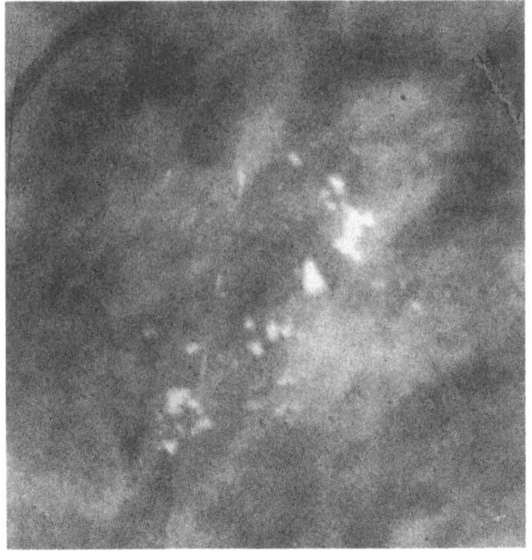

Fig. 5.4. Detail of mammogram (approx. 4 ×): five punctate microcalcifications in a small cluster of indeterminate shape. Histology: fibroadenoma

Fig. 5.5

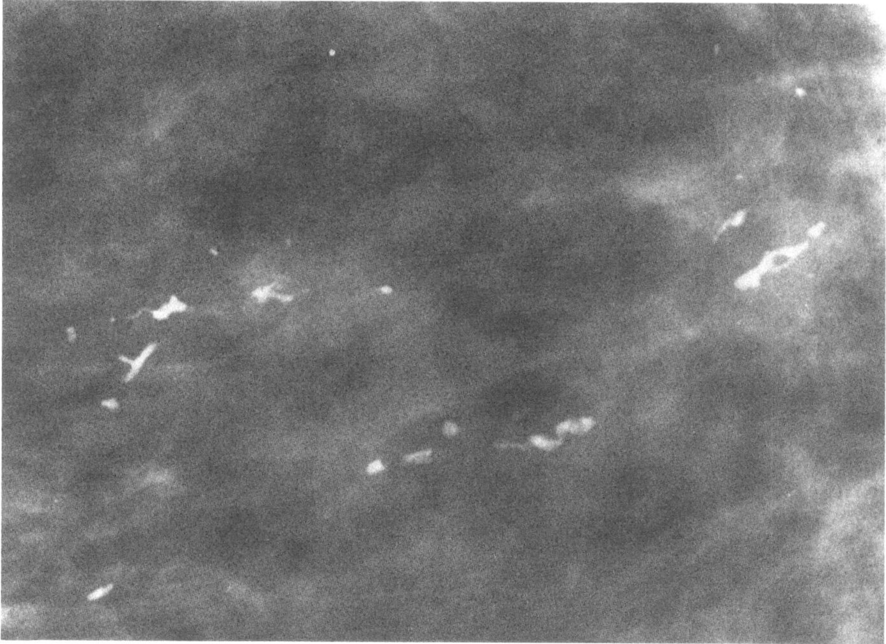

Fig. 5.6. Detail of mammogram (3 ×): polymorphous (punctate, linear, vermiform, y-shaped) microcalcifications in a loose, essentially triangular cluster. There is no soft-tissue shadow. Histology: hyalinized fibroadenoma

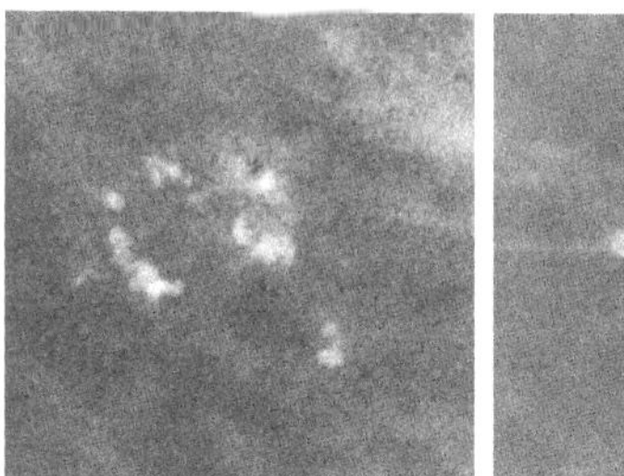

a

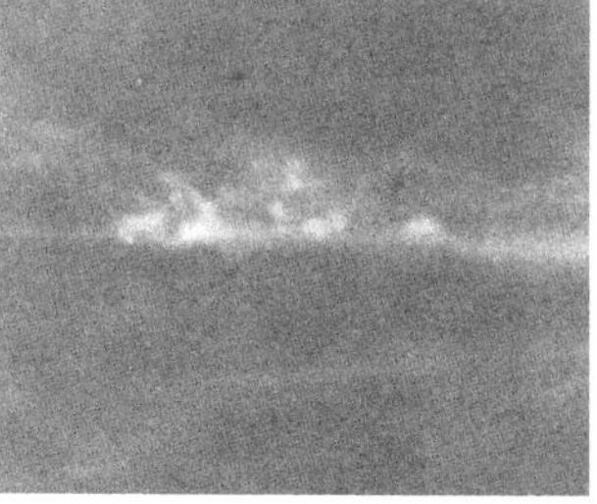

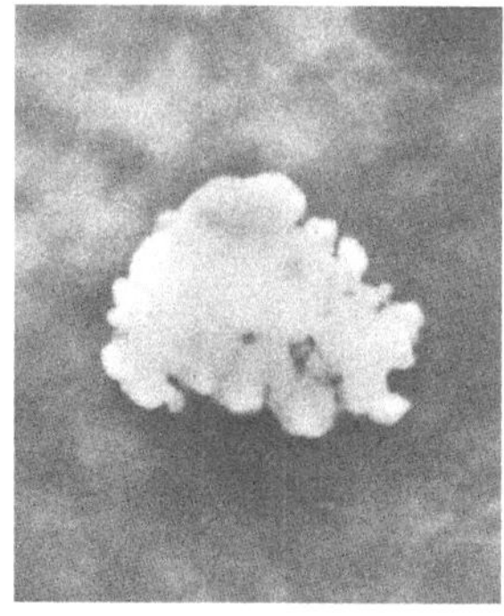

b

Fig. 5.3 a, b. Details of mammogram (approx. 3 ×). **a** Craniocaudad view: rounded cluster of five or six polymorphous (punctate, linear, v-shaped) microcalcifications adjacent to two punctate microcalcifications. **b** On the lateral view the cluster appears triangular, and there is no soft-tissue shadow. Histology: hyalinized and calcified fibroadenoma

Fig. 5.7. Detail of mammogram (original size): dense, ovoid cluster of calcifications separated from one another by fine septa. The calcifications were located in large cavities inside the histologically confirmed fibroadenoma

◁ **Fig. 5.5.** Detail of mammogram (3 ×): triangular cluster of polymorphous (punctate, linear, v-shaped, and irregularly shaped) microcalcifications without a tumor shadow. Pattern is suggestive of intraductal carcinoma. Histology: hyalinized and calcified fibroadenoma. A differential diagnosis cannot be made from the mammographic picture

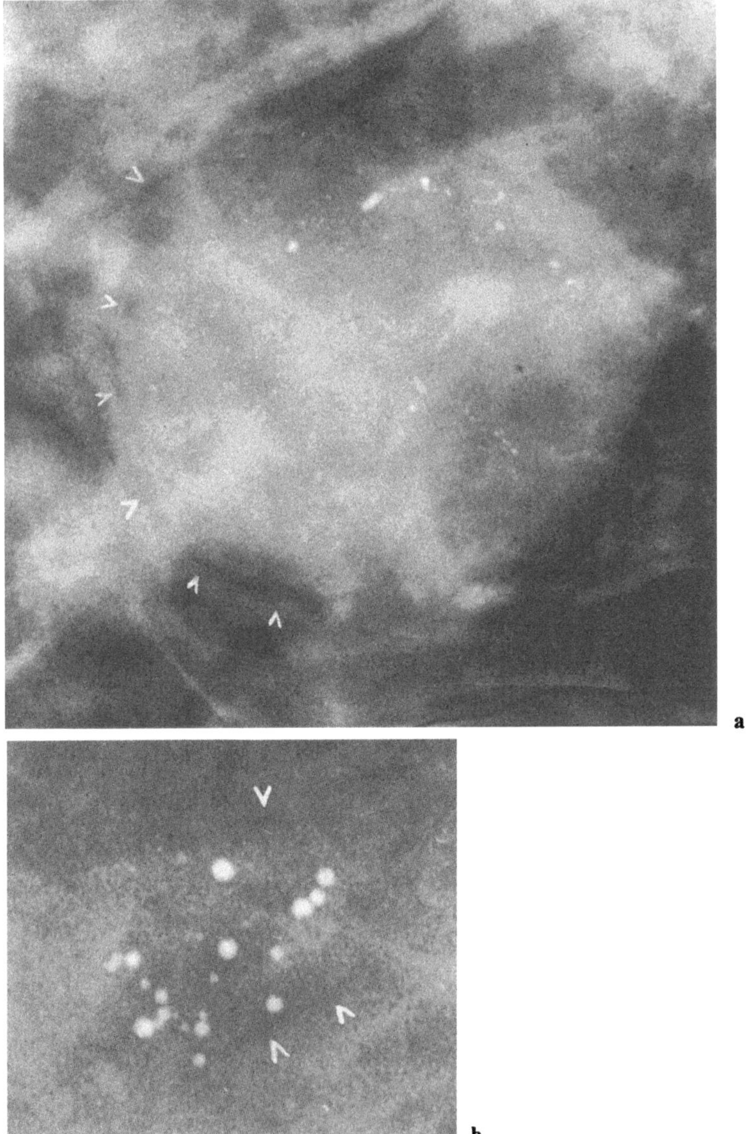

Fig. 5.8a, b. Details of mammograms. **a** Round shadow with partially smooth borders, a fatty margin *(arrows)*, and fine punctate microcalcifications (3×). **b** Round-to-oval cluster of about 30 rounded microcalcifications of variable size. Again, several septa are visible between the calcifications. The impression is that of a faint, oval shadow surrounded by a fine fatty margin *(arrows)*. Histology: fibroadenoma with cystic cavities containing secretions and calcifications (4×)

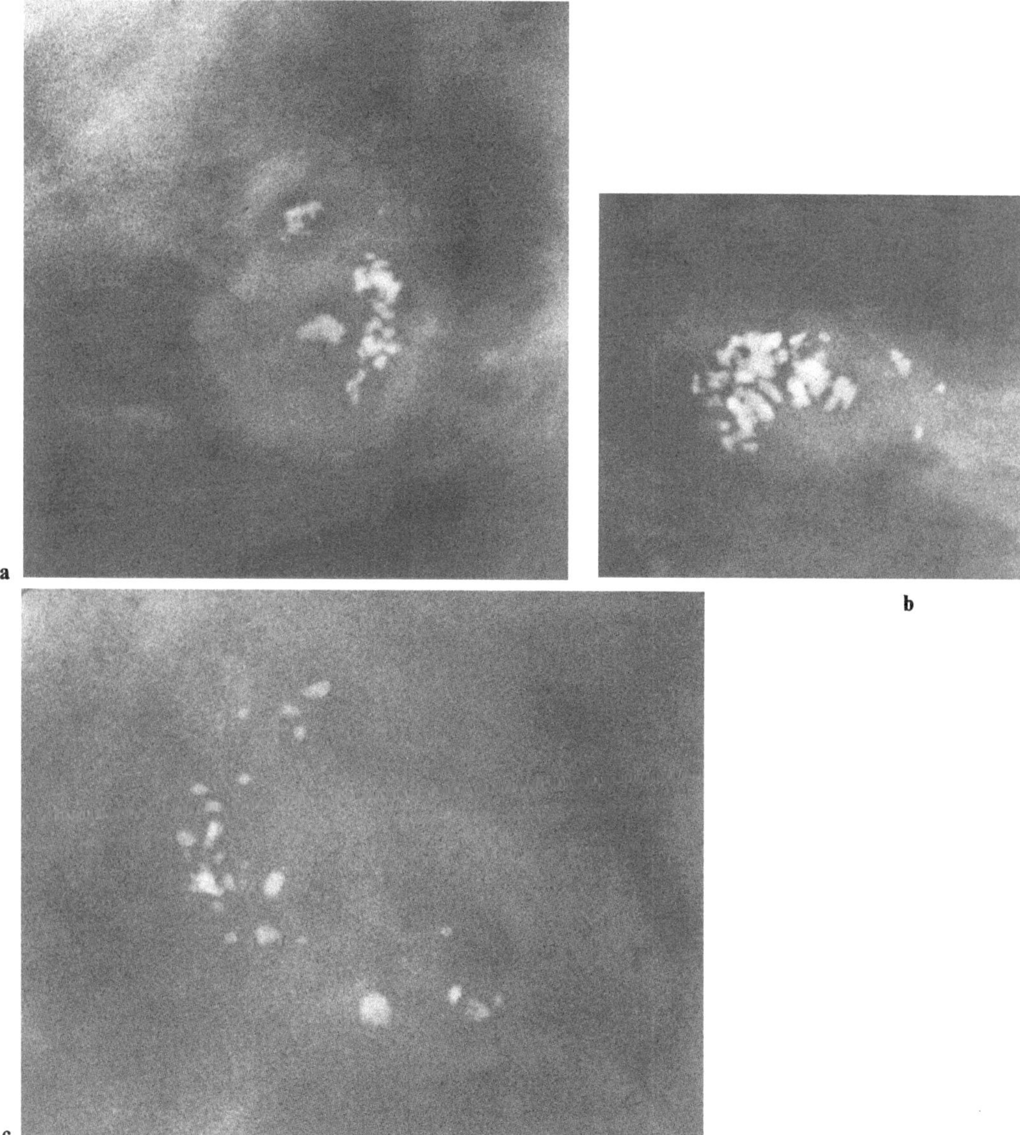

Fig. 5.9 a–c. Details of mammograms. **a** Polymorphous (punctate, linear, V-, and Y-shaped) microcalcifications within a 6-mm shadow. **b** Polymorphous (punctate, linear, v-shaped, irregularly shaped) microcalcifications within a round shadow 1 cm in diameter. The cluster appears to have an ovoid shape. **c** Crescent-shaped cluster, about 1 cm in diameter, of predominantly punctate microcalcifications showing minimal polymorphism (one linear, one V-shaped). A round tumor shadow is faintly visible. Histology established all three cases as fibroadenoma

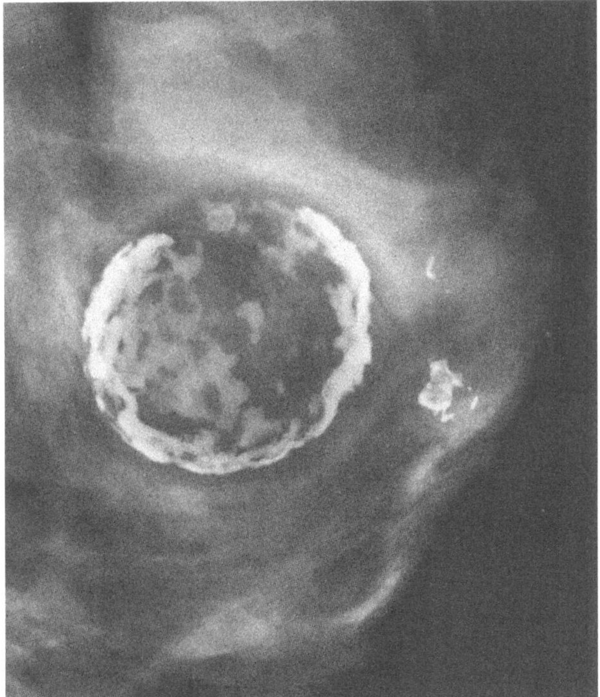
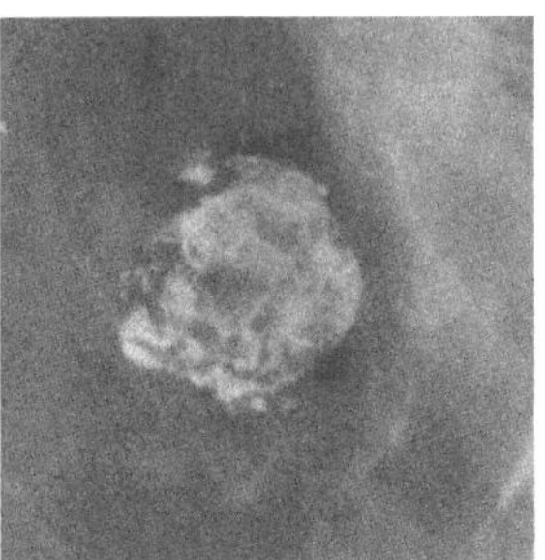

Fig. 5.10. a Detail of mammogram (original size): completely calcified fibroadenoma, showing several large, y-shaped calcifications in addition to a thick, capsulelike calcification. **b** This detail (slightly reduced) shows a completely calcified fibroadenoma resembling an oyster shell. (From HOEFFKEN and LANYI 1973)

Intracanalicular Calcifications. In pericanalicular or predominantly pericanalicular fibroadenomas, the organization of the glandular tree remains largely unaffected. Calcified secretions in these tumors may be manifested by linear, v-, w-, and z-shaped calcifications like those of comedocarcinoma (Figs. 5.3, 5.5, 5.6, 5.9), which is reasonable when we consider that these structures represent "casts" of the ducts that contain them. The intracanalicular calcifications of fibroadenoma tend to be coarser und plumper than those of intraductal carcinoma, however. They might be described as a "poor copy," though in some cases they are remarkably similar to other calcifications, and very small fibroadenomas in particular may be indistinguishable from small cancers. Also, the fine polymorphous microcalcifications typical of carcinoma may betray their true intracanalicular location within a fibroadenoma only by their rounded cluster shape, which is not at all characteristic of carcinoma.

Stromal Calcifications. The necrobiotic calcifications caused by circulatory disturbances and those of the hyalized, sclerosed stroma are not punctate, linear, or branched, but are amorphous and more or less homogenous. The pattern may

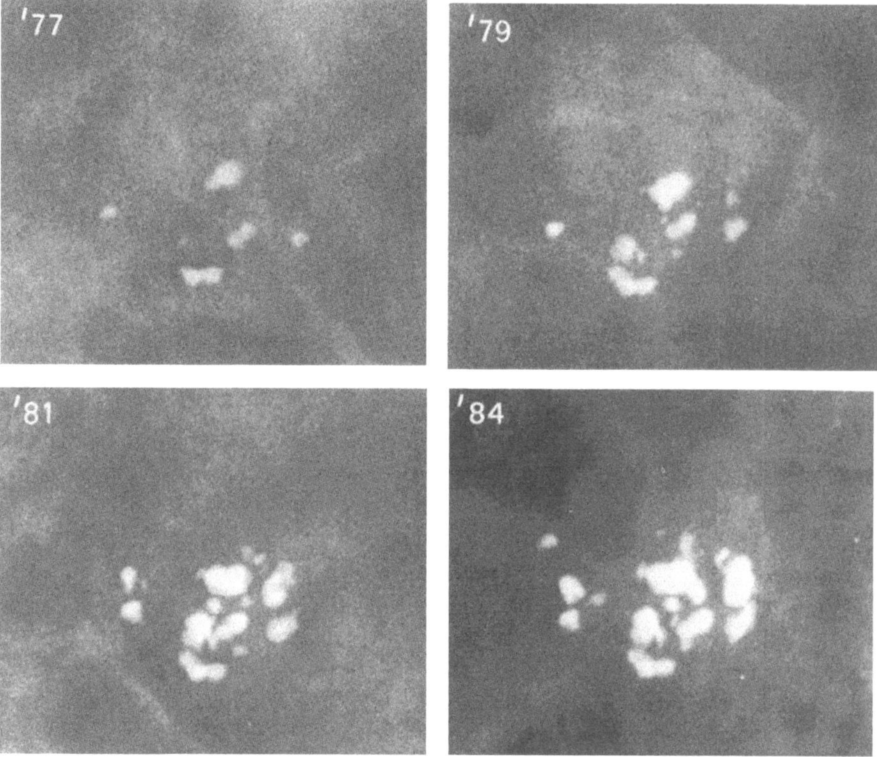

Fig. 5.11. Details of mammograms (4 ×) showing a progressive increase in the number of microcalcifications in a fibroadenoma over a 7-year period. We can observe the evolution of the ovoid cluster shape and polymorphism of the coarse microcalcifications

resemble the outer shell of an oyster (Fig. 5.10b), or it may be crescent-shaped if the calcifications are confined to the fibroadenoma capsule.

Mixed Forms. Mixed forms are common, not infrequently being observed in close proximity to one another (Figs. 5.1 and 5.10a).

Increase of Microcalcifications

The increase in the number of microcalcifications described by MENGES et al. (1976) in intraductal carcinoma is occasionally seen on serial mammograms of fibroadenoma. Usually this is not considered an indication for pathologic evaluation (Fig. 5.11), and it is rare that the finding of an increased number of microcalcifications will lead to biopsy because of suspected comedocarcinoma. In the case shown in Fig. 5.12, the original impression was fibroadenoma (Fig. 5.12a), and reexamination in 6 months was advised, at which time (Fig. 5.12b) the calcifications did not appear to have increased in number. After 1 year (Fig. 5.12c) I thought that I may

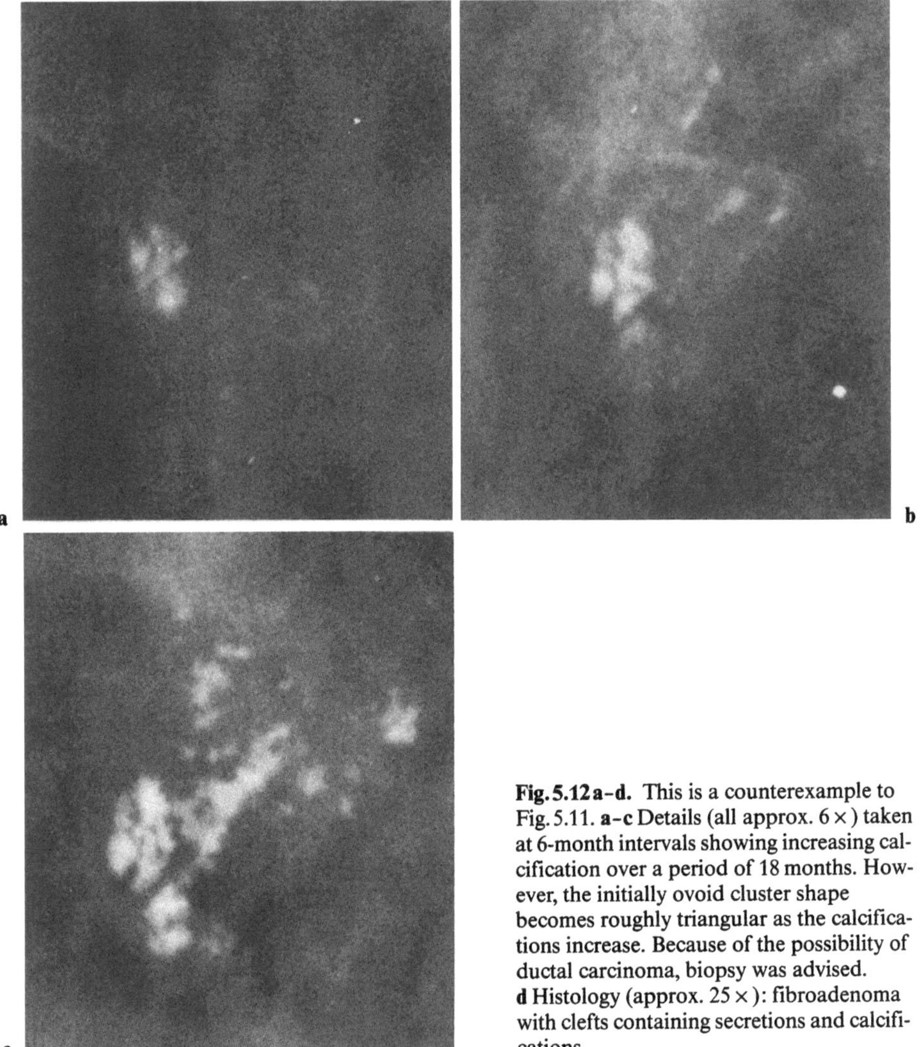

Fig. 5.12 a–d. This is a counterexample to Fig. 5.11. **a–c** Details (all approx. 6 ×) taken at 6-month intervals showing increasing calcification over a period of 18 months. However, the initially ovoid cluster shape becomes roughly triangular as the calcifications increase. Because of the possibility of ductal carcinoma, biopsy was advised. **d** Histology (approx. 25 ×): fibroadenoma with clefts containing secretions and calcifications

Fig. 5.13. Calcified fibroadenomalike tumor of the nipple with chronic osteogenic inflammation of ▷ the skin (4 ×) (Dr. HENDRIKS, Nijmegen, Netherlands)

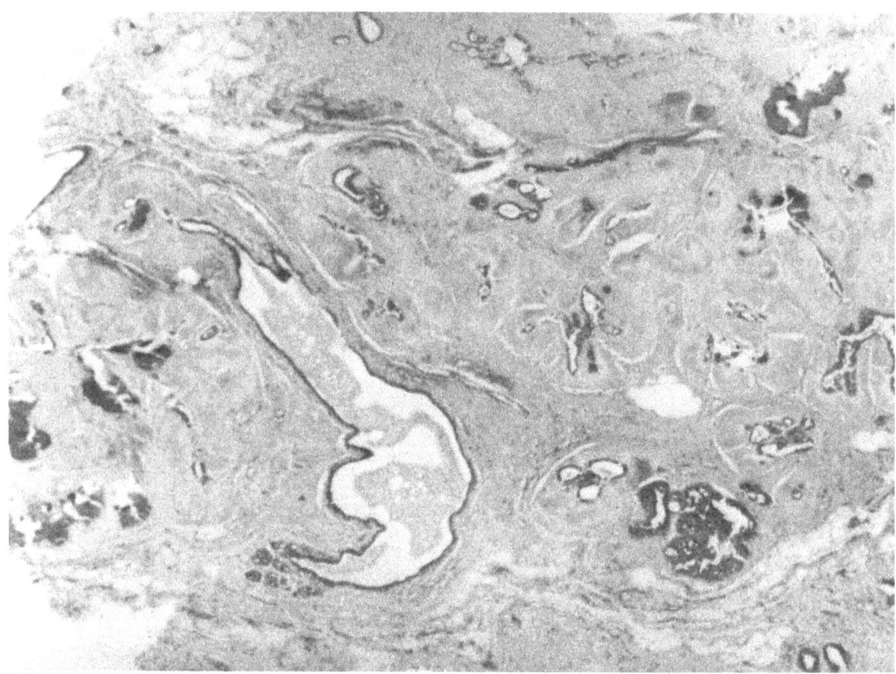

Fig. 5.12 d

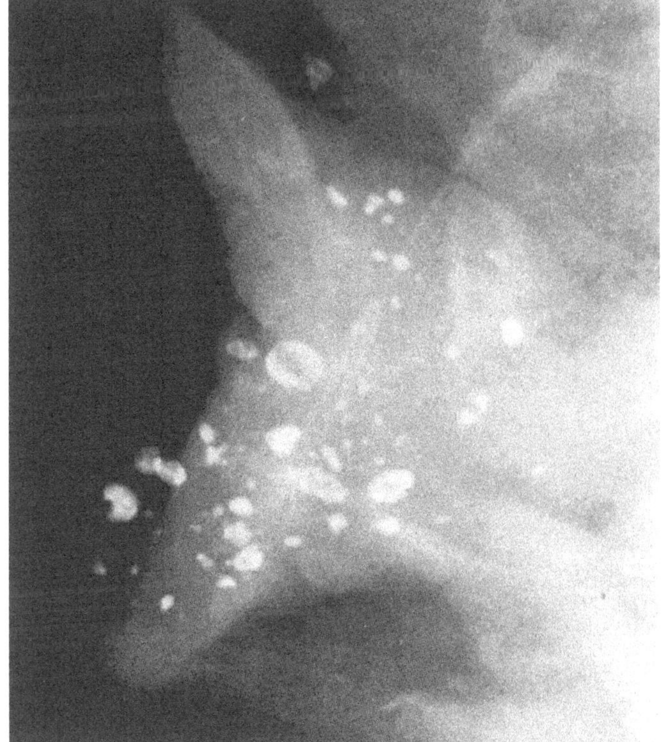

Fig. 5.13

have missed a ductal carcinoma (roughly triangular cluster shape, polymorphism). Biopsy confirmed the original diagnosis of fibroadenoma (Fig. 5.12 d).

Fibroadenoma like Tumor of the Nipple

While adenoma of the nipple is not a particularly rare disease (KINDERMANN and RUMMEL published 199 observations in 1973), fibroadenoma of the nipple or areola is exceedingly rare (Fig. 5.13). It is marked by flaky, round-to-oval calcifications of variable size, primarily with central lucencies in the area of the retracted nipple and areola. Biopsy of the lesion in Fig. 5.13 showed a fibroadenomalike tumor of the nipple associated with a chronic osteogenic skin inflammation (R. HOLLAND, personal communication).

6 Calcifications Outside the Lobular and Ductal System of the Breast

6.1 Calcifications in Fat Necrosis of Varying Etiology

Pathology

Calcifications of mammary fat necrosis always develop according to the same pattern, regardless of the etiologic agent of the necrosis. In the *lesion phase* the membranes of the fat cells become damaged, allowing the leakage of neutral fat from the cells. In the *absorption phase* lipophages remove the liberated neutral fat, leading to the formation of fat vacuoles that are surrounded by macrophages, *plasma cells,* and leukocytes. As the absorption process continues, we enter the *repair phase* in which increasing numbers of fibroblasts appear at the periphery of the vacuoles, walling off the cavity with a relatively dense capsule- or scarlike zone. Calcium salts may be precipitated in the cavity wall; hemosiderosis, birefringent needlelike fatty acid crystals, and macrophage-rich granulomas are also observed.

Radiography

The calcifications of fat necrosis present radiographically either as *calcified macro and microcyst(s)* or as an *amorphous calcification cluster.*
Calcified liponecrotic cysts, first described by LEBORGNE (1967), may occur after
a) trauma from injury, biopsy, primary radiotherapy (BASSETT et al. 1982), or plastic surgery, and
b) bacterial (e.g., acute mastitis with abscess formation) or abacterial inflammations (secretory disease, plasma cell mastitis, ruptured cyst, nonsuppurative panniculitis, Weber-Christian disease).

While all these calcifications present a rounded or ovoid shape on mammograms, they differ significantly in number, size, and homogeneity.

Liponecrotic Microcysts

In the series of 1044 consecutive mammograms there were a total of 90 liponecrotic microcysts (8.6%). This is therefore a common lesion. In the great majority of cases (73), the liponecrotic microcysts were solitary; in seven cases they were arranged in clusters, and in nine they were scattered. There was only one case where we saw a cluster of liponecrotic microcysts associated with an area of scar (Fig. 6.1). One patient in this series cited a recent blunt trauma as the presumed cause of the liponecrotic microcysts discovered in a follow-up examination. But in all other cases the patient could give no history of trauma or other event that might account for the formation of these almost uniformly sized (2–3 mm diameter) calcifications. The large number of cases makes it extremely unlikely that we are dealing with "silent

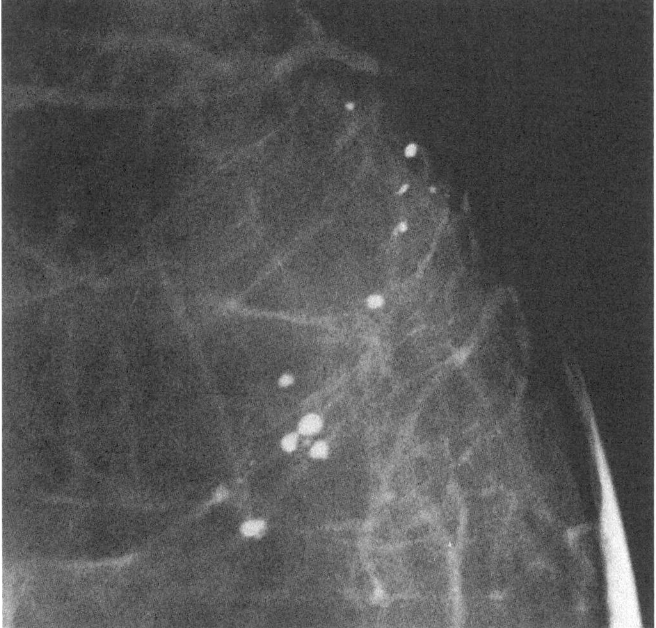

Fig. 6.1. Detail of mammogram (slightly magnified): liponecrotic microcysts arranged linearly along the scar from a previous biopsy

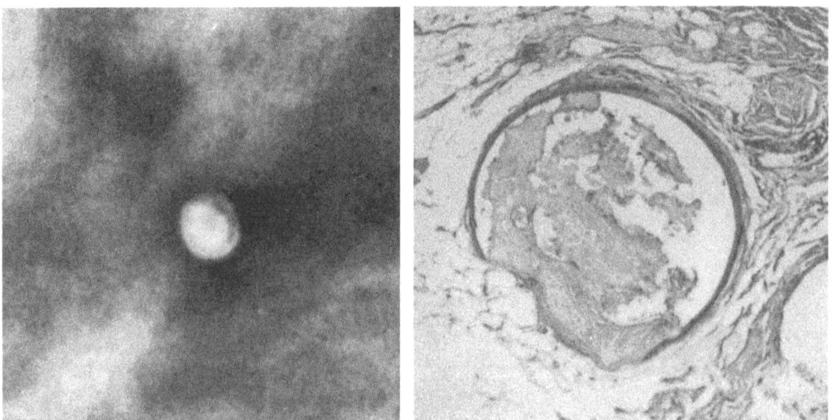

Fig. 6.2. **a** Specimen radiograph (3 ×). This liponecrotic microcyst was found adjacent to a radiographically suspicious area of clustered microcalcifications (histology: severe papillomatosis). **b** The mammographic and histologic presentations of the cyst are identical: the ring-shaped calcification on the X-ray corresponds to the calcified capsule, and the intracystic amorphous calcification to granulation tissue within the lesion (approx. 40 ×)

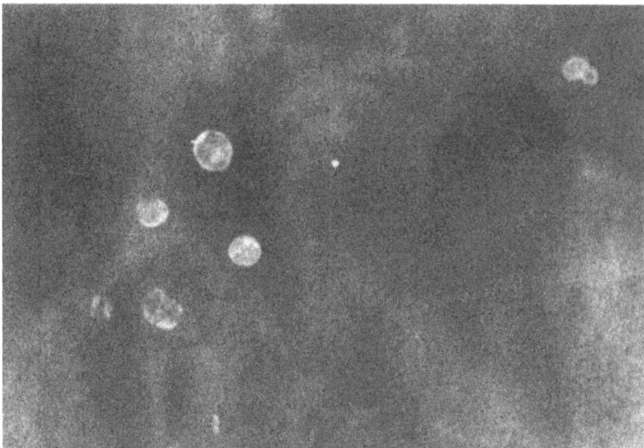

Fig. 6.3. Detail of mammogram (slightly magnified): clustered liponecrotic microcysts with no history of trauma. Roughly equal-sized calcified rings with more or less pronounced intracystic calcifications of the granulation tissue

trauma" that has been forgotten by the patient, and suggests that these vesicular, calcified zones of fat necrosis may have formed from the spontaneous rupture of microcysts in cystic breast disease or as a sequel to "retention syndrome" analogous to plasma cell mastitis (see p. 131). However, this still makes it difficult to explain why a liponecrotic microcyst was found in exactly the same location in the upper outer quadrant of the right breast in a pair of twin sisters. Liponecrotic microcysts may be solitary (Fig. 6.2), clustered (Fig. 6.3), or scattered (Fig. 6.4). Usually they present a central lucency or show several punctate or amorphous calcifications within the calcified ring.

These lesions are very difficult to examine histologically because of their hard consistency; the microtome tends to "pry" them out of the paraffin block. CITOLER obtained the specimen in Fig. 6.2b by first softening the calcium salt crust of the liponecrotic cyst with ultrasound so that histologic sections could be prepared. The section identifies the amorphous central calcification on the radiograph as calcified intracystic granulation tissue.

Sometimes the disappearance or reappearance of liponecrotic microcysts may be noticed on follow-up mammograms. Also, the formation of liponecrotic microcysts is occasionally seen following surgery (Figs. 6.5-6.7). The vesicular, sometimes slightly ovoid calcifications found in the vicinity of linear calcified secretions likewise represent liponecrotic microcysts. They are caused by secretions extravasating through the duct wall into the surrounding tissue and inciting a circumscribed, "chemical," abacterial inflammation (Fig. 6.8). The older term "plasma cell mastitis" for the combined presence of calcified secretions and liponecrotic microcysts on mammograms is something of a misnomer, because plasma cell infiltration is not always seen histologically. LEBORGNE, in 1967, postulated a link between liponecrotic microcysts and the development of carcinoma, but this has not yet been confirmed. We have seen one case in which a cluster of liponecrotic microcysts occurred in association with a tubular carcinoma (Fig. 6.9).

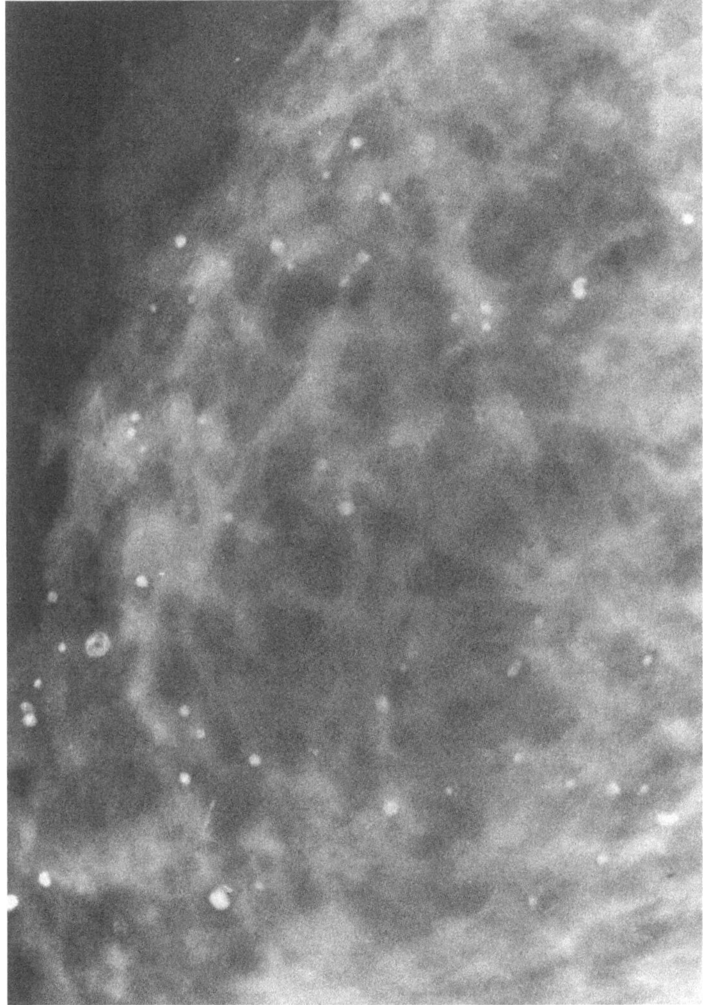

Fig.6.4. Detail of mammogram: numerous scattered liponecrotic microcysts of roughly equal size, some completely calcified. The lesions were bilateral, and the patient gave no history of trauma

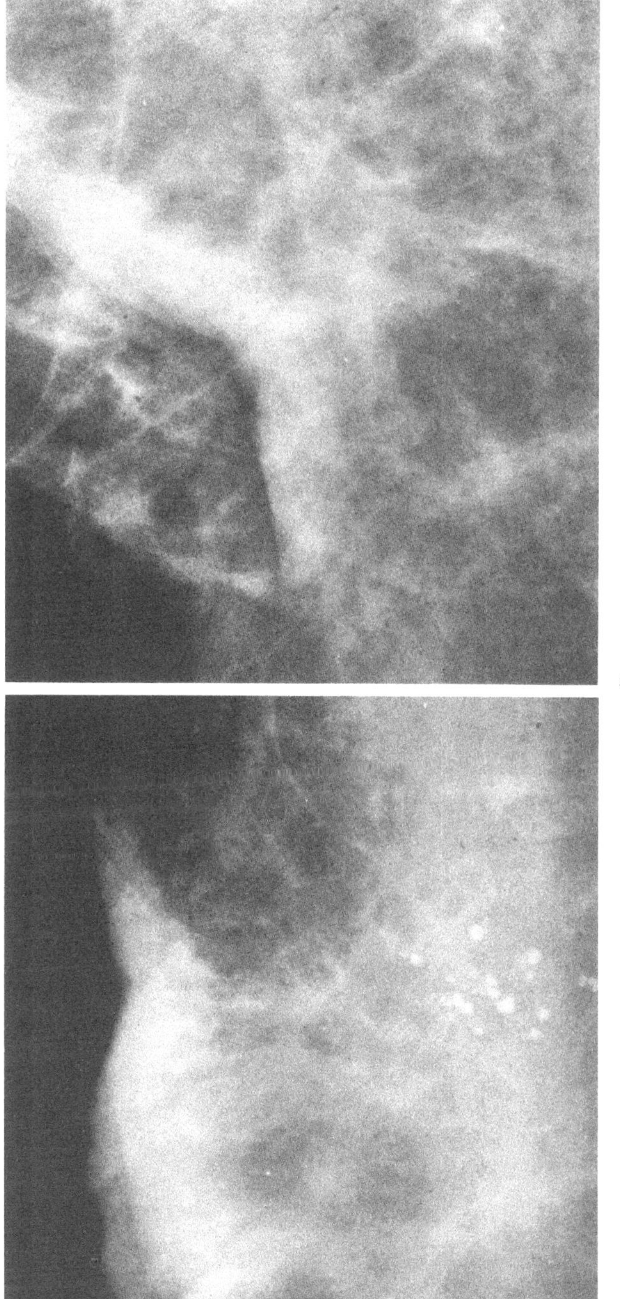

Fig. 6.5 a, b. Details of mammograms (approx. 3 ×).
a Tissue behind the nipple had been removed for biopsy 6 months previously. Cicatricial changes with nipple retraction. **b** Three years later, numerous liponecrotic microcysts are present in the biopsied area

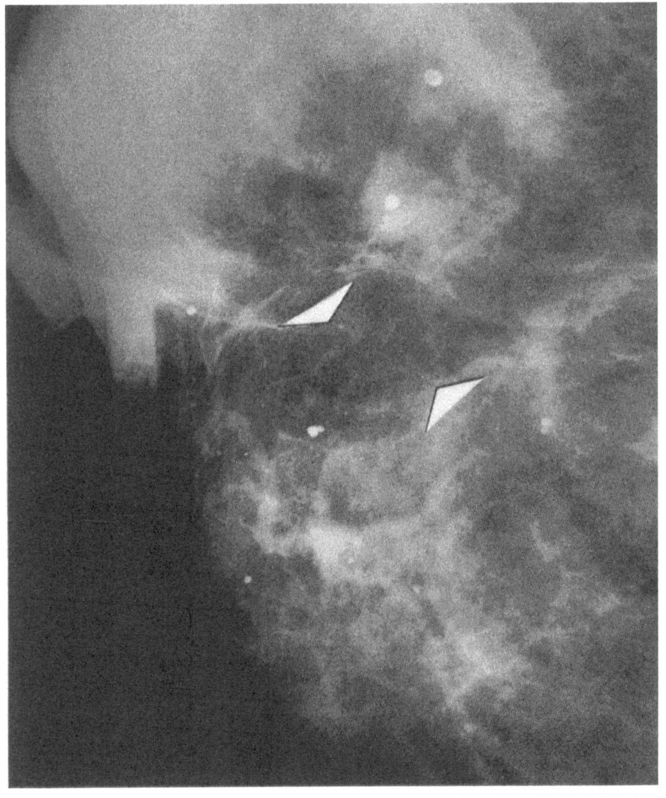

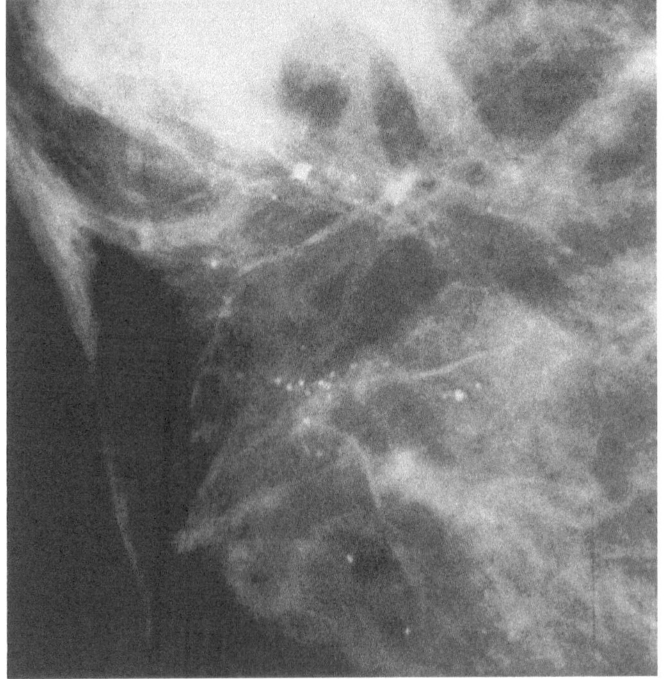

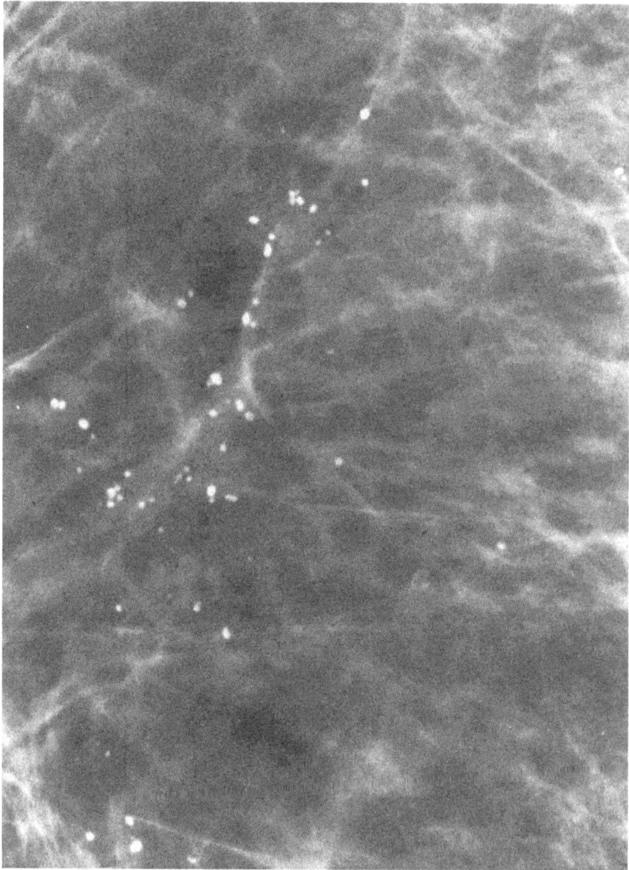

Fig. 6.7. Detail of mammogram (slightly magnified): numerous calcified liponecrotic microcysts of approximately equal size in a patient who had undergone reduction mammoplasty. Similar findings in the contralateral breast

◁ **Fig. 6.6a, b.** Details of mammograms (slightly magnified). **a** Bandlike parenchymal defect *(arrows)* with several liponecrotic microcysts 1 year after biopsy. **b** Two years later the calcified liponecrotic cysts are more numerous

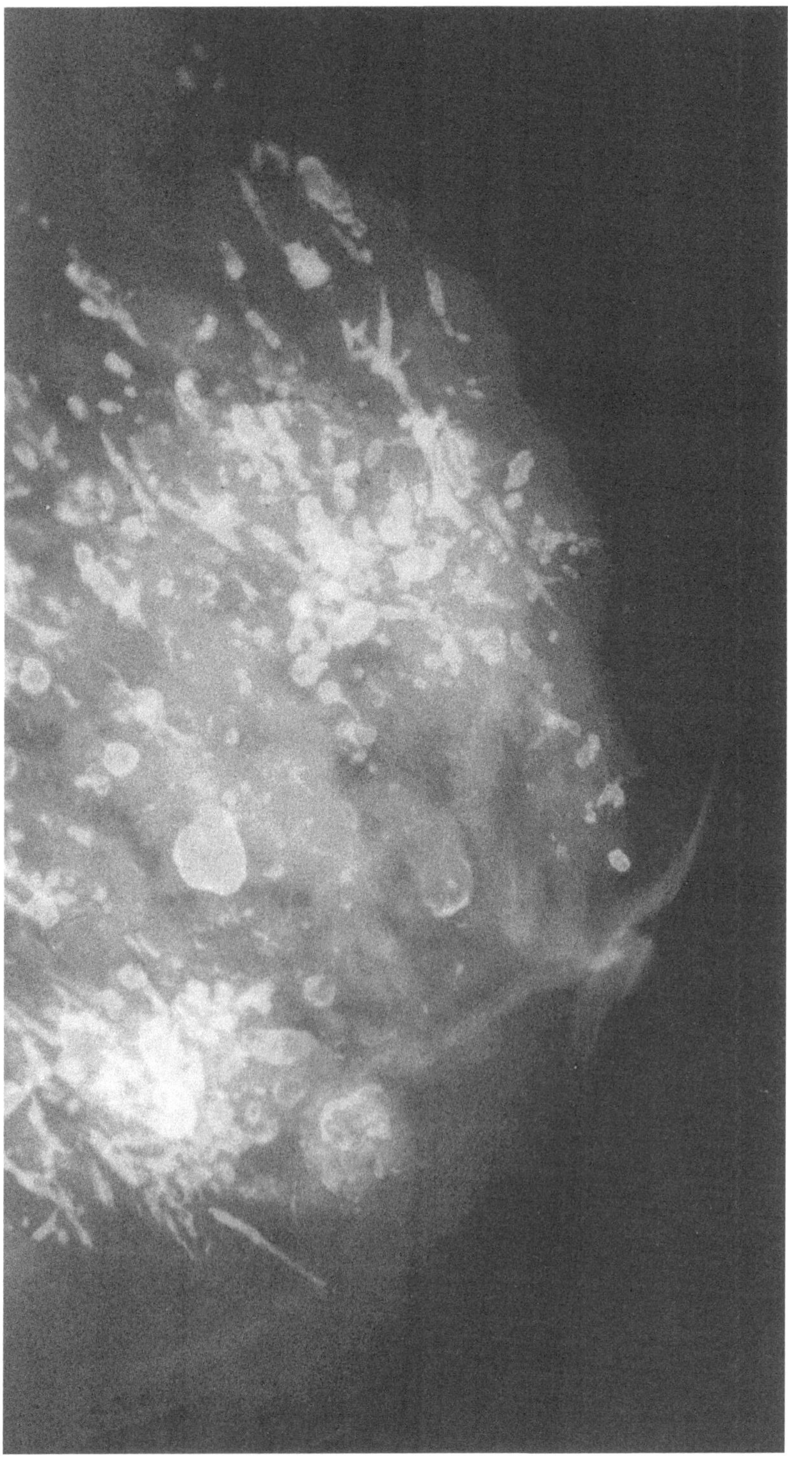

Liponecrotic Macrocysts

Five liponecrotic macrocysts were found in the above-mentioned series of 1044 consecutive mammograms (0.5%), demonstrating the rarity of the gross liponecrotic cyst. The majority of macrocysts are oil cysts (ANDERSSON et al. 1977) that have formed in a scarred area; they have a fibrous capsule that may calcify (Fig. 6.10). Liponecrotic micro- and macrocysts may coexist in the area of an operative scar (Fig. 6.11).

Silicone injection for breast augmentation may be followed by the appearance of small, spherical bodies with calcified shells resulting from encapsulation of the foreign material (Fig. 6.12). This is probably based on an abacterial inflammatory reaction. Because silicone injection does not leave a cutaneous scar, differential diagnosis can be quite difficult if the patient does not disclose that she has had a mammoplasty (INOUE et al. 1978). Calcifications can also form after paraffin injection (THIELS and DUMKE 1977; KOIDE and KATAYAMA 1979). The calcification of implant capsules after augmentation mammoplasty has been reported by REDFERN et al. (1977) and by BENJAMIN and GUY (1977). Figure 6.13a was obtained in a breast augmented with dermatofat grafting. The location of the bizarre, linear calcifications visible on both planes could not be determined radiographically (in the capsule? in the implanted fat?). Only when a similar implant had to be removed was it discovered that the calcifications were located in the shell-like capsule of the implant, and that the implanted fat itself was filled with oil. Thus, calcified dermatofat grafts actually may be regarded as calcified oil cysts (Fig. 6.13). Calcifications of fat grafts have been reported by HERMANUTZ and MÜLLER (1970) and by REINHARDT (1974).

The usually multiple, round to-oval calcifications that form in the subcutaneous fatty tissue (Fig. 6.14) in the setting of nonsuppurative nodular panniculitis also are regarded as fully calcified liponecrotic macrocysts (LEONHARDT 1968; HOEFFKEN and LANYI 1973; BERNSTEIN 1977). This disease, named after Weber and Christian, belongs to the rheumatic group of diseases. Its clinical features include rheumatoid arthritis and recurring painful nodules of the trunk, breast, and extremities, with erythema and fever. The histologic picture is one of inflammatory, nodular fat necrosis of an essentially traumatic form, accompanied by the infiltration of leukocytes, lymphocytes, and macrophages with the formation of multiple granulomas (BÄSSLER 1978). The author observed three such cases over a period of 10 years. *None* could be identified clinically or from patient's history as nonsuppurative panniculitis by the above definition, and they were diagnosed as idiopathic fat granulomas (Fig. 6.14) or as idiopathic disseminated calcified steatonecrosis (Fig. 6.15).

◁ **Fig. 6.8.** Pronounced plasma cell mastitis. Elongated linear and branched ductal calcifications coexist with vesicular calcifications of varying size, representing liponecrotic cysts. The latter resulted from the extravasation of secretions into the interstitium, inciting an abacterial mastitis and causing circumscribed liquefaction of the fatty tissue

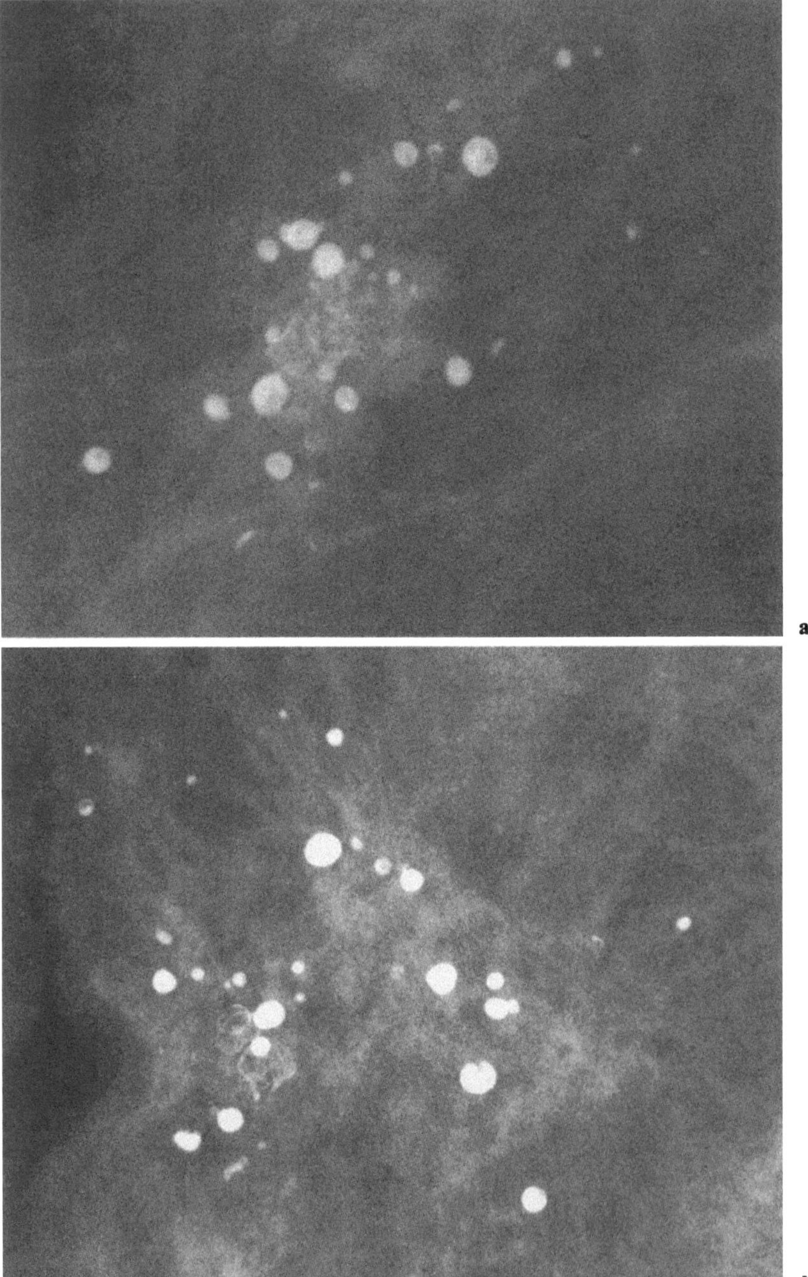

Fig. 6.9. a Detail of mammogram (4 ×): clustered liponecrotic microcysts showing varying degrees of calcification in a biopsy scar. After several follow-ups, fine linear and v-shaped microcalcifications appeared at the center of the cluster. Biopsy was performed because of suspected comedocarcinoma. **b** Detail of specimen radiograph (4 ×). It is evident that the suspicious linear and v-shaped microcalcifications represent newly formed liponecrotic microcysts; the linear and v-shaped microcalcifications on the mammogram were simulated by the thin cystic calcifications. Histology: 4-mm tubular carcinoma coexisting with liponecrotic changes. The malignancy bore no causal relationship to the radiographic signs; the tubular carcinoma was an incidental finding.

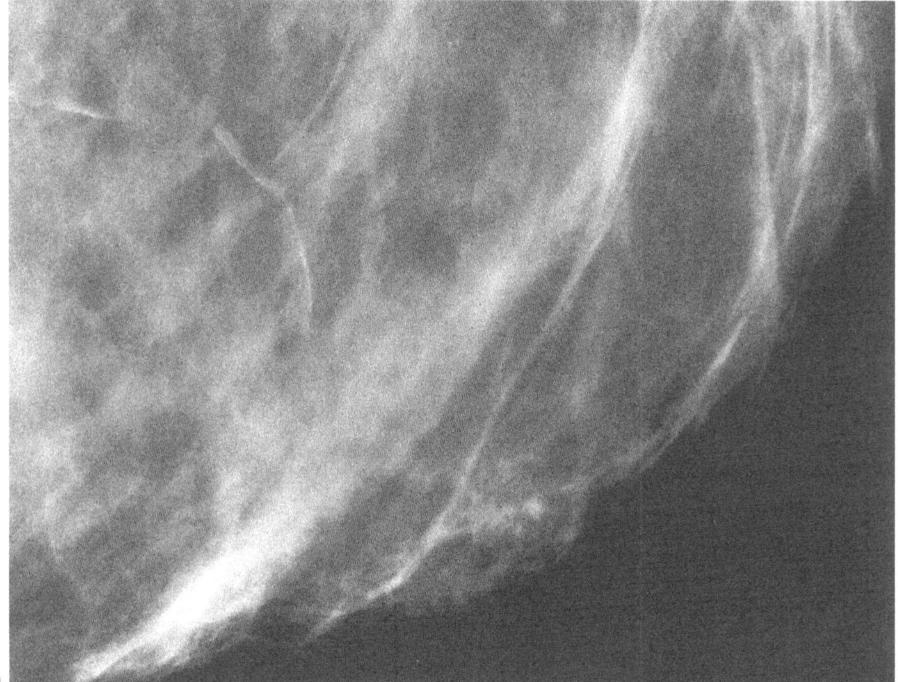

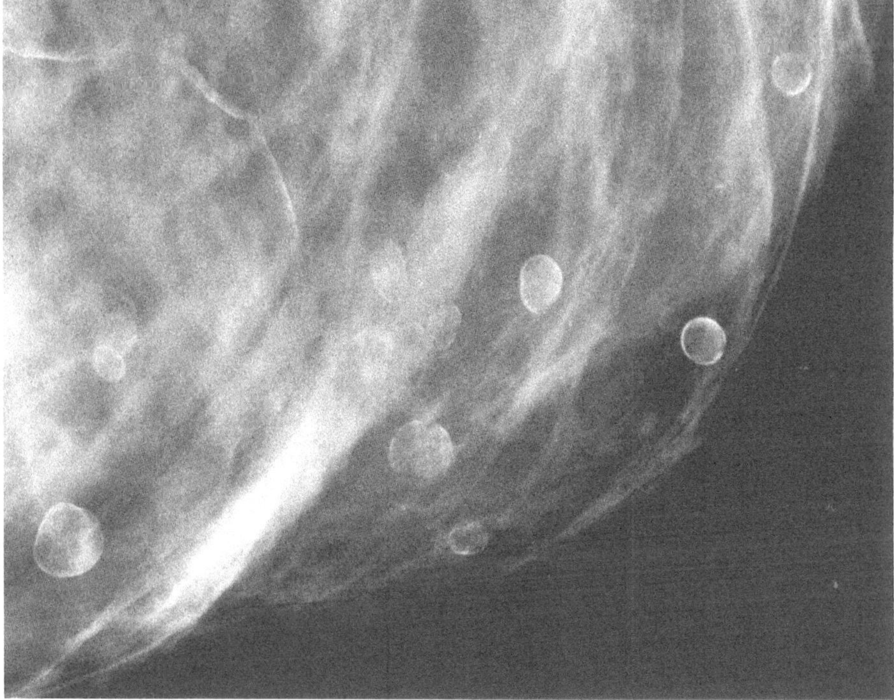

Fig. 6.10 a, b. Details of mammograms (slightly magnified). **a** Arterial calcification in a breast with cystic disease. **b** Three years later, following an automobile accident 2 years before that had caused a hematoma of the breast: multiple calcified liponecrotic macrocysts in the area of the former hematoma

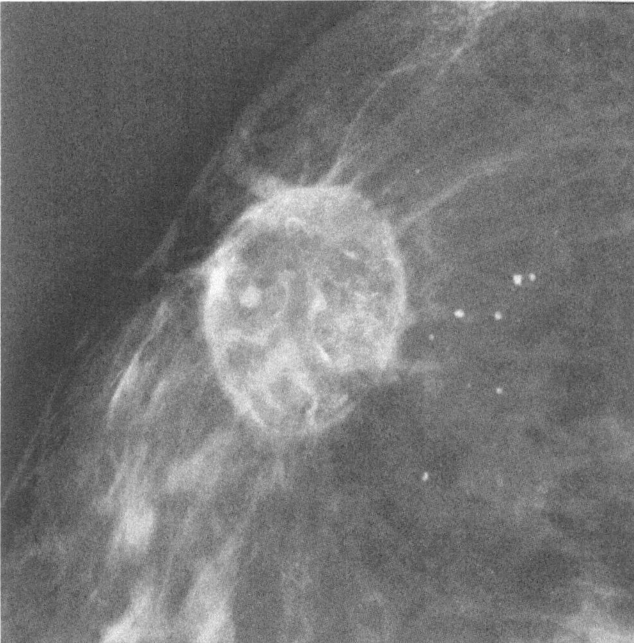

Fig. 6.11. Detail of mammogram (slightly magnified) from a biopsied breast. The scarred area contains a large, ovoid oil cyst with peripheral calcification and tortuous linear calcifications. Multiple liponecrotic microcysts are also present

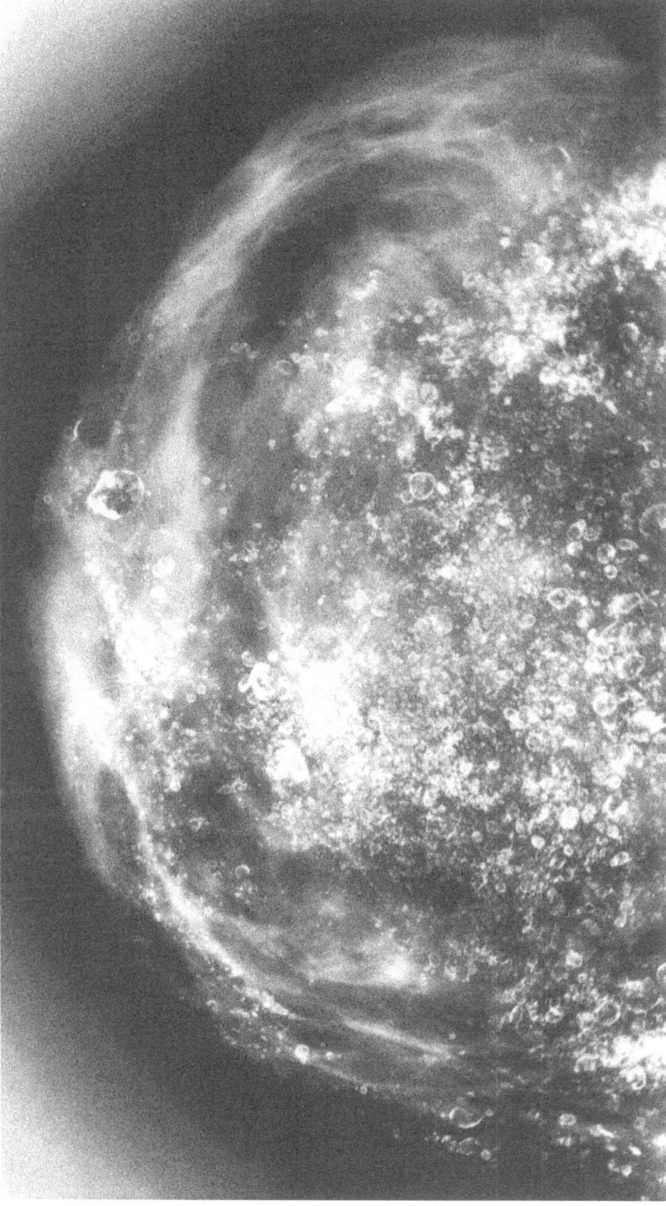

Fig. 6.12. Innumerable, densely arranged liponecrotic micro- and macrocysts forming calcified rings in a breast previously augmented by silicone injection (Dr. M. RADO, Bergheim)

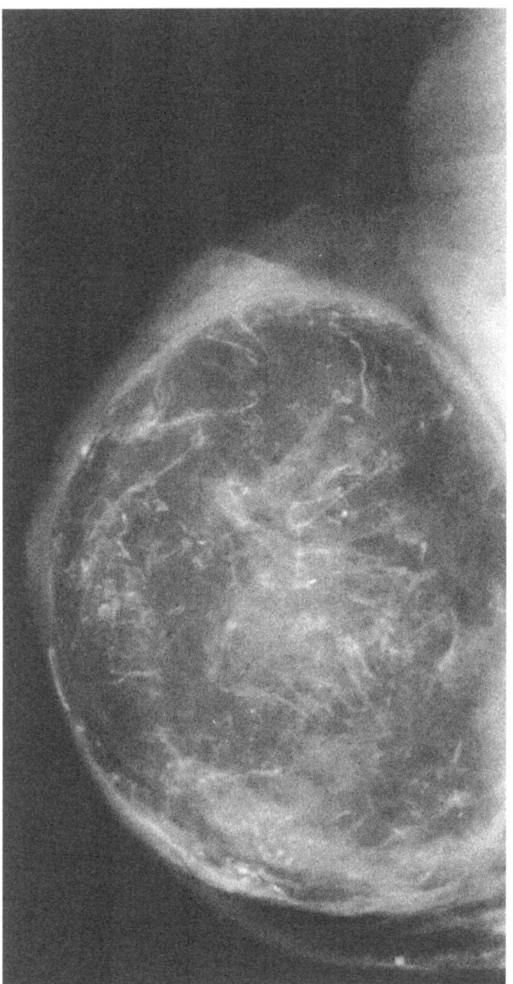
a

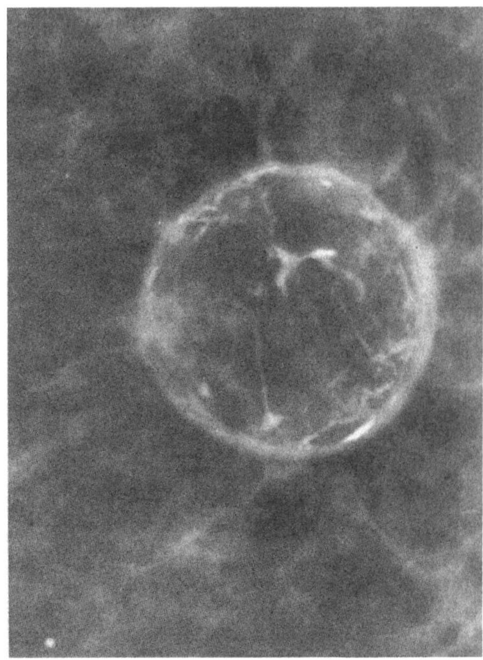
b

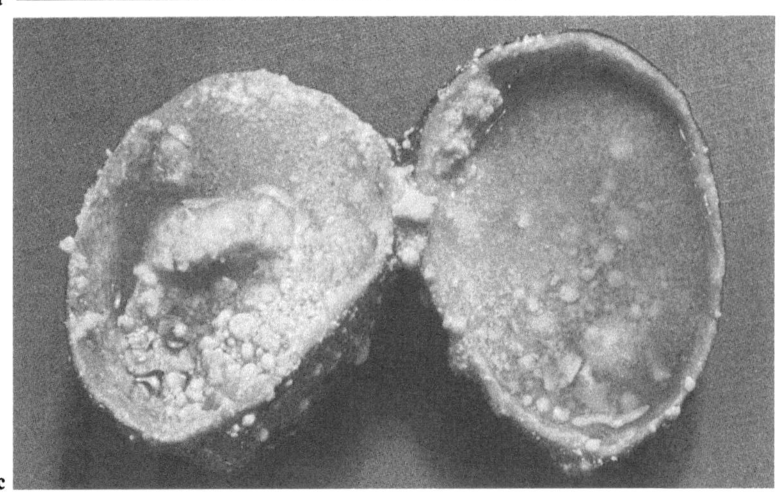
c

Fig. 6.13 a–c

Fig. 6.14. Clinical examination showed subcutaneous, movable, painless, stony hard nodules in both breasts. Detail of mammogram (1.5 ×): calcifications of varying size, characteristic of calcified liponecrotic macrocysts. The contralateral picture was similar. There was no history of surgery, trauma, or rheumatic disease. Radiographic diagnosis: multiple systemic (because bilateral), idiopathic, calcified, subcutaneous fat necrosis

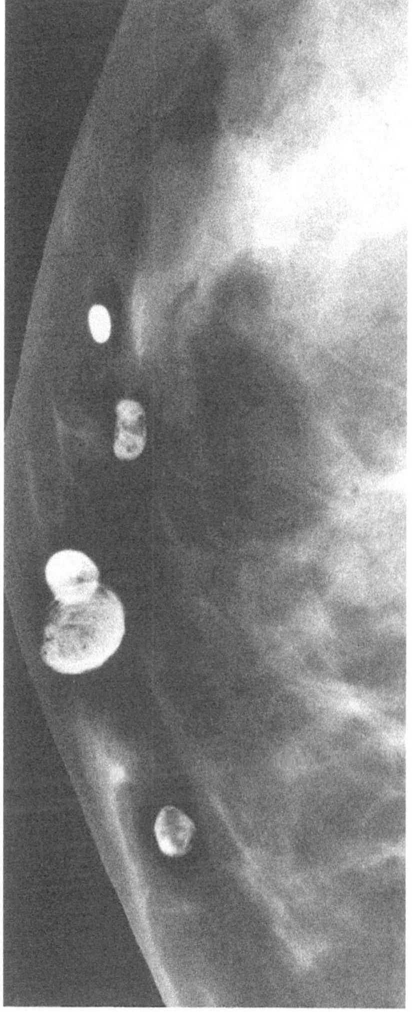

◁ **Fig. 6.13. a** Lateral mammogram (slightly reduced). A dermatofat graft had been implanted several years previously. The implant is encapsulated by numerous linear, y-shaped, and tortuous calcifications (from HOEFFKEN and LANYI 1973). **b** Detail of mammogram (slightly magnified). An unusually large oil cyst has formed in the area of a previous biopsy. Again we see encapsulation and calcifications of the type seen in **a**. **c** Photograph of a removed dermatofat graft that has been cut in half. Most of the calcifications are located in the capsule, and some are in the granulation tissue that protrudes into the lumen of the oily implant (Professor HOEFFKEN, Cologne) (cf. Fig. 6.2b)

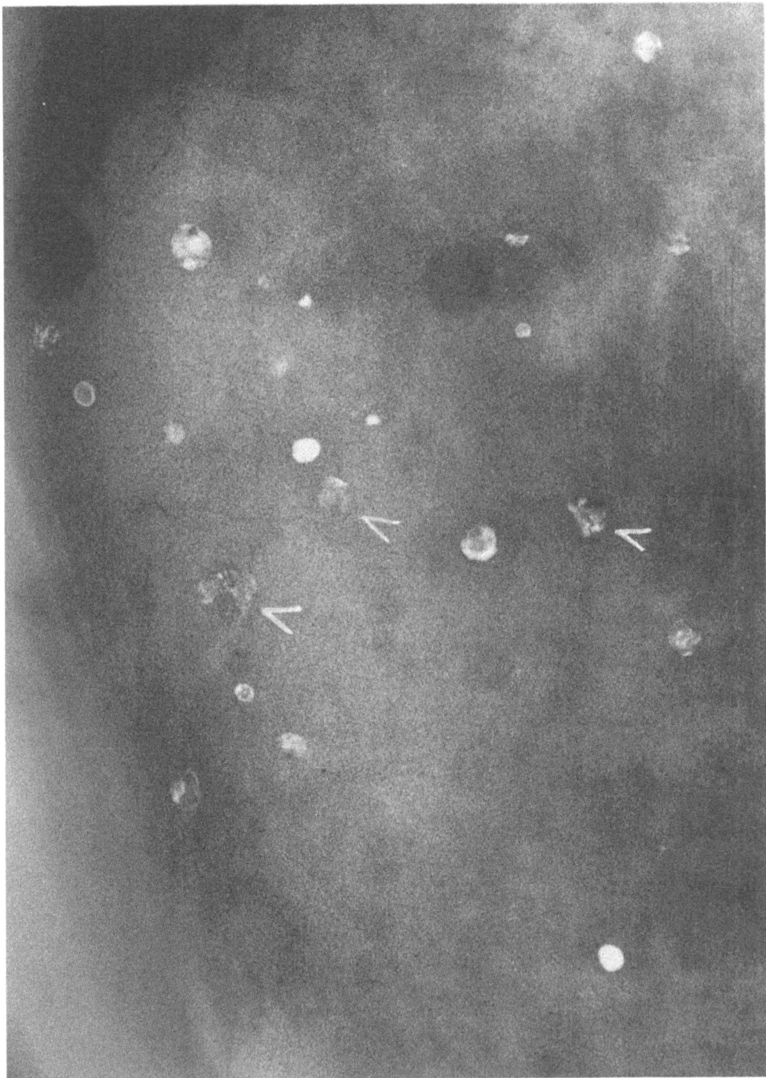

Fig. 6.15. Detail of mammogram (3.5 ×). Preoperative mammography before plastic surgery showed circumscribed, rounded lucencies, liponecrotic microcysts, and small clumps of amorphous microcalcifications in both breasts *(arrows)*. No history of trauma, mastitis, or rheumatoid arthritis. Histology: cavities with partly calcified contents; old, cystic encapsulated, and partly calcified foci of fat necrosis (bilateral)

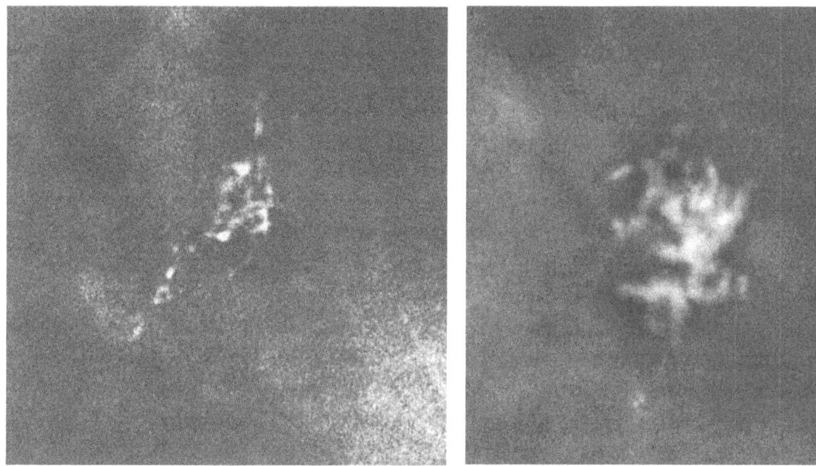

Fig. 6.16 a, b. Details of mammograms (4.5 ×). **a** Triangular cluster of polymorphous (punctate, linear, v-, and y-shaped) microcalcifications in the area of a biopsy incision. Radiographic diagnosis: suspicion of ductal (comedo) carcinoma. Histology: nodular lipomatosis with clumpy calcifications. **b** Picture similar to **a**, also in the area of a biopsy incision. Histology: fat necrosis with calcifications

Amorphous, Clustered Calcifications in the Area of a Scar. Amorphous, branched, rod-shaped, angular, densely packed calcifications arranged in a roughly triangular pattern, as in Fig. 6.16, are infrequently seen in the area of a biopsy scar. The author has personally observed four cases of this type. Differentiation from intraductal carcinoma can be difficult (BASSETT et al. 1978) but is easier if calcified liponecrotic microcysts are found in the vicinity of this unusual lesion.

6.2 Malignant Mixed Tumors with Osseous Metaplasia

Pathology

Mixed tumors are malignant growths that contain mesenchymal (sarcomatous) and epithelial (carcinomatous) elements in varying proportions. They are similar to tumors of the salivary gland. They are most common in the mammary glands of dogs (INGLEBY and GERSHON-COHEN 1960) and are quite rare in the human breast. Most of these tumors contain areas of cartilaginous, osteoid, or osseous metaplasia. The predominance of mesenchymal or epithelial elements determines whether the tumor is classified as an osteochondrofibromyxosarcoma, osteosarcoma, or carcinosarcoma with osseous metaplasia.

It is not unusual for components of a fibroadenoma or cystosarcoma phyllodes to coexist with sarcoma, leading the pathologist to conclude that the lesion developed from a preexisting fibroadenoma or cystosarcoma. Immature spindle cells, fibrochondroblasts, osteoblasts, chondroblast-rich cartilage tissue, and/or well-differentiated bone, possibly containing hematopoietic marrow, can be demonstrated histologically in the same lesion.

Osteogenic mixed tumors are extremely rare. Their reported prevalence is 0.2%–1.0% (SCHÖNER and GUTGESELL 1981). Among the patients examined by the author one such tumor was found among 499 malignant neoplasms.

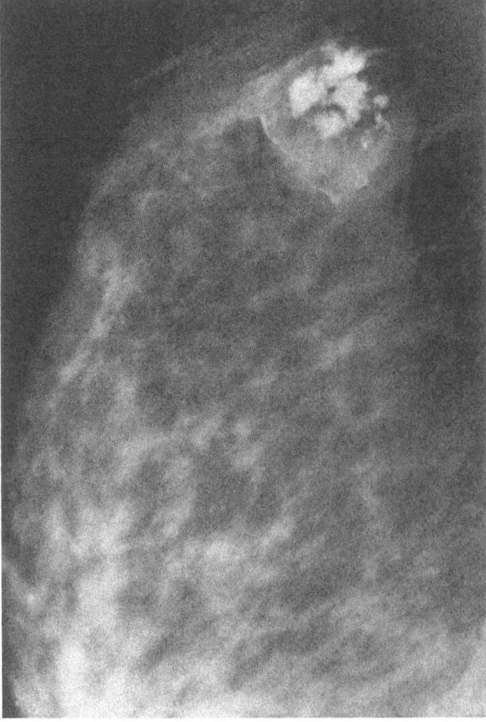

Fig. 6.17. Detail of mammogram (original size): round shadow with very smooth margins containing bizarre calcifications that do not resemble those of fibroadenoma and may cause problems of differential diagnosis on superficial examination. Careful analysis identifies these calcifications as osseous tissue, however. Histology: osteogenic sarcoma (From HOEFFKEN and LANYI 1981)

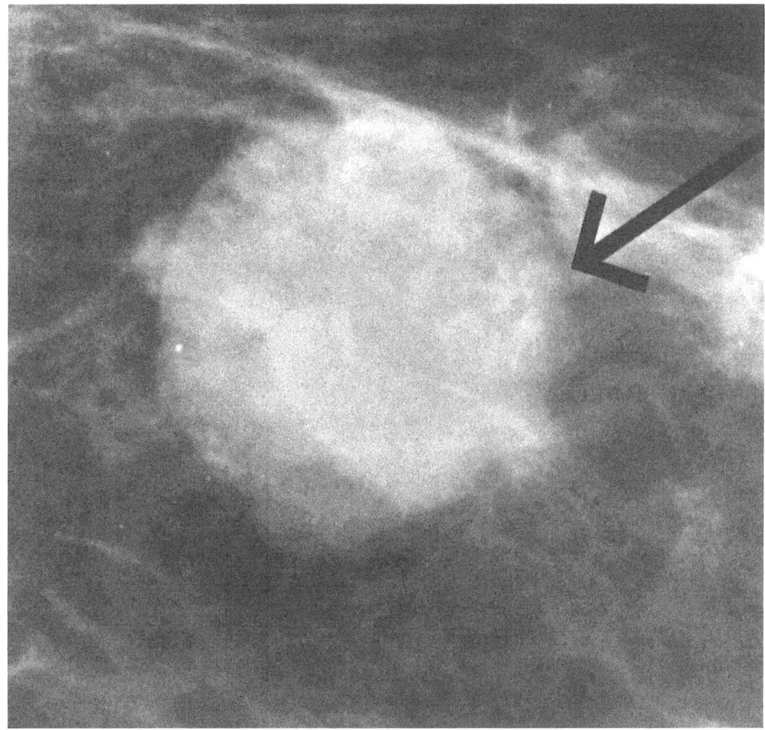

Fig. 6.18. Detail of mammogram (2 ×). Palpable breast nodule presents radiographically as a round shadow with partly lobulated and partly indistinct margins and a faint area of calcification *(arrow).* Histology: osteogenic carcinosarcoma

Radiography

The round, sharply marginated tumor shadow is distinguishable from fibroadenoma only if the trabecular architecture of the well-differentiated osseous tissue is recognized (Fig. 6.17). In the case seen by the author, the site of osseous metaplasia presented only as a somewhat denser area because the well-differentiated bone was too sparse to be identified radiographically (Fig. 6.18).

6.3 Calcified Arteries and Thrombi

The arteries of the breast are distinguishable from veins on mammograms only if their walls contain sclerotic deposits. Calcified arteries are demonstrated in approximately 3% of cases (37 of 1044 mammograms). They are not peculiar to the elderly, and the author found bilateral arterial calcifications in an 18-year-old woman who had no hypertension or other symptoms of generalized arteriosclerosis. Neither were any abnormalities found in clinical examinations of other young women, recommended because of calcified mammary arteries (such recommendations are no longer made). The link between calcified breast arteries and diabetes is controversial: while BAUM et al. (1980) claim that intramammary arterial calcifications are suggestive of diabetes, SCHMITT and THREATT (1984) deny that this relationship exists. McDOUGAL and LUKERT (1977) made the interesting observation that vascular calcifications of the breast in patients with secondary hyperparathyroidism resolved after renal transplantation.

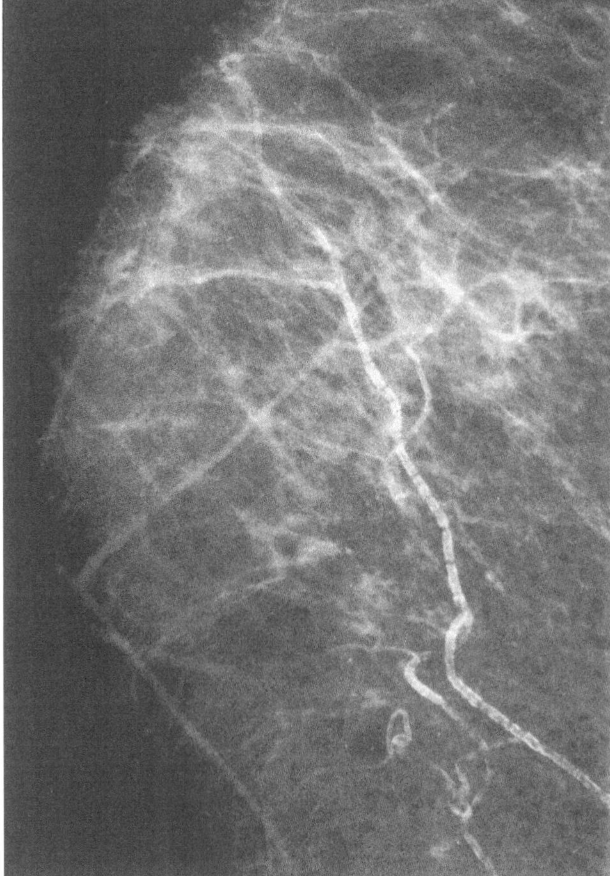

Fig. 6.19. Mammogram (slightly reduced): calcified arteries in a woman 65 years of age

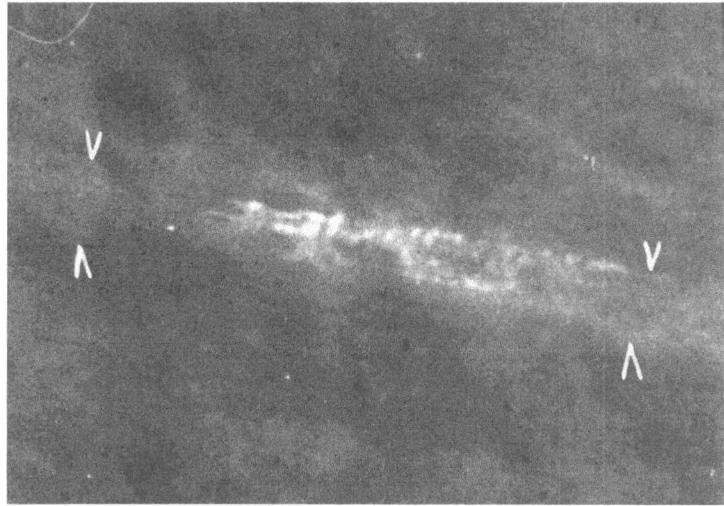

Fig. 6.20. Detail of mammogram (4 ×): oblong cluster of punctate and some linear microcalcifications. The first impression is that the lesion is indistinguishable from an early ductal carcinoma. But analysis of the calcifications shows that they are arranged largely in two parallel lines, and that a vascular shadow is visible in line with the cluster *(arrows)*. Partial calcification of an artery

Mammograms show *parallel* calcifications that vary in length (and may be punctate). The pattern resembles that of bronchial calcifications (Fig. 6.19). The complete calcification of an entire artery poses no problems of differential diagnosis, unlike cases where only a short arterial segment is involved and the calcifications appear to be clustered (Fig. 6.20). The parallel position of the linear and punctate calcifications serves to distinguish this lesion from intraductal carcinoma.

Calcified thrombi in the breast are extremely rare or very rarely diagnosed as such. We have seen one case in which a calcification adjacent to a carcinoma gave the impression of a completely calcified liponecrotic microcyst and was identified histologically as a calcified thrombus. It is likely that a certain percentage of cases diagnosed radiographically as solitary calcified liponecrotic cysts are actually calcified thrombi (Fig. 6.21).

Calcified hemangiomas are also extremely rare. An interesting case was described by Tabár and Dean (1983), who saw fibroadenomalike calcifications inside a slightly lobulated soft-tissue shadow about 4 cm in diameter with sharp margins and a "halo." The lesion is mammographically indistinguishable from a calcified fibroadenoma.

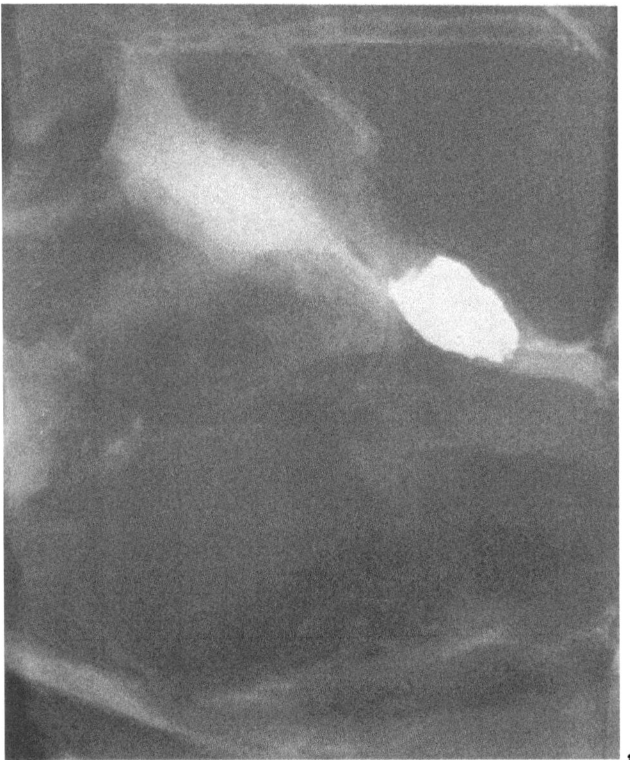

a

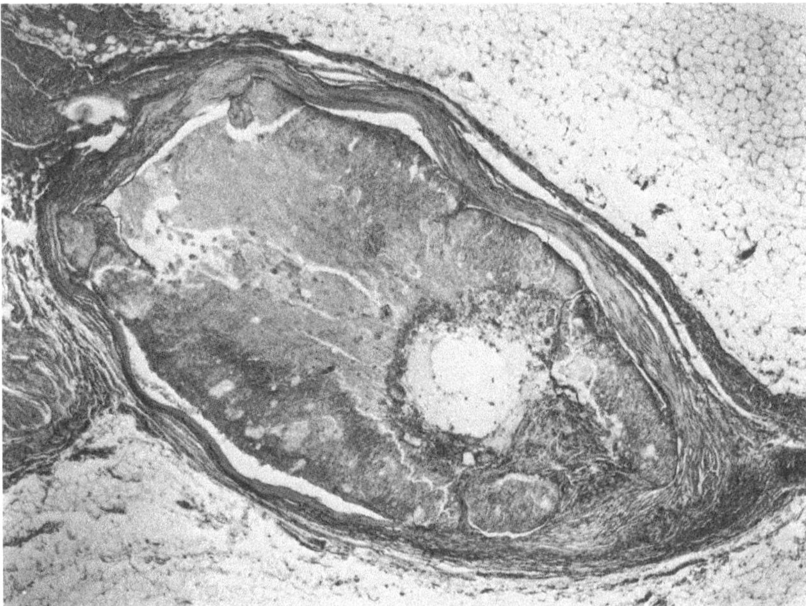

b

Fig. 6.21. a Specimen radiograph (10 ×): ovoid, homogeneous, very intense calcification occurring in a bandlike soft-tisue shadow. A calcified vessel wall is seen above this area. **b** The decalcified histologic section (80 ×) shows circumscribed luminal dilatation with a sclerosed intima and calcified media. An organized thrombus fills the lumen. (Professor BARTH, Esslingen)

6.4 Calcifications in Parasitic Diseases

Hydatid disease of the breast is rare even in countries where *Echinococcus* parasitisms are endemic. In the breast, as elsewhere, it may be marked by cystic calcifications.

Filariasis of the breast can elicit the formation of foreign body granulomas. Figure 6.22 shows the mammogram – unique in the world literature – of a woman believed to have filariasis of the breast. We see a number of scattered, fine, elongated, wavy, or tortuous calcifications that are distinguished from the "worms" of intraductal carcinoma by their localization in the *inter*ductal connective tissue outside the mammary ducts.

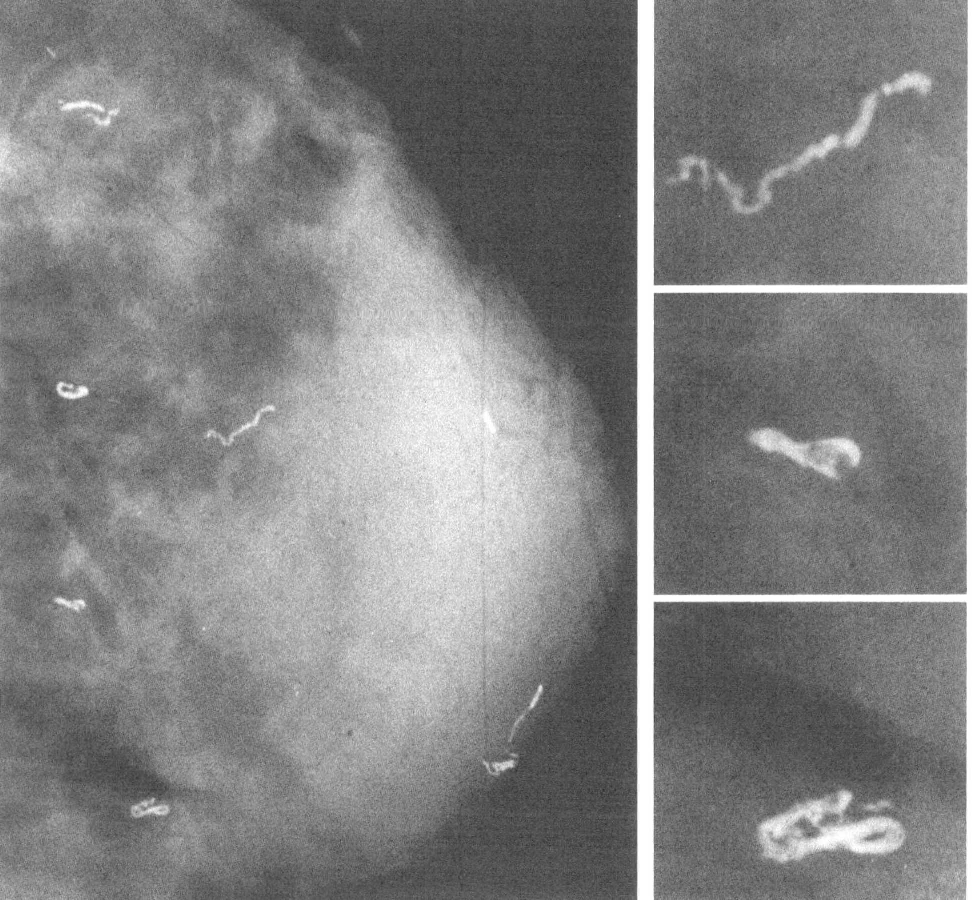

Fig. 6.22. a Mammogram (original size) of a young black African woman showing seven vermiform calcifications that are definitely outside the lobular and ductal system of the breast. **b** Details (approx. 4×). Diagnosis: filariasis (Professor KIEFER, Wiesbaden)

6.5 Calcified Foreign Bodies

Foreign bodies left in the breast after open biopsy may become calcified. Calcified suture material accounts for 0.66% of intramammary calcifications (Fig. 6.23). Calcifications around drains are seen even less frequently (Fig. 6.24).

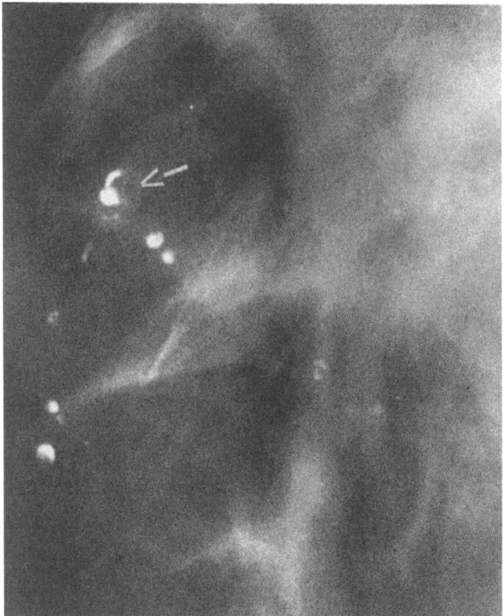

Fig. 6.23. Detail of mammogram (2 ×): calcified suture material coexisting with liponecrotic microcysts following biopsy. The knot and cut end of the suture are easily recognized *(arrow)*

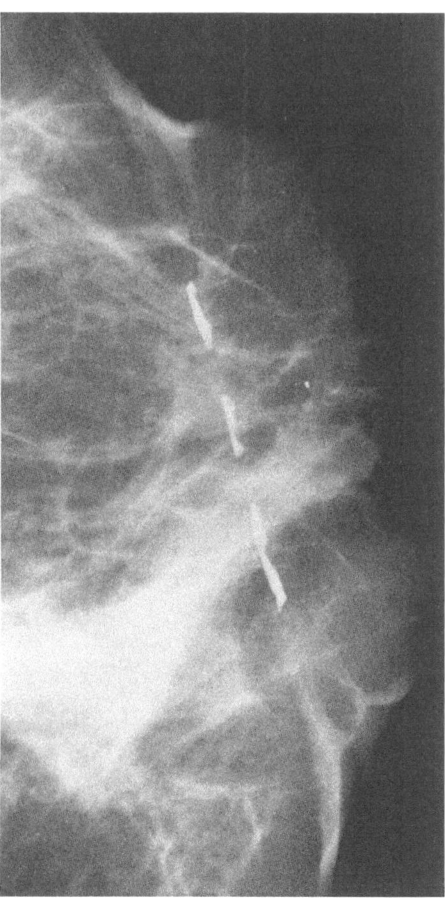

Fig. 6.24. Detail of mammogram (original size): linear calcifications and areas of skin retraction associated with the placement of a rubber drain after biopsy

6.6 Calcified Sebaceous Glands

The sebaceous glands are accessory organs of the hairs (free sebaceous glands independent of hair follicles occur only in the areolar region). The secretory activity of the sebaceous cells is stimulated by androgenic hormones and appears to be inhibited by estrogens. When the glandular ducts become obstructed, the secretions accumulate together with exfoliated epithelial cells, and a retention cyst or comedo forms.

Small retention cysts of the sebaceous glands of the mammary skin are a common clinical finding. They present as yellowish or black, gritty, intracutaneous nodules that project slightly above the level of the surrounding skin (Fig. 6.30b).

They are most visible radiographically when they are calcified (HOEFFKEN and LANYI 1973). This is the case in almost 3% of all mammograms examined, with 30 calcified sebaceous glands being detected in 1044 consecutive examinations - 8 solitary, 5 scattered (Fig. 6.25), 15 clustered (Fig. 6.26), and 2 scattered and clustered. The calcifications are approximately 1-1.5 mm in size. Usually they are ring-shaped, slightly angular, or dumbbell-shaped and have central lucencies. Less frequently they are punctate or linear without central lucencies. When calcifications of this type occur in dense clusters, they can present problems of differential diagnosis. These problems vanish if the intradermal localization of the sebaceous gland calcifications can be confirmed (Figs. 6.27 and 6.30).

Occasionally we find clustered sebaceous gland calcifications whose intracutaneous localization cannot be established with either of the standard two-plane views. This phenomenon is explained by the hemispheric shape of the breast: all four quadrants of the surface contain points that appear to be located within the breast on standard biplane compression mammograms (Figs. 6.28 and 6.29). Generally this problem can be solved by obtaining tangential images (Fig. 6.30). Because the clustered calcifications of sebaceous glands often give the impression of microcystic adenosis due to the shape of the individual calcifications, it would still be appropriate to elect follow-up over biopsy in cases where an intracutaneous localization cannot be established.

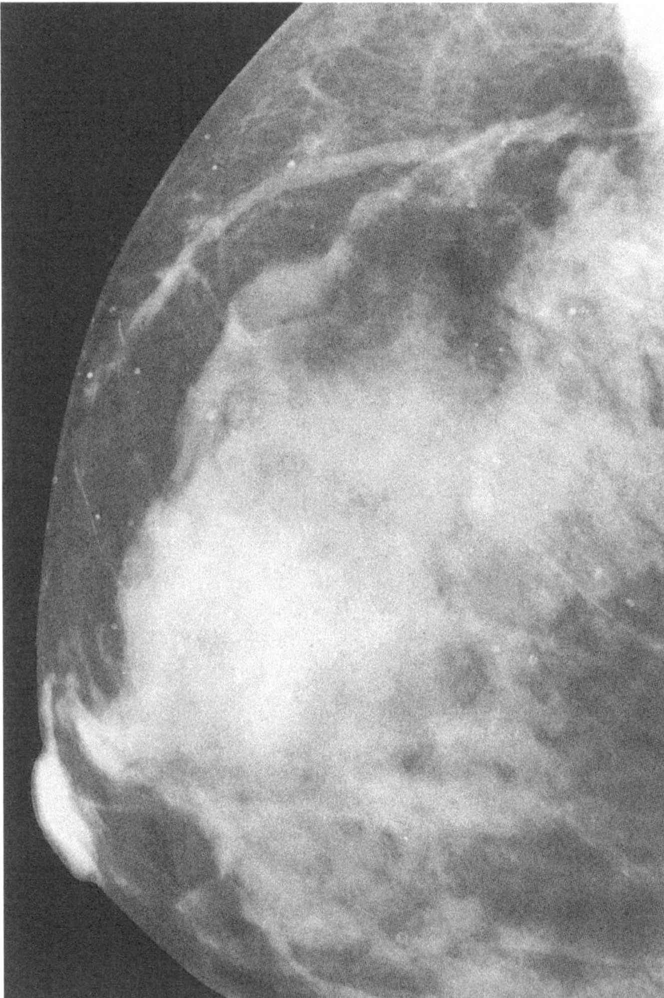

Fig. 6.25 a. Legend on opposite page

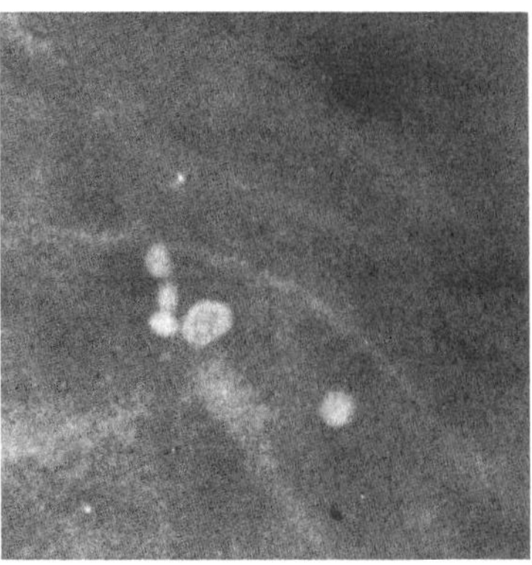

Fig. 6.26. Detail of mammogram (4 ×): triangular cluster of five rounded microcalcifications, one with central lucency. The three that are closest together show septa (similar to microcystic adenosis). Clustered sebaceous gland calcifications

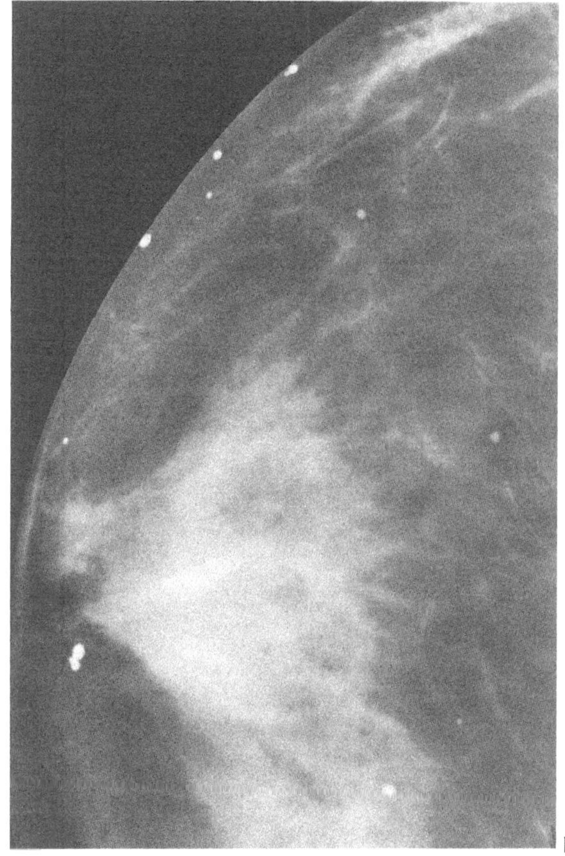

b

Fig. 6.25 a, b. Details of mammograms (original size). **a** Lateral view: scattered, punctate micro-calcifications of approximately equal size, most with central lucencies. **b** Craniocaudad view: some of the calcifications show an intracutaneous localization

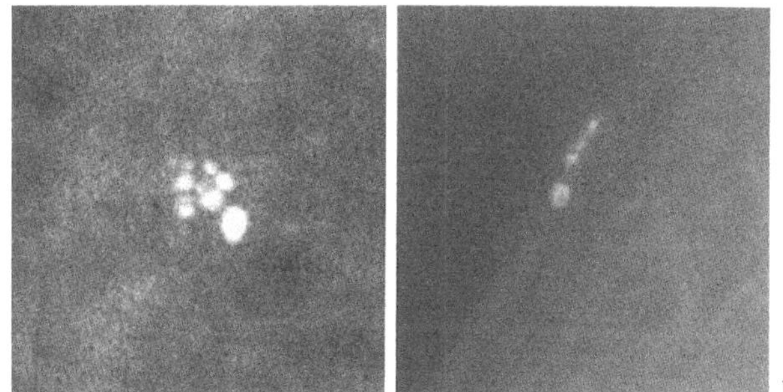

a   b

Fig. 6.27 a, b. Details of mammograms (approx. 3 ×). **a** Craniocaudad view: tight cluster of eight rounded microcalcifications separated by fine lines, suggestive of microcystic adenosis. **b** Lateral view: the calcifications are intradermal, and one shows a central lucency. Diagnosis: calcified seba-ceous glands

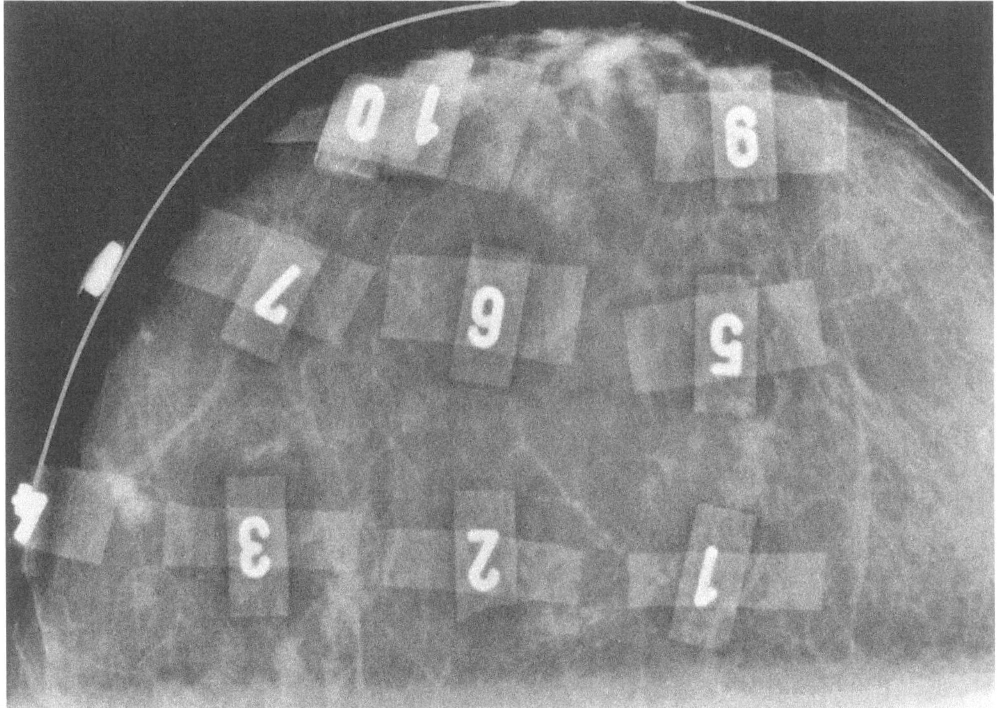

a

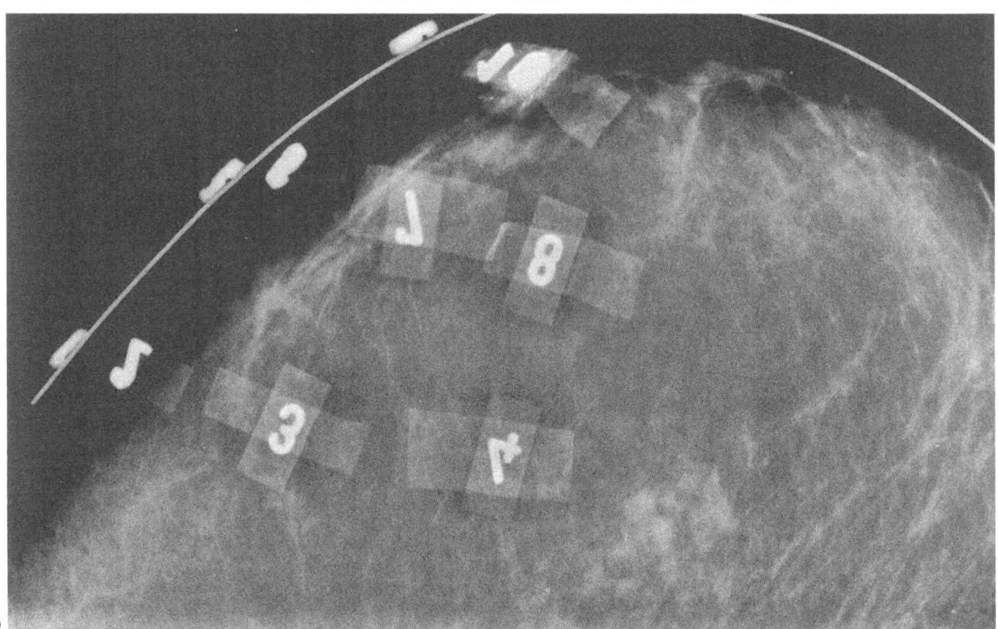

b

Fig. 6.28 a, b. Model experiment. Lead numbers 1–10 were taped to the upper outer quadrant of the breast and radiographed in two views (**a** craniocaudad, **b** mediolateral). Numbers 3 and 7 appear to be located within the breast on both planes

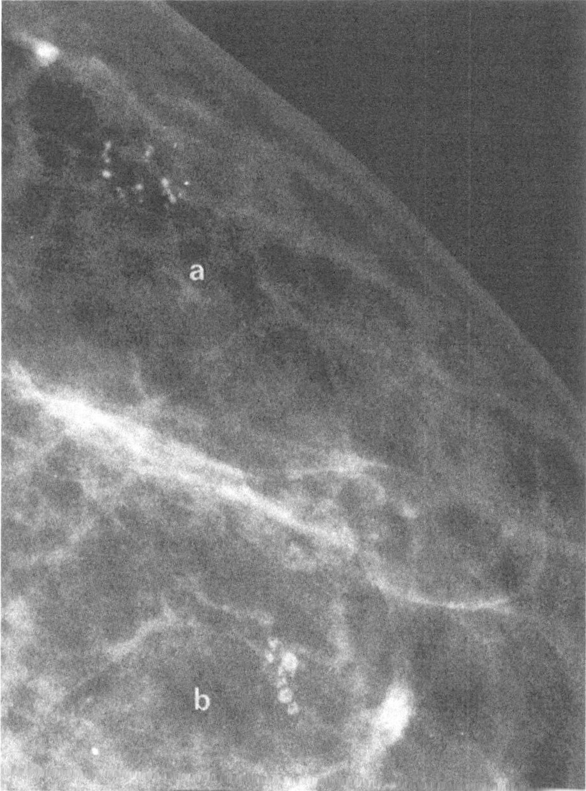

Fig. 6.29. Detail of mammogram (2 ×). Lateral view: two clusters of calcified sebaceous glands. Cluster *a* is obviously close to the skin, while cluster *b* appears to be within the breast on both planes

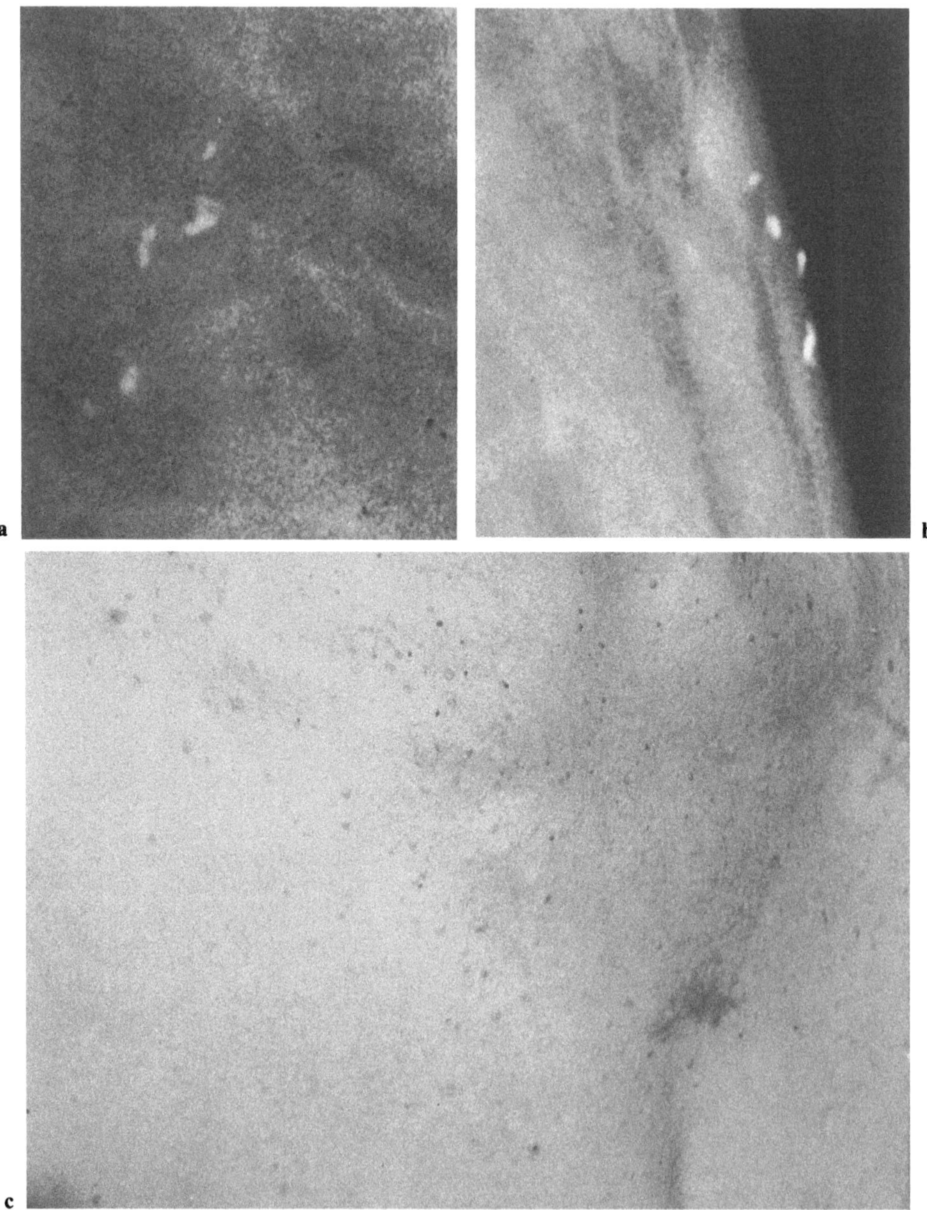

Fig. 6.30 a–c. Patient had previously undergone contralateral mastectomy for carcinoma. **a** Detail of craniocaudad mammogram (4 ×): five linear and punctate microcalcifications in a triangular or diamond-shaped cluster. Patient's history raised the suspicion of early ductal carcinoma of comedo type, especially since the cluster appears to be intramammary on the lateral projection as well. **c** Clinical examination showed numerous sebaceous glands above and on the breast, directing suspicion toward calcification of them. Multiple tangential films were taken until finally the microcalcifications were localized to the skin (**b**), i.e., identified as harmless sebaceous glands. An unnecessary biopsy was avoided

6.7 Scattered Calcifications and Ossifications of the Stroma, Subcutaneous Tissue, and Skin

Calcifications and ossifications of the stroma, subcutaneous tissue, and skin are a rarity. FRANCE and O'CONNELL (1970) described bilateral hyalinosis with calcification and dermal ossification as a sequel to bilateral nonspecific mastitis. Mammograms showed extensive focal ossification throughout both breasts. BÄSSLER (1978) does not accept this explanation, because chronic inflammations are common in the breast, yet diffuse hyalinosis of the stromal tissue with calcification and ossification is rare.

BROKS (1976) described a case of generalized subcutaneous and cutaneous mammary calcification (Fig.6.31) whose etiology could not be determined. Previously the patient had developed hypoparathyroidism following a strumectomy. (This is contradictory, since parathyroidectomy is the accepted treatment for calcinosis.) The author assumed that the condition was related to a vasculopathy or to dihydrate or prednisone medication.

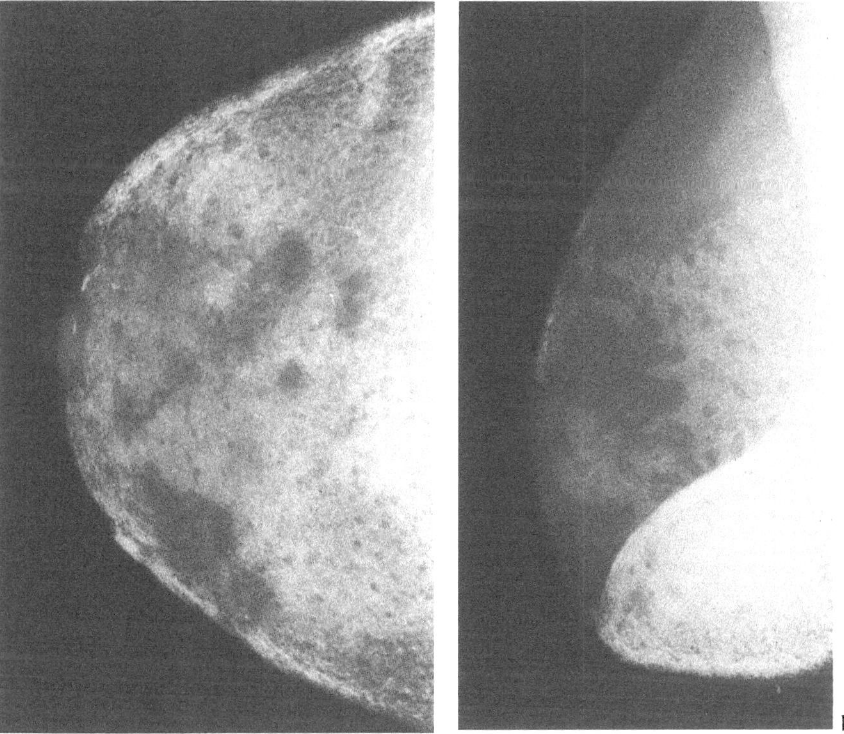

Fig.6.31. a Craniocaudad mammogram of left breast: scattered, nonhomogeneous, maplike subcutaneous/cutaneous calcifications of the breast. b Lateral mammogram of right breast: similar but less extensive calcifications. Bilateral calcinosis cutis. c See p.244 (Dr.BROKS, Utrecht, Netherlands)

6.8 Calcifications in the Axillary Lymph Nodes

The finding of a calcified lymphadenoma, while common in the region of the pulmonary hilus or mesentery, is decidedly rare in the lymphatic drainage of the breast. BJURSTAM (1978) reported finding microcalcifications in metastatic carcinoma of the axillary lymph nodes. Figure 6.32 shows an enlarged metastatic lymph node with polymorphous microcalcifications. The author has seen similar although larger lymph node calcifications in a man with the histological diagnosis of a "necrotic, reticular-histocytic lymphadenitis with abscess formation – cat scratch disease (?)" (CREMER, Cologne) (Fig. 6.33 a, b).

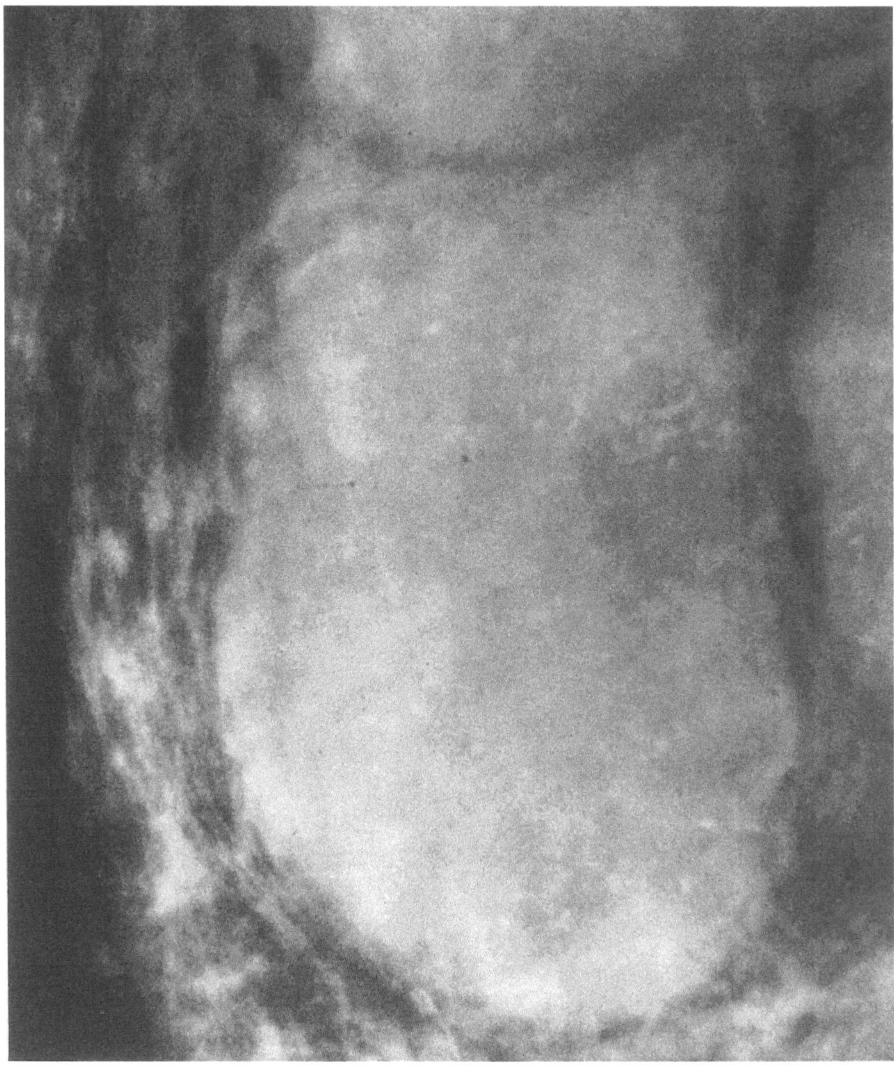

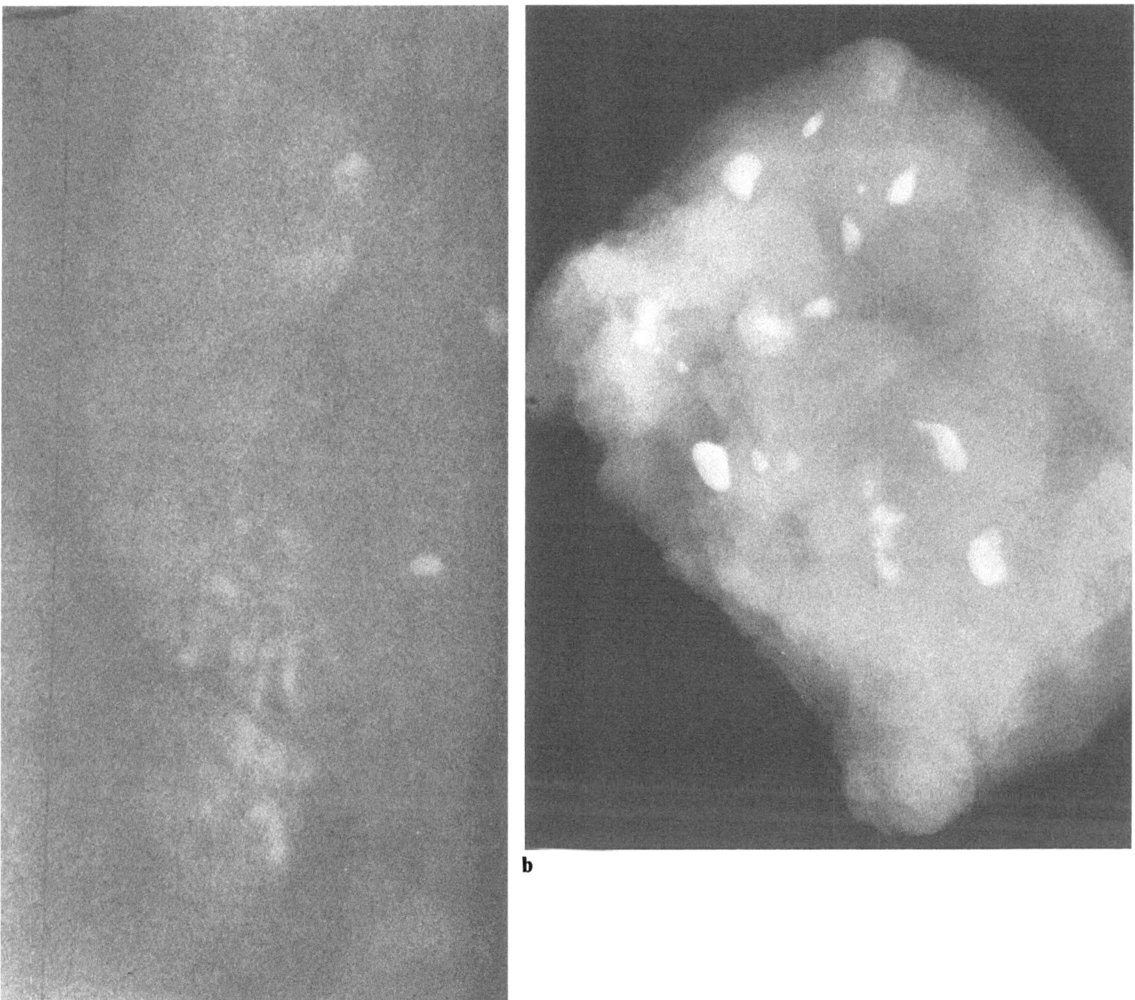

6.33. a Soft-tissue radiograph of the axilla (approx. 3 ×). Multiple oblong, clumpy, faint calcifications are visible within an enlarged lymph node. **b** Specimen radiograph (approx. 3 ×): rounded, teardrop-shaped, and amorphous calcifications of the lymph node

◁ **Fig. 6.32.** Soft-tissue radiograph of the axilla (approx. 25 ×). Polymorphous microcalcifications within an enlarged metastatic lymph node. The impalpable primary tumor appears to be an intraductal cluster a few millimeters in diameter on mammography. Cytology showed carcinomatous pleurisy (Professor LENZ, Eschweiler).

6.9 Artifacts That Mimic Calcifications

Artifacts that resemble intramammary calcifications may occur
1) on the skin or
2) within the imaging and developing system.

Concerning materials on the skin, an ointment or powder containing a radiopaque substance (e. g., zinc ointment) (Fig. 6.34) or spilled contrast material used for galactography (Fig. 6.35) can give the false impression of clustered microcalcifications. BROWN et al. (1981) reported a case in which tattoo marks on the skin simulated microcalcifications within the breast.

Dust particles or metal filings left from repair work on the cone mounting can leave tiny spots on the mammogram that resemble microcalcifications. Water-soluble contrast material used in galactography may leak onto the film-holder table from the lactiferous duct and be picked up by the breast of the next patient to be examined. Dirt particles on the cassette or on the screen (Fig. 6.36), or fingerprints on the film (Fig. 6.37) can all mimic intramammary microcalcifications. Even with automated processing, dirty rollers can produce groups of spots that resemble calci-

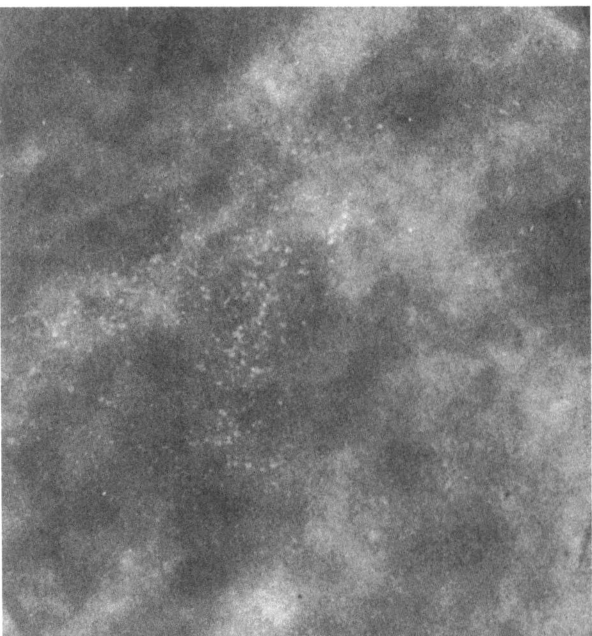

Fig. 6.34. Detail of mammogram (3 ×). Case referred for a second opinion: extensive microcalcifications were seen only on the craniocaudad projection. None were visible on reexamination 1 week later. The patient has the habit of dusting herself with powder when she perspires heavily

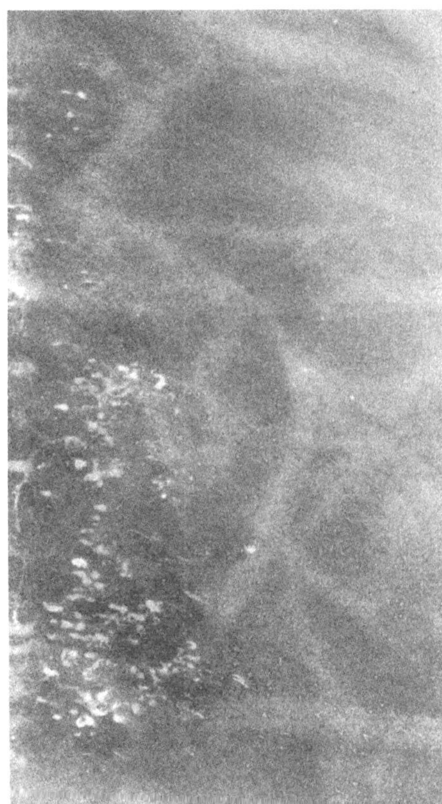

Fig. 6.35. Detail of mammogram (3.5 ×). Galactography had been performed previously in this breast. The very intense punctate, comma-shaped, and v-shaped features were not visible on the plain films taken before galactography, and they disappeared after the breast was washed. Contamination of the skin surface with contrast medium

fications. Artifacts, regardless of their origin, rarely mimic intramammary lesions on two different planes of the same breast. If an artifact is suspected or some other doubt exists, the questionable mammogram should be repeated after first attempting to eliminate the presumed cause (e. g., wash the breast thoroughly with water, and clean the tube, cassette, screen, and film-holder table).

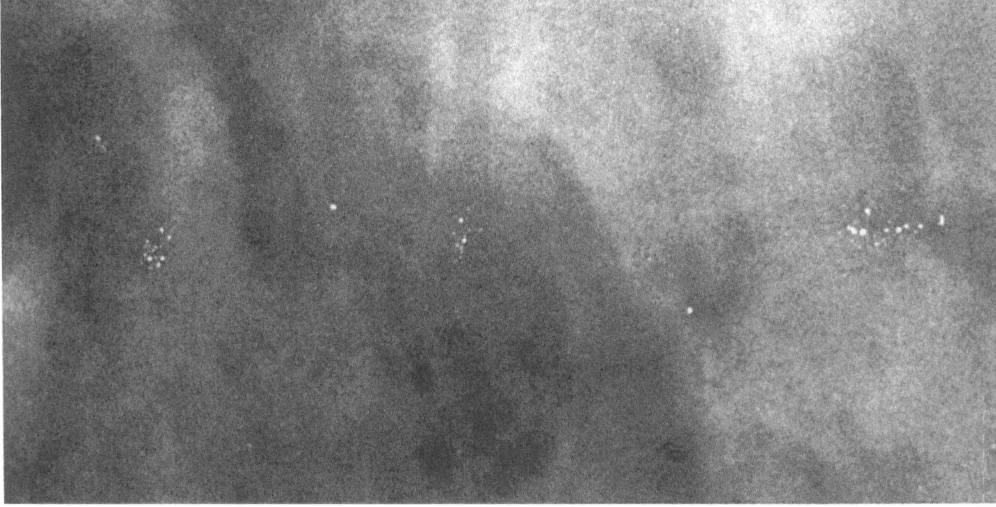

Fig. 6.36. Detail of craniocaudad mammogram (2 ×): these diamond-shaped, amorphous, and ovoid clusters of high-density, punctate shadows occurred repeatedly on the same cassette. They disappeared after the screen was cleaned

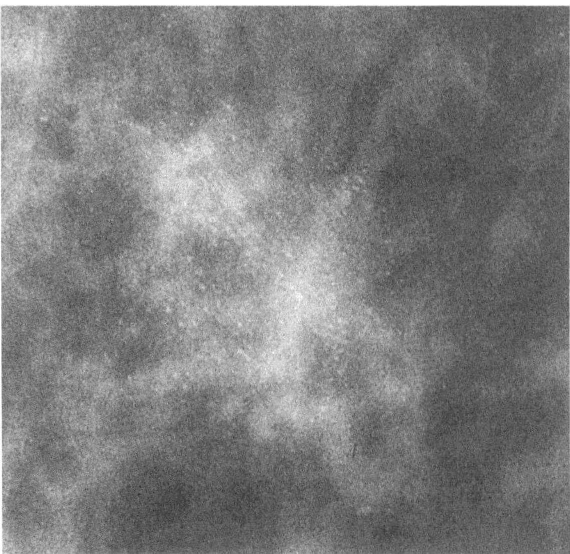

Fig. 6.37. Fingerprints resemble clustered microcalcifications and are visible in one view only (4 ×)

7 Differential Diagnosis of Microcalcifications

The radiologist should understand that there is more to differential diagnosis than just listing all conceivable diagnoses and leaving it to the pathologist to solve the problem. Admittedly, there are cases in which there is no better solution than to recommend biopsy. However, to recommend biopsy indiscriminately for all clustered microcalcifications, doing so more or less automatically, is an admission of incompetence.

Scarring and disfigurement of the breasts (Fig. 7.1) because of innocuous microcalcifications cannot always be justified by claiming that the surgery was necessary to establish the nature of a suspicious lesion. Also, it should be remembered that intramammary scars can cause later problems of differential diagnosis.

A proper differential diagnosis in general, and the differential diagnosis of microcalcifications in particular, must rely on the following:

Knowledge of Pathologic Anatomy. Clearly, if the examiner is not familiar with all relevant pathologic processes, he will be unable to formulate an effective differential diagnosis.

History Taking. A cluster of 5–6 microcalcifications that are not obviously "malignant" or "benign" discovered in a high-risk patient (e.g., family history, prior contralateral mastectomy) has to be interpreted quite differently from a similar cluster found in a patient not at risk. Comparison with any previous mammograms can also influence our assessment: the appearance of new microcalcifications is always suspicious!

Clinical Examination. The clinical picture is essential for differential diagnosis. It can be critically important to know whether or not the microcalcifications are associated with a palpable tumor, or whether the nipple manifests eczematous changes (Paget's disease?).

Technical Image Quality. High image quality is a sine qua non for the successful differential diagnosis of microcalcifications.

Biopsy or Follow-up? Many times it is useful diagnostically to recall the patient at a later date for a repeat mammogram. In patients with microcalcifications, reexamination in less than 6 months is unlikely to show a perceptible change that would be of any further diagnostic value. The classic example is a biopsy scar containing several microcalcifications that are not obviously characteristic of carcinoma or of liponecrotic microcysts. In this case the physician must decide whether to have the patient undergo a repeat biopsy or follow the microcalcification "to the bitter end." Follow-up may even be recommended in women over 65 with questionable microcalcifications, provided the cluster is small (about 1 cm in diameter) and clinically occult. However, this recommendation is not acceptable when there is a small cluster exhibiting the features of ductal carcinoma described earlier. A number of leading mammographers in the United States consider the follow-up of nonpalpable clustered microcalcifications to be inappropriate under any circumstances and believe that immedaite biopsy is indicated. At the same time, however, several of them describe carcinoma cases in which the number of microcalcifications did not increase until the 3rd year, indicating that they indeed must have followed microcalcifications for a prolonged period (HOMER 1981).

Diagnostic Humility. The final element of differential diagnosis is the "diagnostic humility" of the physician. He must know his limitations, but also he must seek constantly to expand his capabilities. He must learn, and not just from books, but from personal experience. The physician should keep records of cases that were referred for biopsy and of the histologic results. Analysis of one's own correct diagnoses and misdiagnoses is the best training!

Beginning on p. 198, we present mammograms showing clustered and scattered microcalcifications of varying etiology. As a self-evaluation quiz, the reader should try to identify those cases in which biopsy should be recommended, and those in which it should not.

7.1 Checklist

History

Self-history:	*Contralateral breast cancer?* (high risk!)
	How many pregnancies? (nulliparity means a higher risk!)
Previous biopsies:	If so, check previous histologic findings! An unequivocal microcalcification cluster must be interpreted differently if the patient had previously had a true proliferative cystic disease possibly with atypia, than if the lesion had been completely innocent.
Other trauma?	*Iatrogenic trauma?* (e. g., plastic surgery?)

Clinical Examination

Palpation:	If a palpable mass is found, is it assignable to the visible microcalcification cluster? For example, a patient referred for evaluation of a simple cyst may be found also to have a microcalcification cluster suggesting intraductal carcinoma.
Nipple changes?	Any kind of eczematous changes, even minimal exfoliation, may raise suspicion of Paget's disease, in which case even minimal or uncharacteristic microcalcifications will assume importance.
Discharge:	Nipple discharge is of little help diagnostically, because it occurs in both benign and malignant conditions. Even a bloody discharge is not pathognomonic for intraductal carcinoma. Galactography can be used to determine whether the questionable microcalcification cluster is related to the secreting duct.

Mammographic Interpretation

Mammograms are routinely taken and evaluated on two planes. (Hereafter, lack of reference to the second plane means that that view contained no useful information.)
Answer the following questions:

1. *Is only one type of microcalcification seen, or are several different patterns present together?* (e.g., fibroadenoma and sebaceous gland, fibroadenoma and carcinoma, etc.). The examiner is cautioned not to overlook an intraductal carcinoma because of an easily diagnosed coexisting lesion (e.g., a "classic" calcified fibroadenoma)!

2. *Where are the microcalcifications located?*
Extramammary localization? If so, is there an artifact on the film? on the skin? intracutaneous?
Intramammary localization?
Is an *intraductal* localization suggested by the cluster shape (see p. 91)?
What is the appearance of the cluster contours (see p. 95)?
If the calcifications are not intraductal, are they:
a) *intralobular?* (cluster shape, see p. 42, 59)
b) *inside a fibroadenoma?* (cluster shape, see p. 146)
c) *in connective tissue? fatty tissue?* (history of trauma or previous surgery?) (see p. 157)
d) *intra-arterial?* (see p. 176)

Mixed localization? For example, *intraductal* and *intralobular* (as with coexisting milk of calcium cysts and carcinoma), *intraductal* and *interductal* (interstitial) connective tissue localization (e.g., calcified secretion and liponecrotic cysts; plasma cell mastitis), or *intraductal* and *intracutaneous* localization (e.g., carcinoma and calcified sebaceous glands).

3. *What is the shape of the microcalcifications?*
Monomorphous? Polymorphous?
If *monomorphous:*
a) Are they in both views? ("teacup sign"? see p. 51)
b) Is septation present? (see p. 42)
If *polymorphous:*
a) Does the polymorphism increase in accordance with the number of microcalcifications? *Caution:* The more extensive a ductal carcinoma, the larger its comedo component and thus the greater the polymorphism (see p. 108). *Even minimal polymorphism is suspicious!*
b) Is the cluster shape consistent with an intraductal process? Consider that polymorphous microcalcifications are found not only in intraductal lesions and in carcinoma but also in fibroadenoma (see p. 152), in sclerosing adenosis (see p. 48), in obliterative comedomastitis (see p. 133) and, rarely, in fat necrosis (see p. 173). Remember also that the cluster shape is sometimes difficult to evaluate in very small lesions (3–4 mm in size).

4. *Is the change unilateral or bilateral?*
If *homogenous,* predominantly punctate, slightly polymorphous microcalcifications
are present *bilaterally,* an intraductal carcinoma is unlikely. (The author has not personally seen a case of simultaneously occurring bilateral duct carcinomas with associated microcalcifications, though he has seen extensive bilateral papillomatosis).

5. *How should microcalcifications adjacent to a soft-tissue shadow be interpreted?*
When microcalcifications are seen in the vicinity of a soft-tissue shadow suggestive
of carcinoma, there is a tendency to draw a connection between the two radiographic signs. But soft-tissue shadows typical of carcinoma can both facilitate and
hamper the differential diagnosis of microcalcifications. A microcalcification cluster in proximity to a scirrhus, for example, is not necessarily malignant in nature.
Neither does a confirmed carcinoma on one side necessarily mean that a microcalcification cluster in the opposite breast also signifies carcinoma. Conversely, an
incipient carcinoma marked by a small microcalcification cluster may be discovered incidentally in the vicinity of a wholly benign lesion.

A rounded, slightly lobulated shadow with smooth margins and a "halo sign"
(fatty margin) establishes the diagnosis of a calcifying fibroadenoma even if the
microcalcifications visible within this shadow are polymorphous. Microcalcifications in cyst walls are infrequent, and they are usually localized at the periphery of
the round, smooth-bordered shadow on one plane. They are easily identified as
cyst-wall calcifications on the pneumocystogram.

7.2 Questions and Answers

Questions

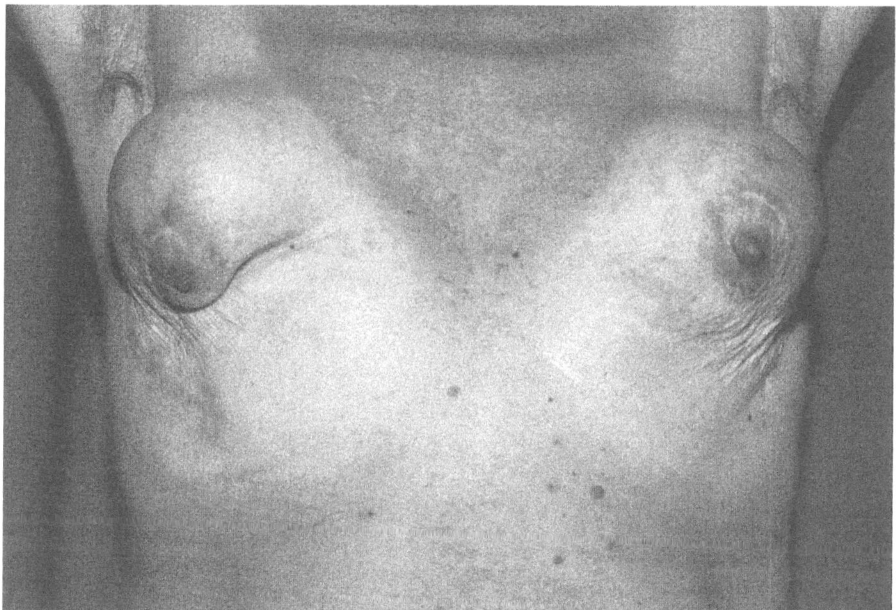

Fig. 7.1. Woman 42 years of age who has undergone a total of three biopsies because of microcalcifications. Both breasts are disfigured, and the woman reports sexual problems and rejection by her partner

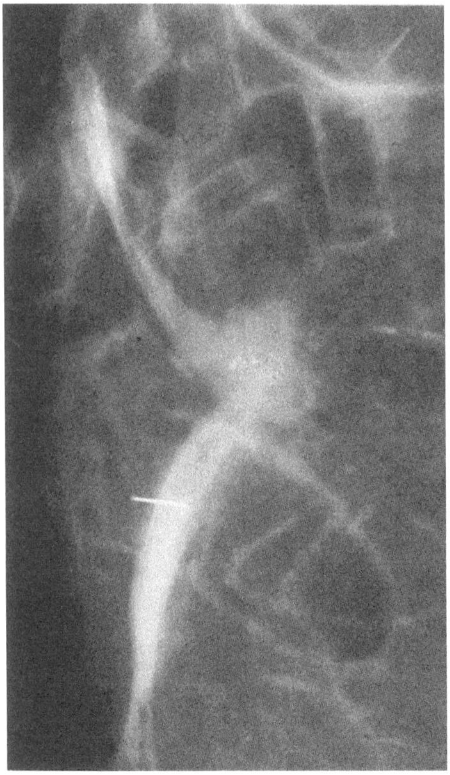

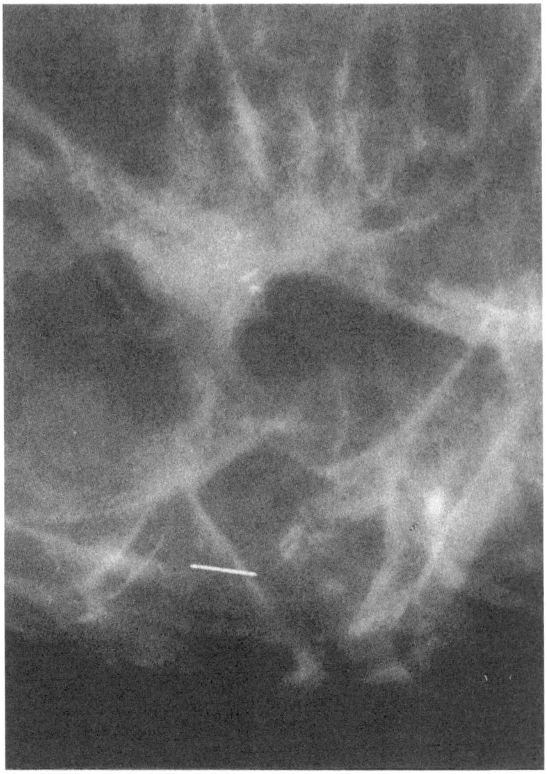

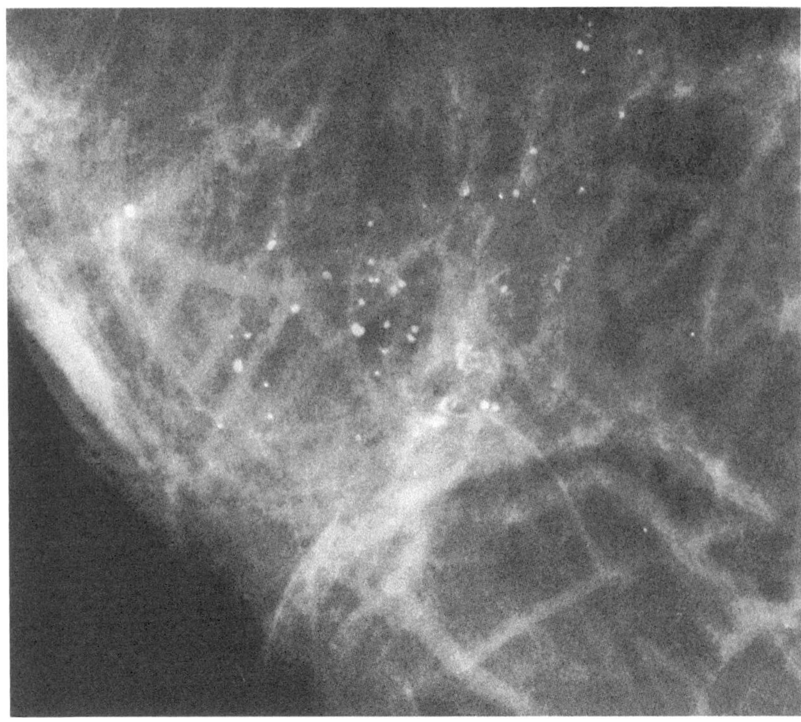

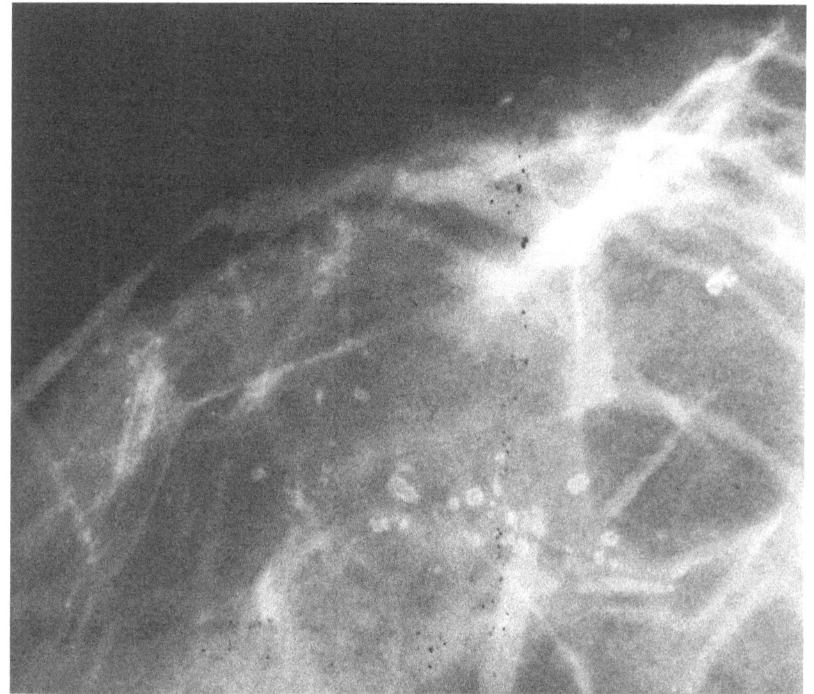

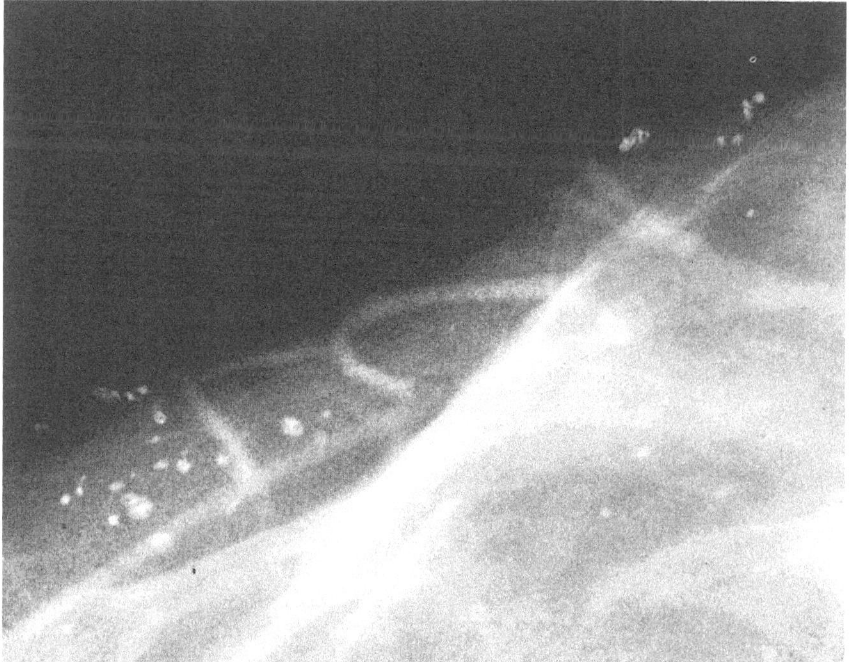

Fig. 7.2. Microcalcifications in biopsy scars.
Case 1: **a** Lateral view, **b** craniocaudad view. Biopsy was done 6 years ago;
no microcalcifications were visible 4 years ago.
Case 2: **c** Plastic surgery was performed 10 years previously.
Case 3: **d** Craniocaudad view, **e** lateral view. Biopsy was done 6 months ago because of
microcalcifications.
In which case is biopsy indicated?

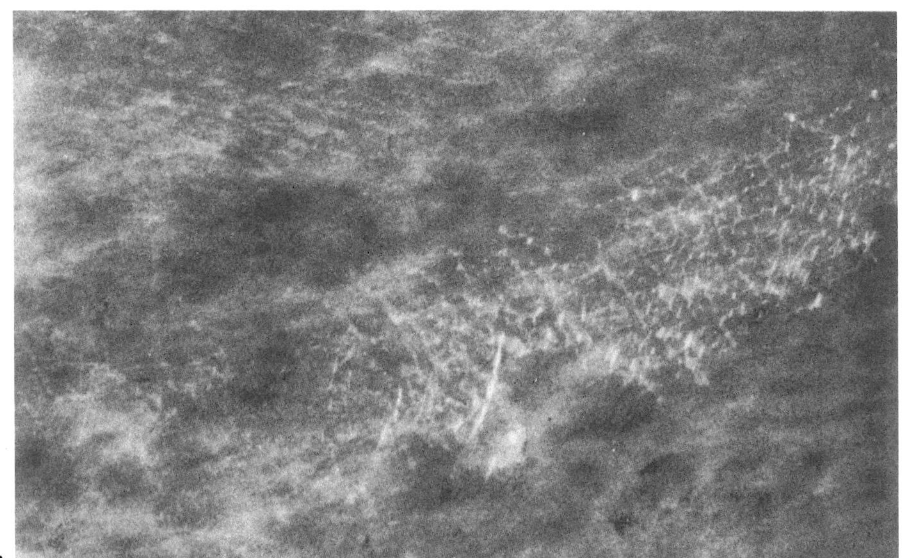

a

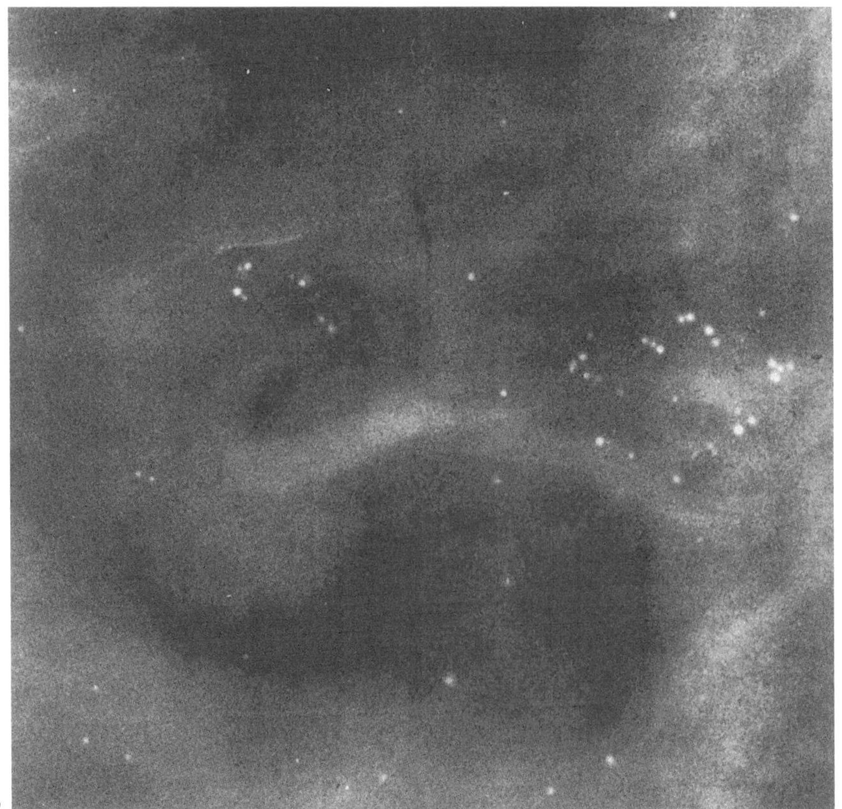

b

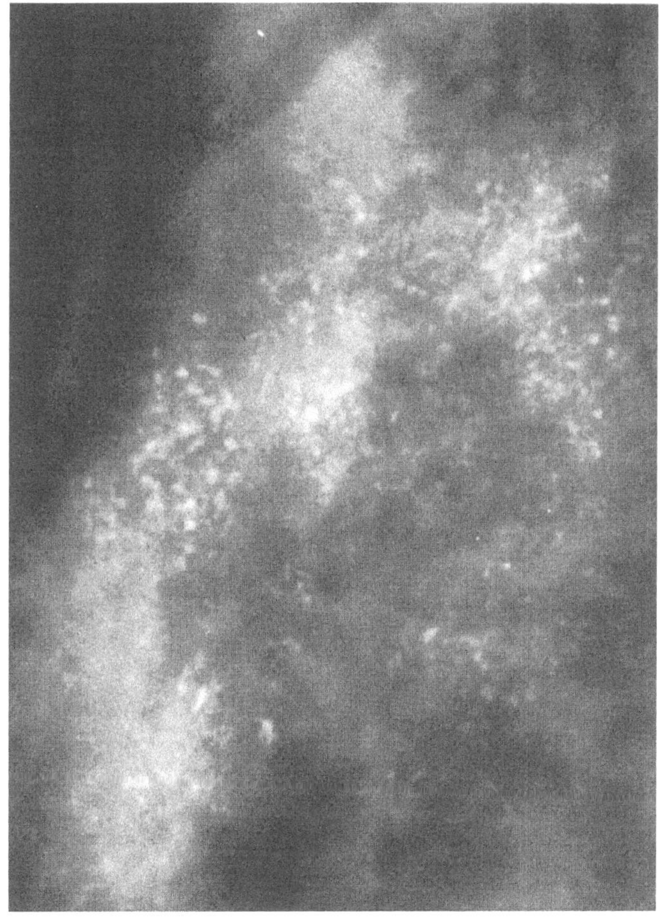

c

Fig. 7.3. None of these patients has a palpable mass
Case 1: **a** Craniocaudad view; this change is not visible on the lateral view.
Case 2: **b** Craniocaudad view; findings on the lateral view are similar.
Case 3: **c** Lateral view; findings on the craniocaudad view are similar.

In which case(s) is biopsy indicated?

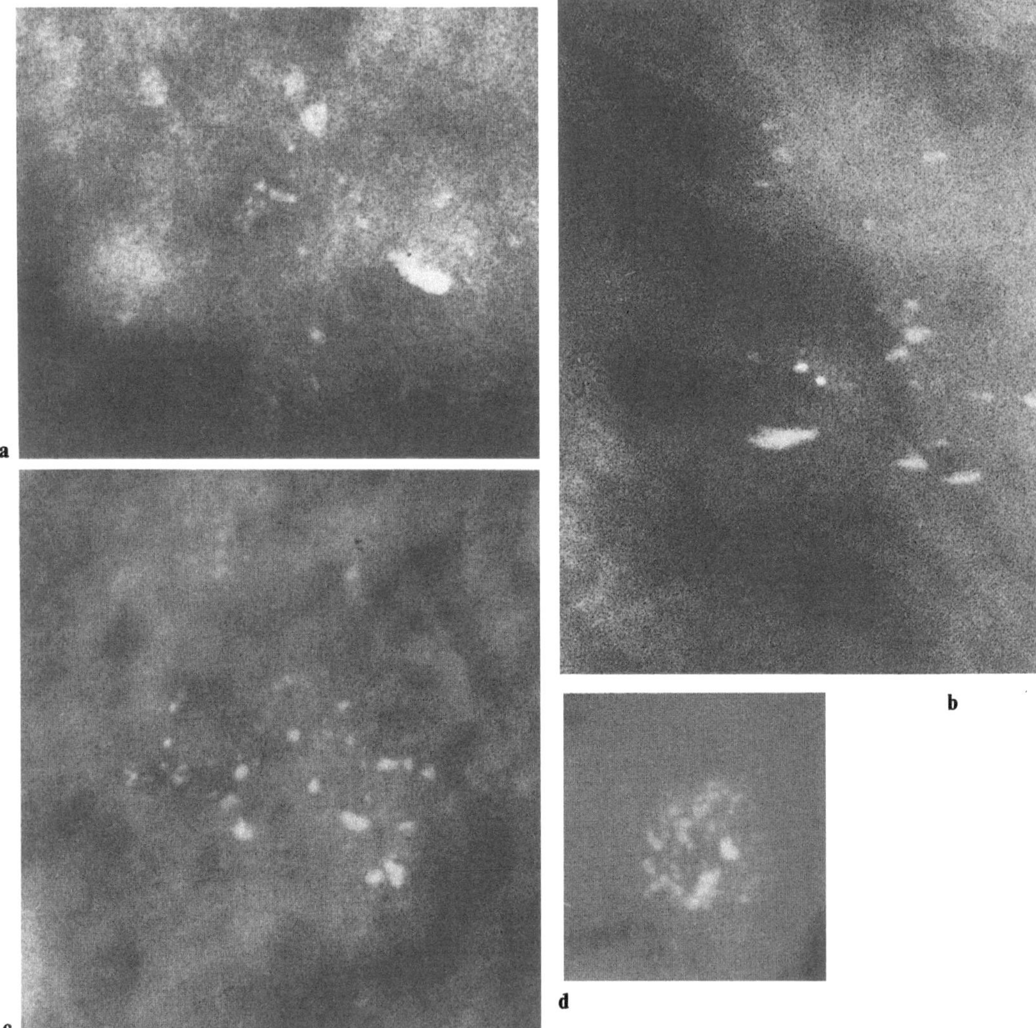

Fig. 7.4
Case 1: **a** Craniocaudad view; **b** lateral view.
Case 2: **c** Lateral view.
Case 3: **d** Lateral view.
Case 4: **e, f** Follow-up mammogramms show an increase in the number of microcalcifications over a 4-year period.

In which case would you recommend biopsy?

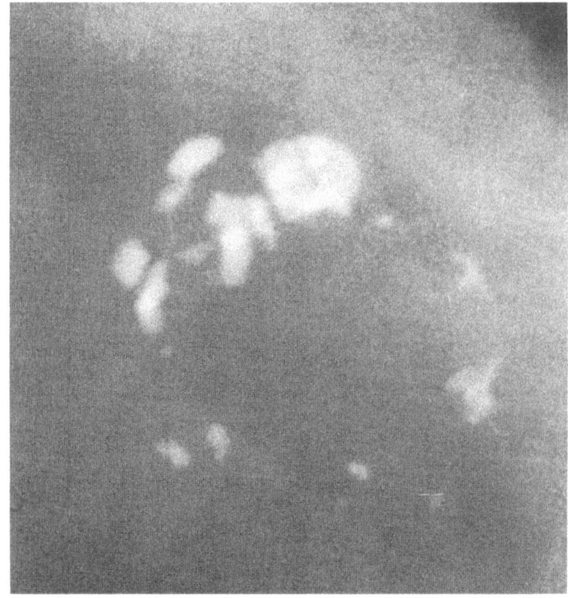

e

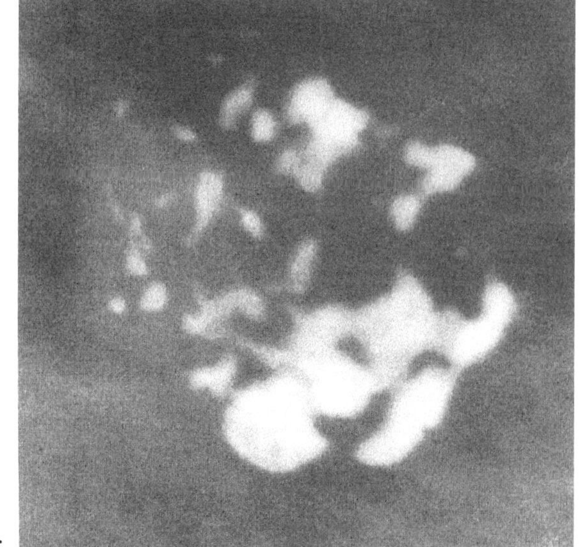

f

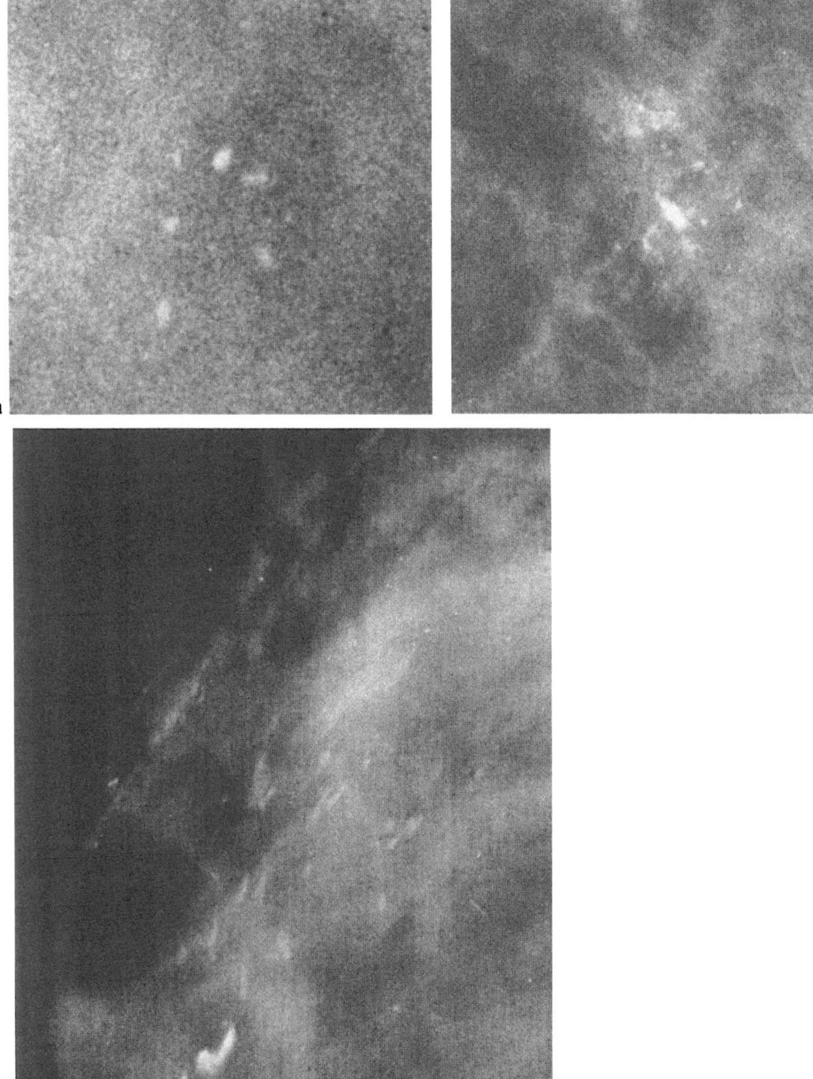

Fig. 7.5

Case 1: **a** Lateral view

Case 2: **b** Lateral view; no changes are visible on the craniocaudad view.

Case 3: **c** Craniocaudad view.

Case 4: **d** Lateral view, highly magnified. Patient had a prior contralateral mastectomy for carcinoma. No microcalcifications were visible 6 months previously.

Case 5: **e** Lateral view in 1980, **f** lateral view in 1984.

Case 6: **g** Lateral view.

In which case(s) would you recommend biopsy?

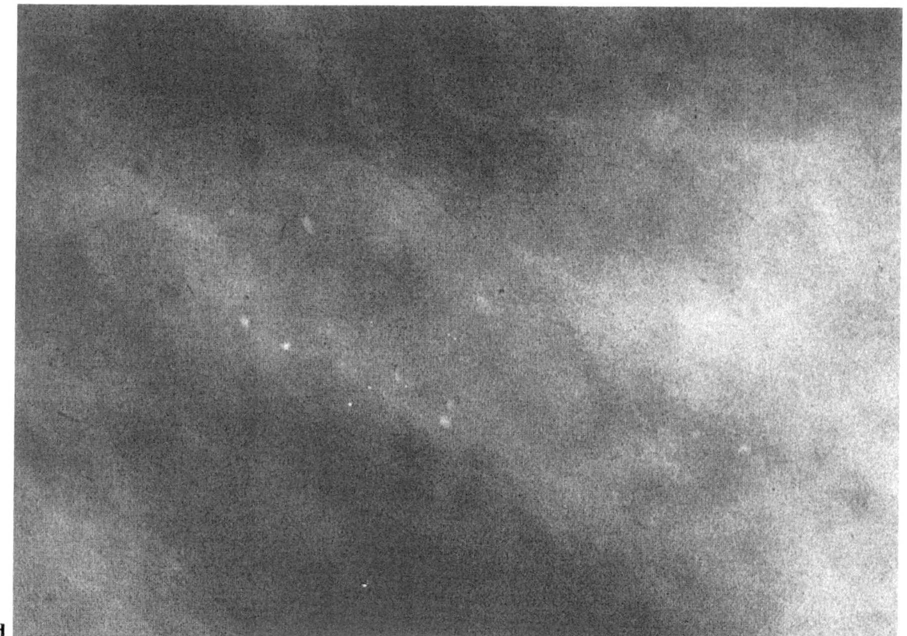

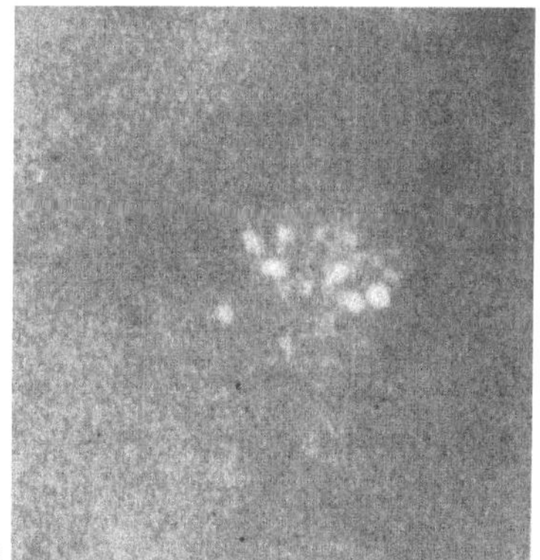

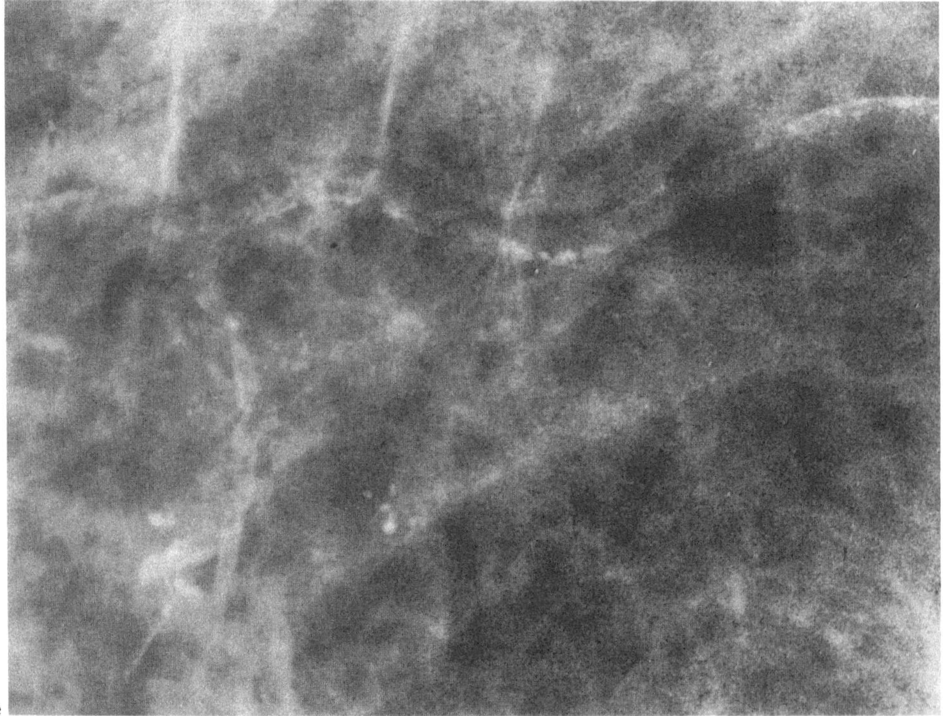

e

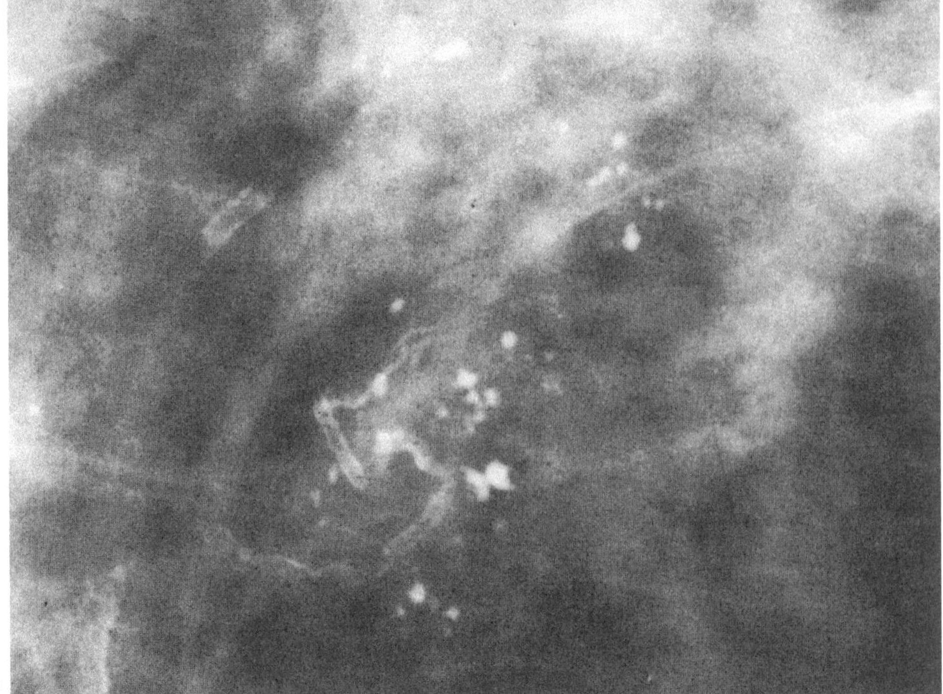

f

Fig. 7.5e, f. Legend on p. 204

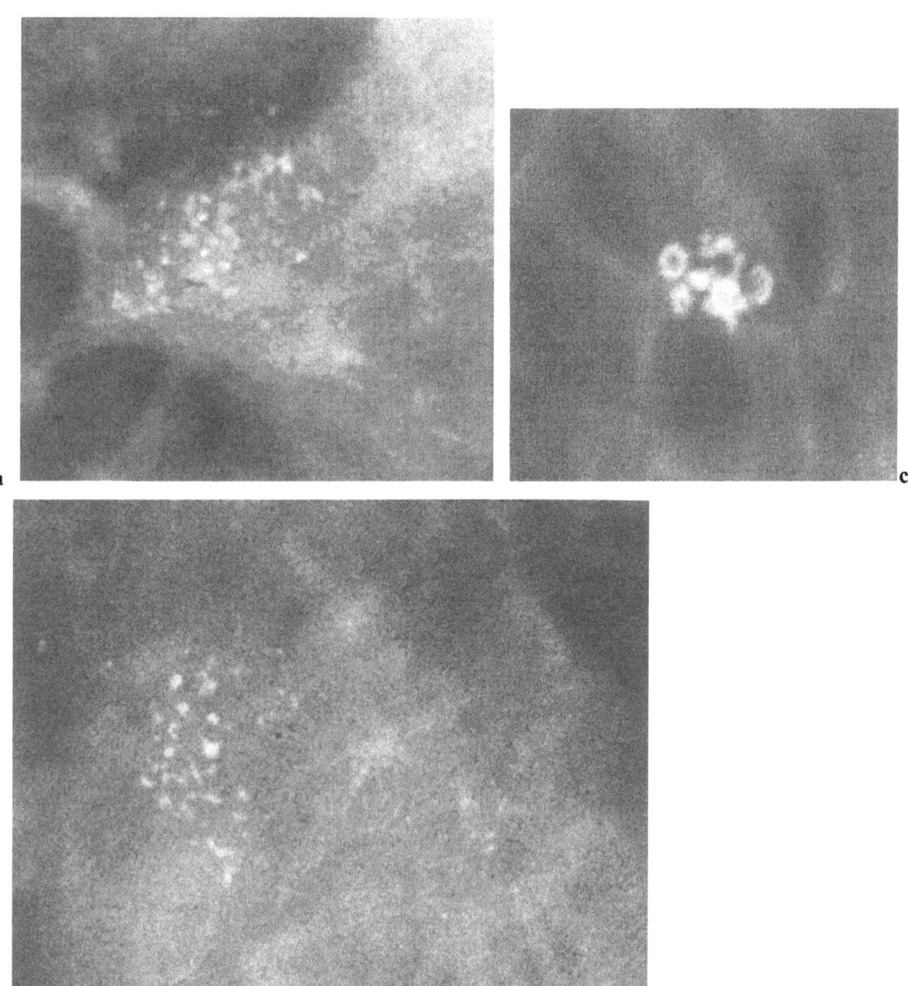

Fig. 7.6
Case 1: **a** Lateral view.
Case 2: **b** Lateral view.
Case 3: **c** Craniocaudad view; **d** lateral view.
Case 4: **e** Craniocaudad view; **f** lateral view.

In which case(s) is biopsy indicated?

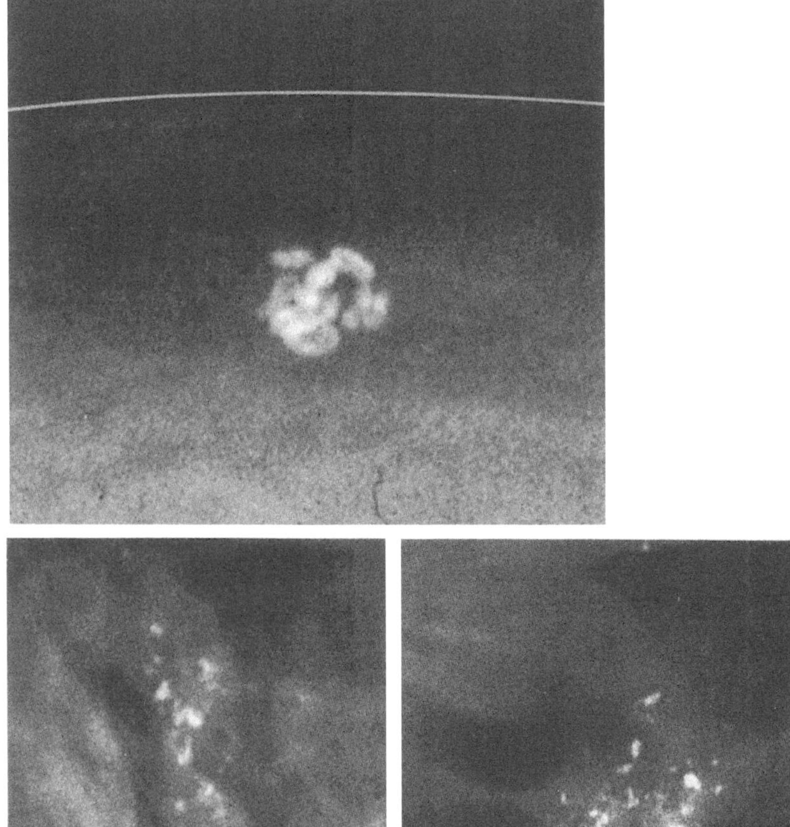

Fig. 7.6 d–f. Legend see p. 207

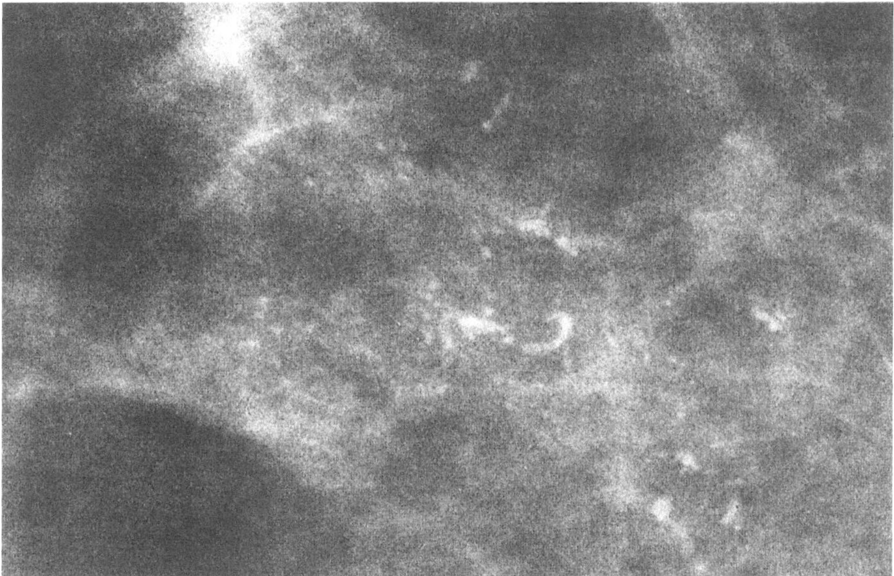

Fig. 7.7. You recommended biopsy on the basis of this microcalcification cluster. Histology: type A and B lobular neoplasia.

Questions:
1. *Do you agree with the histologic diagnosis, and do you recommend reexamination in 1 year?*
2. *Do you disagree with the histologic diagnosis, and do you recommend reexamination in 6 weeks to make certain that the microcalcification cluster has been removed and microscopically examined?*

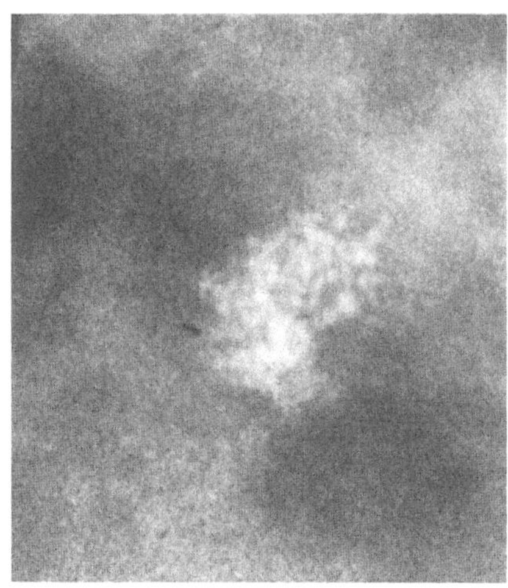

Fig. 7.8. Detail of mammogram (4 ×). You recommended biopsy on the basis of these microcalcifications. Histology: type A lobular neoplasia. Sclerosing adenosis.

Questions:
1. *Do you agree with the histologic diagnosis?*
2. *Do you disagree, and do you call the surgeon and say, "I'm sorry, but you have to operate again. The mammogram shows unmistakable evidence of carcinoma!"?*

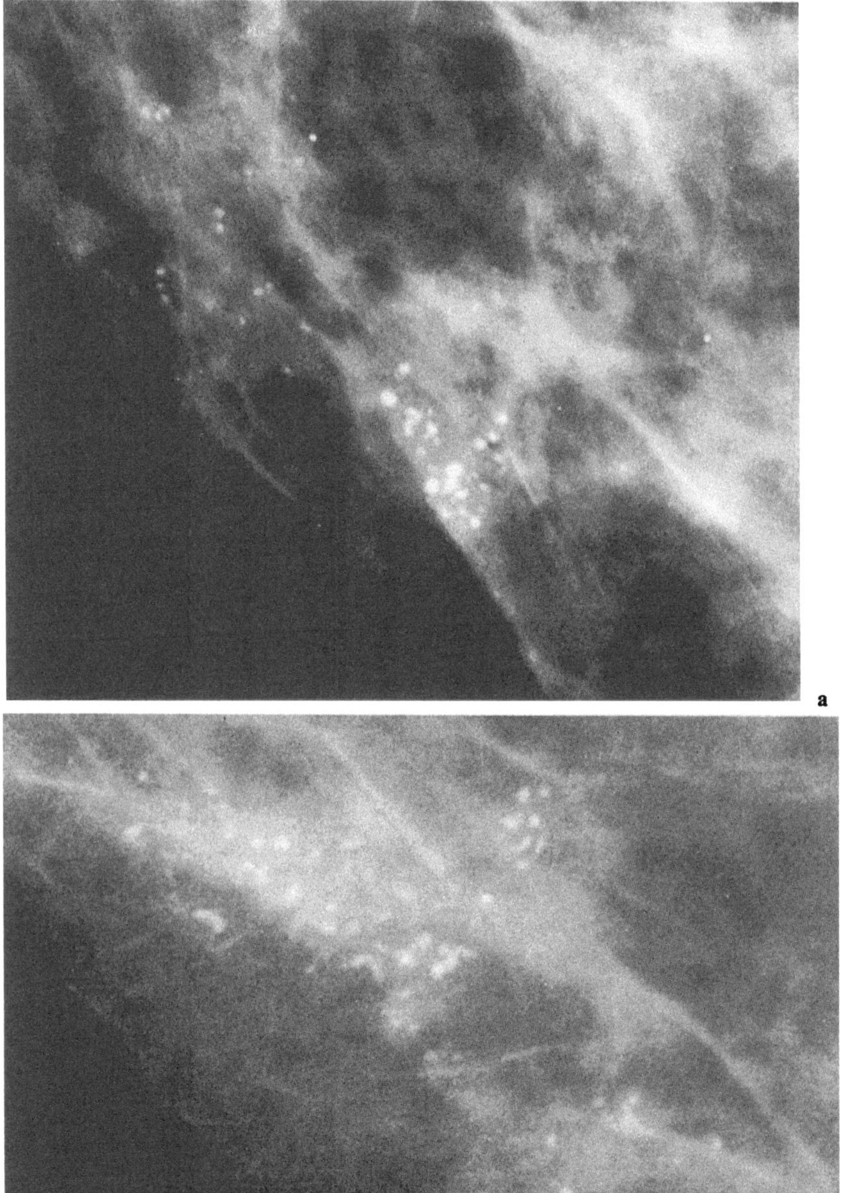

Fig. 7.9 a, b

Fig. 7.10. The wife of a friend and colleague has a cluster of microcalcifications in her right breast. She has already had two biopsies of the left breast for cystic disease. Her mother had breast cancer.

Question:
1. *Would you recommend a third operation?*
2. *Would you say, "Don't worry, we're dealing with a .... We'll reexamine you in 6 months"?*

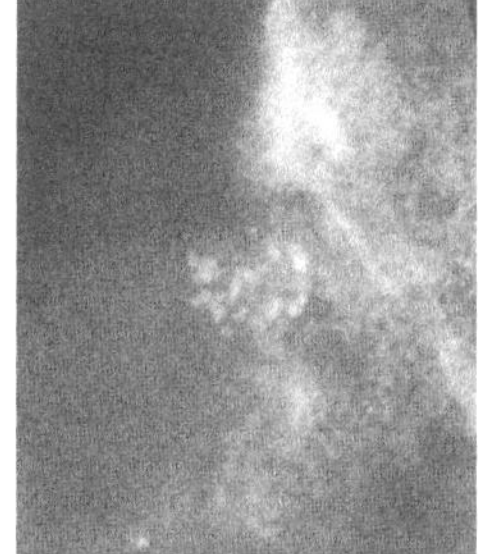

◁ **Fig. 7.9. a** The mammogram shows microcalcifications in a scar 2 years after a biopsy. You learn that another radiologist advised the patient to have the biopsy because of microcalcifications. You review the old films (**b**) and find no appreciable increase in the number of microcalcifications. What do you tell the patient?

1. *You have benign calcifications; we'll reexamine you in 2 years.*
2. *Unfortunately, the suspicious area was not removed 2 years ago, and we'll have to repeat the biopsy.*

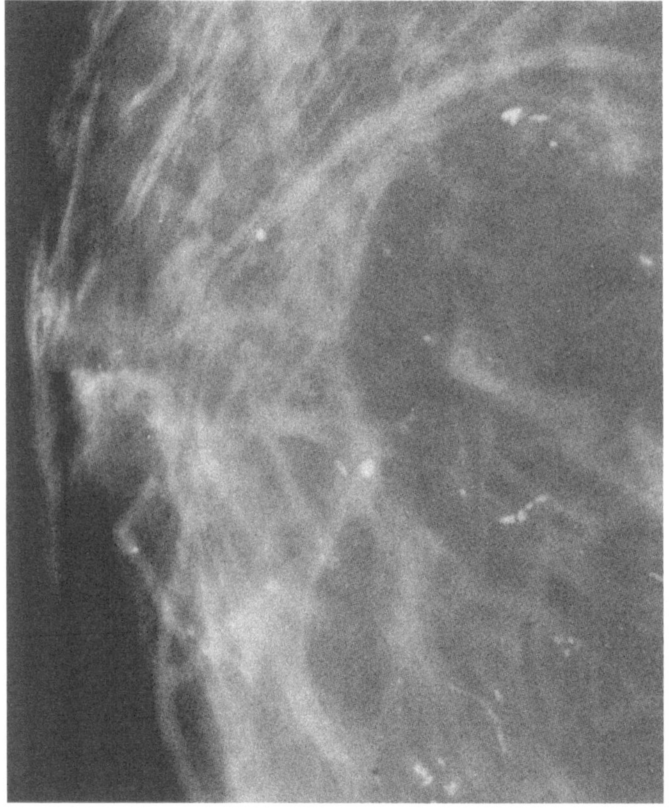

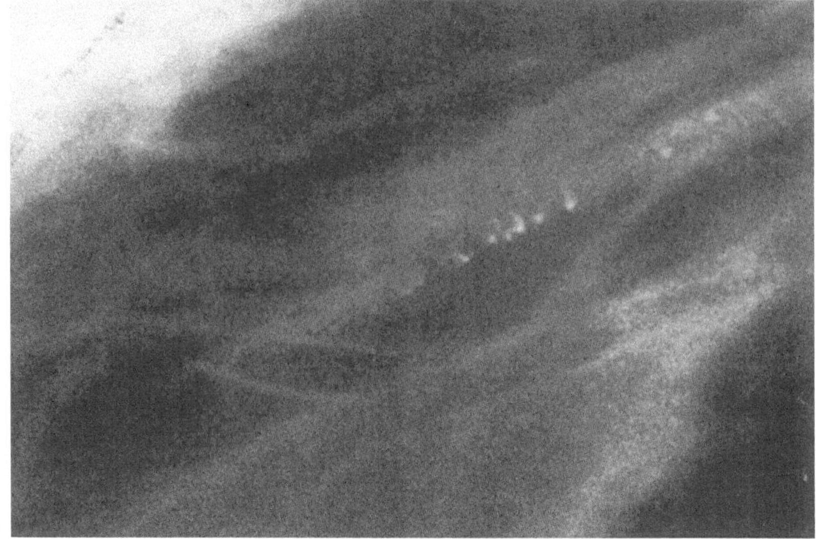

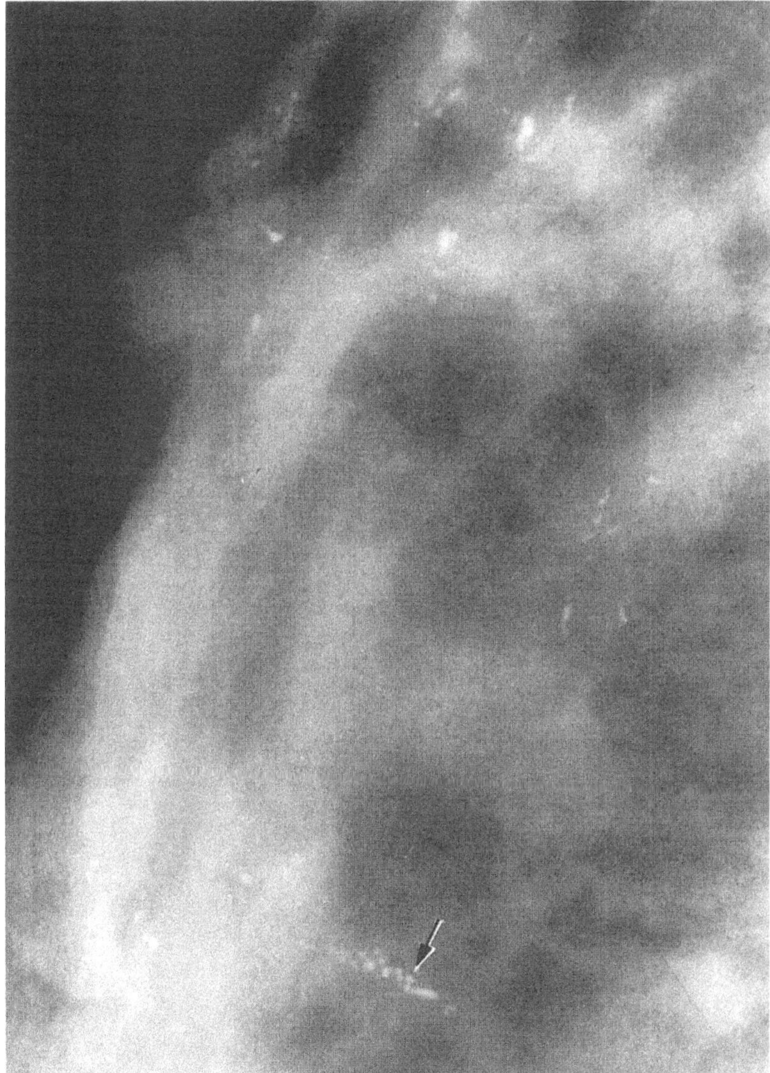

Fig.7.11. Three women were referred for mammography with suspected Paget's disease. None have palpable masses. You find more or less extensive microcalcifications in all three women.

*In which patient(s) (**a, b,** or **c**) would you presume a causal relationship between the microcalcifications and the nipple eczema in the sense of a ductal carcinoma that has spread to the nipple?*

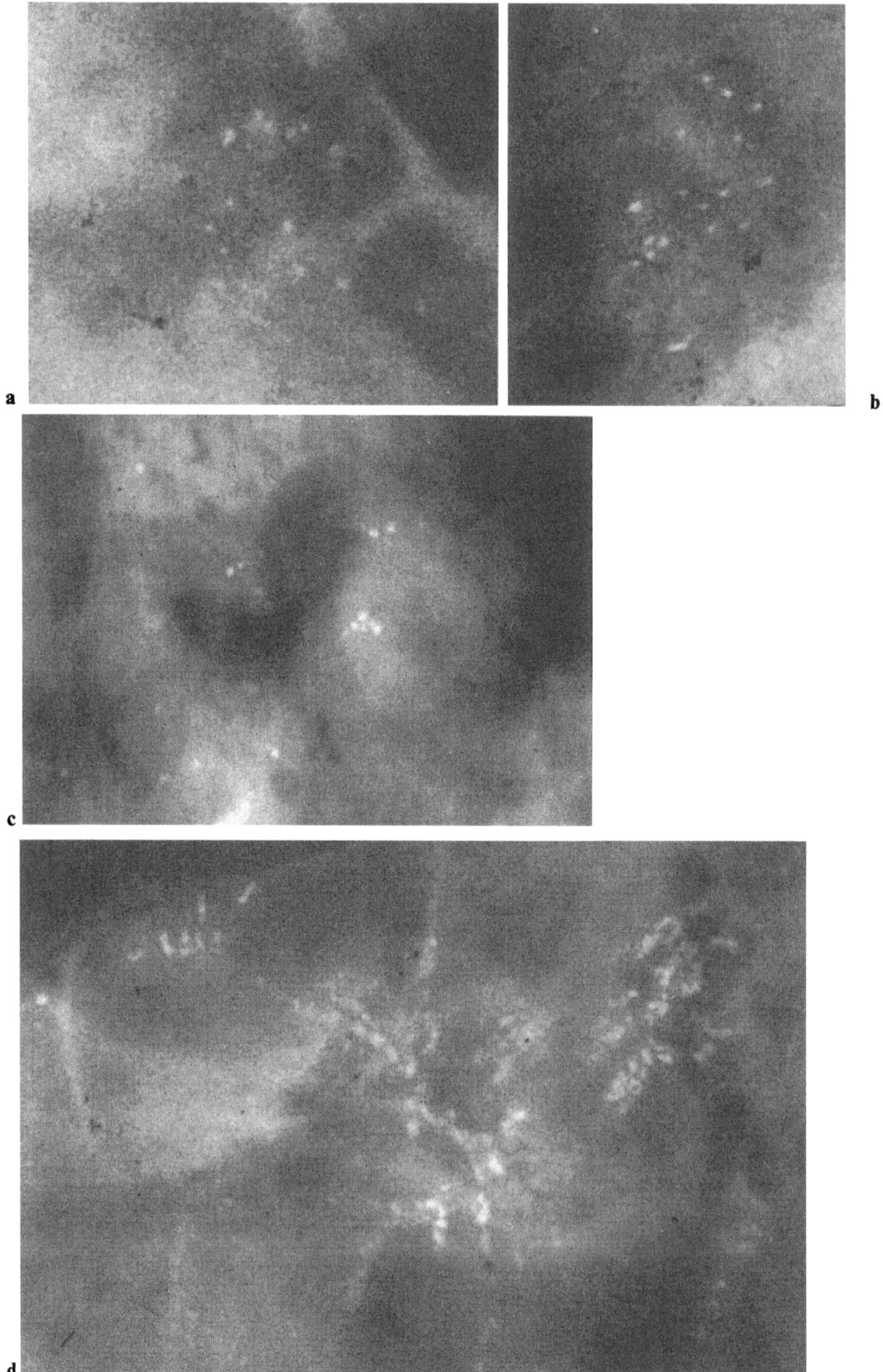

◁ **Fig. 7.12.** You are a budding radiologist and are present while your supervisor discusses mammographic findings. You see three different cases of clustered microcalcifications, and he recommends biopsy in all three.

*What would you think of case 1 (**a** craniocaudad, **b** lateral), case 2 (**c**), and case 3 (**d**)? For example, "My supervisor is right; all these cases should be biopsied." Or, "He has 'overdiagnosed' in these cases; I would not recommend biopsy!"*

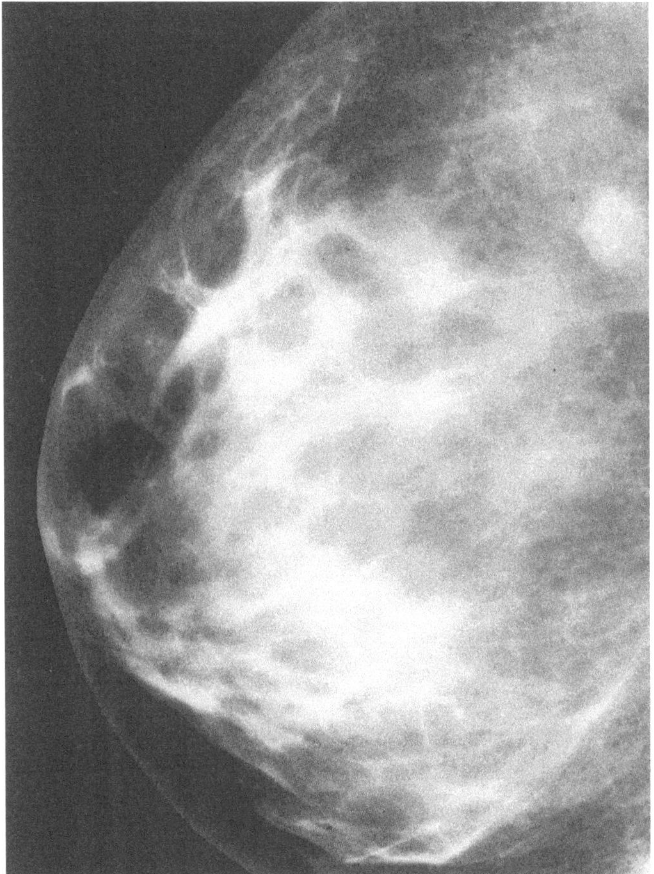

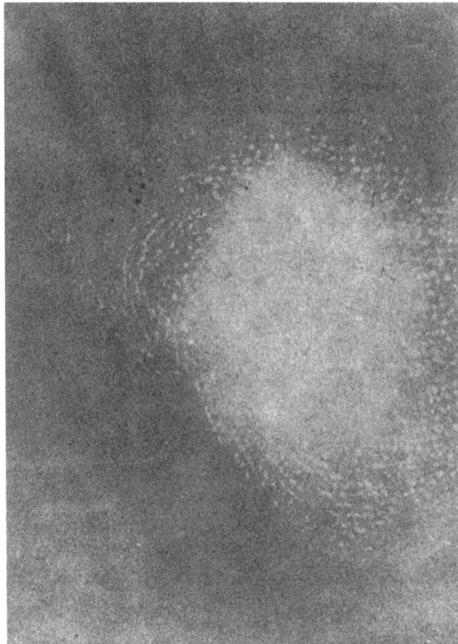

Fig. 7.13. This case has been referred to you for a second opinion. **a** Mammogram (reduced). **b** Detail of mammogram (3 ×). The accompanying sheet notes that "the lateral view shows a cherry-sized density in the upper portion of the left breast situated close to the chest wall and containing microcalcifications. There is no palpable mass at that location, and the lesion is not visible on the craniocaudad view. The remaining areas of the breast are unremarkable, and no skin changes are apparent. Conclusion: It cannot be established with certainty that the questionable finding is benign, and enucleation is recommended."

Do you agree or disagree with the findings of your colleague and his conclusion?

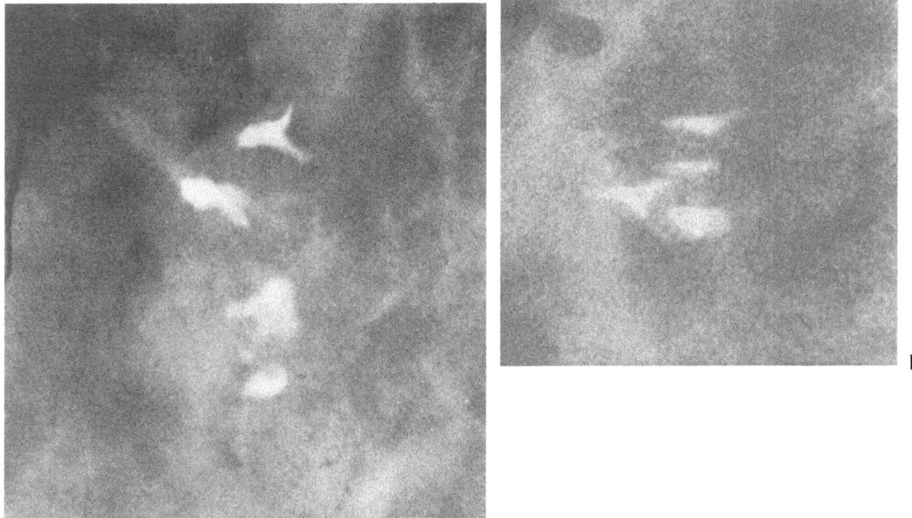

Fig. 7.14. Lateral mammograms, highly magnified. **a** *Case 1*. **b** *Case 2;* no microcalcifications are visible on the craniocaudad view.

Which of the two lesions is of intraductal (canalicular?) and which of lobular origin?

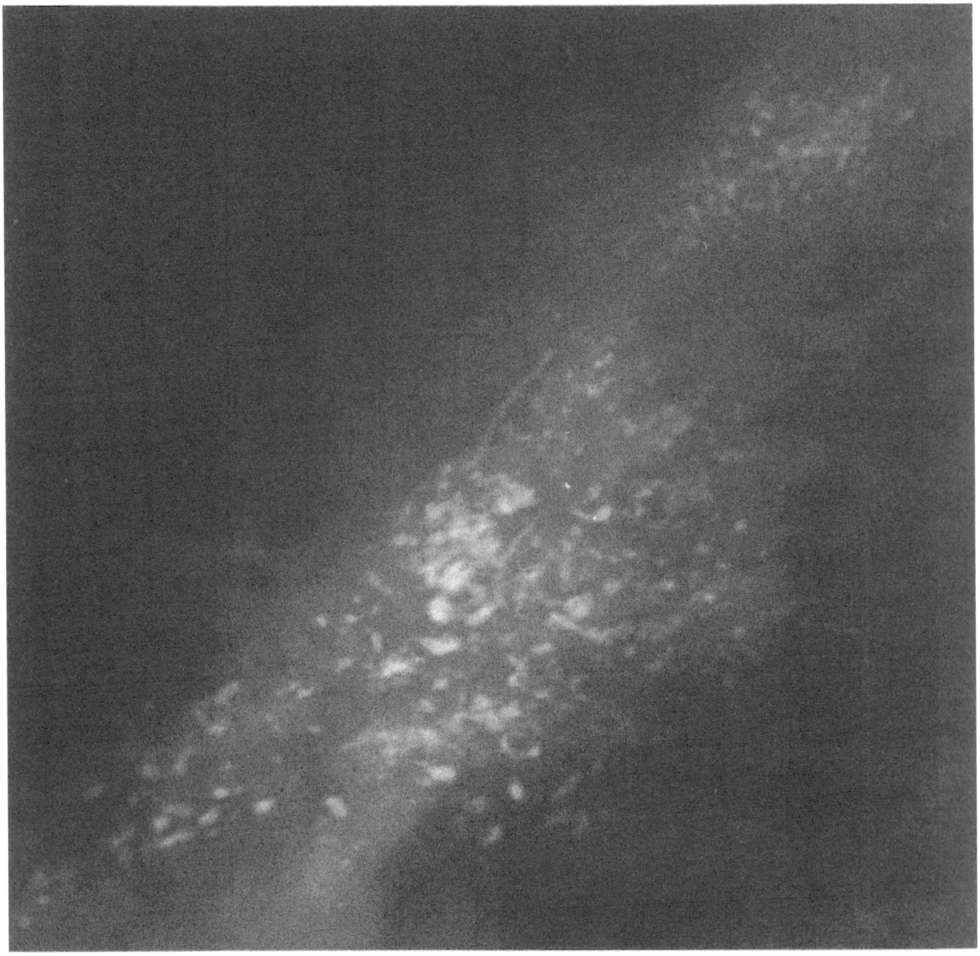

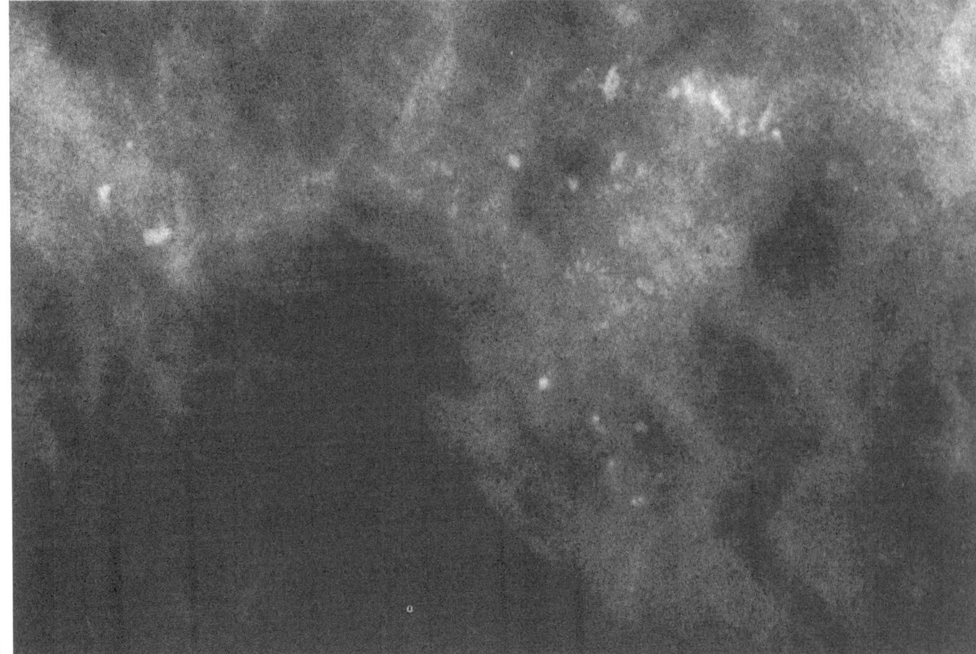

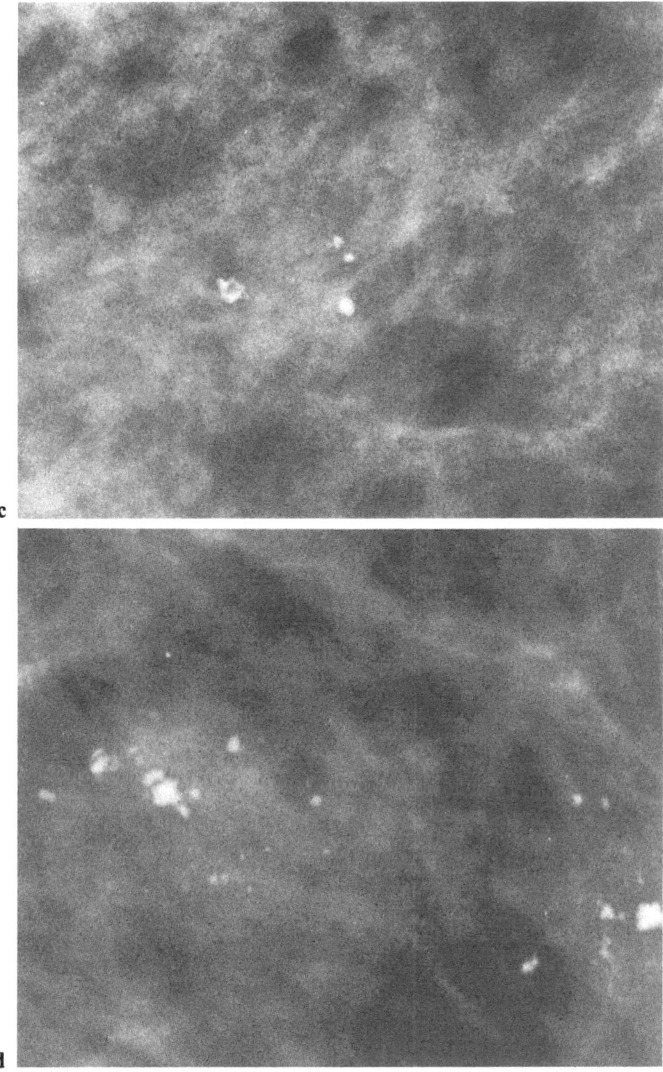

Fig. 7.15. There are three cases of clustered microcalcifications. *Case 1:* **a** (5×); *Case 2:* **b** (4×); *Case 3:* **c, d** (4×). The microcalcifications in case 3 (**c, d**) increased markedly in number over a 2-year period.

One case is benign. Which one?

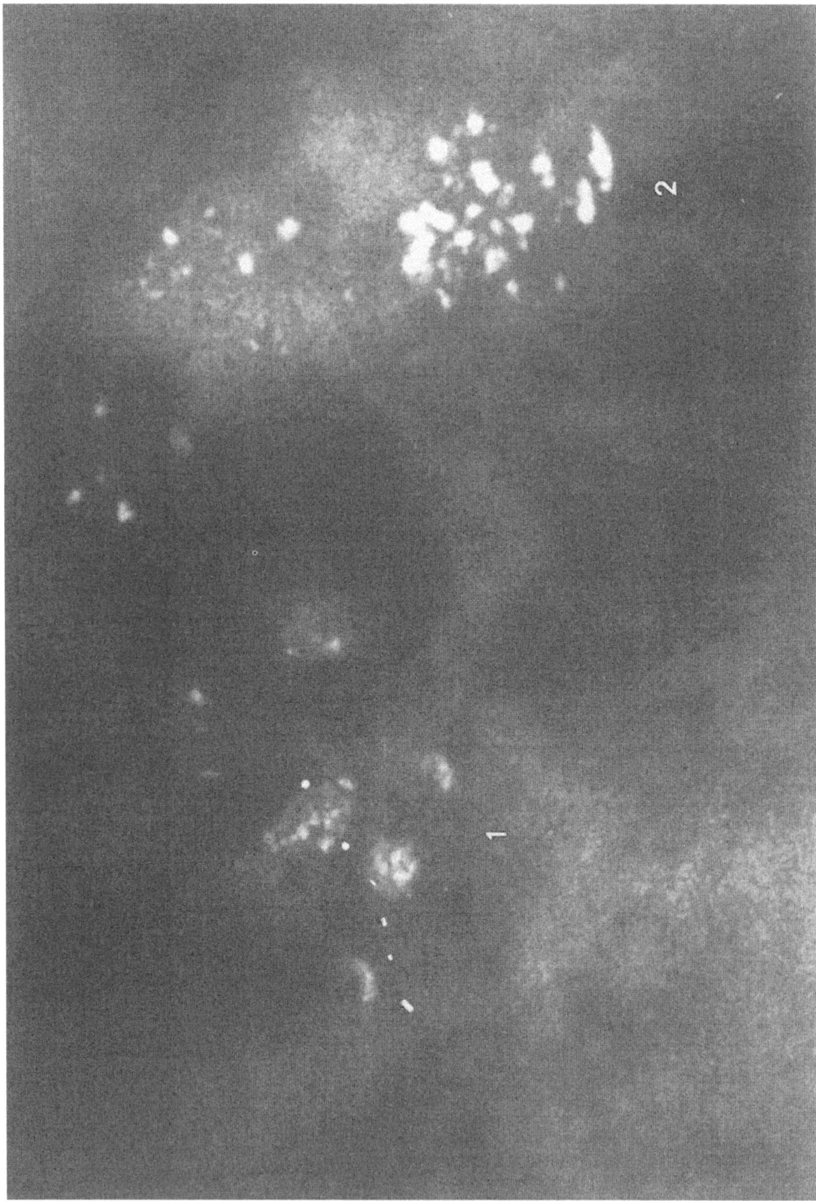

Fig.7.16. Two microcalcification clusters of different etiology in the same breast (lateral view, 15 ×).

Would you recommend biopsy? If so, would it be because of cluster 1 or cluster 2?

Fig. 7.17. Although the lesion is magnified 3 times, please examine this figure with a hand lens!

Would you recommend biopsy?

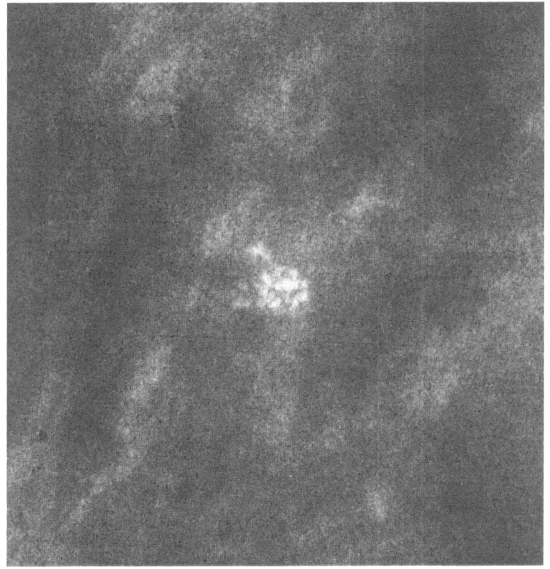

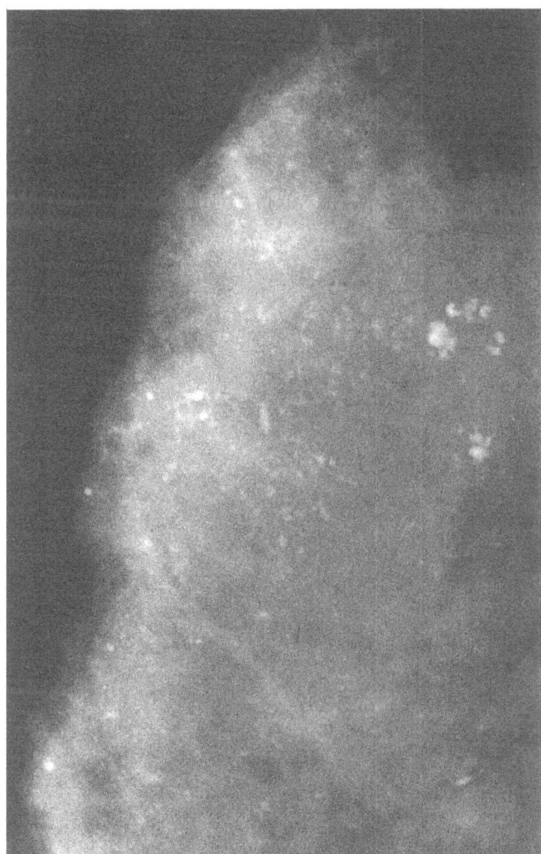

Fig. 7.18. Two different microcalcification patterns are visible on this slightly magnified view.

Can you identify them?

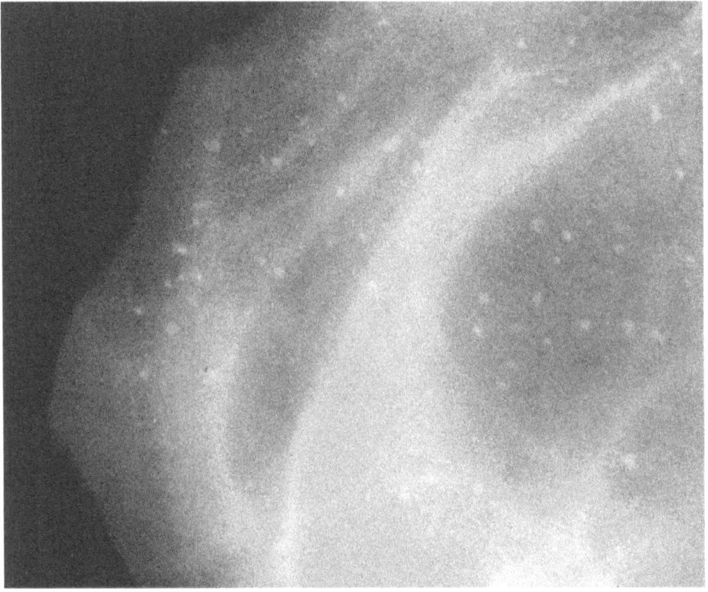

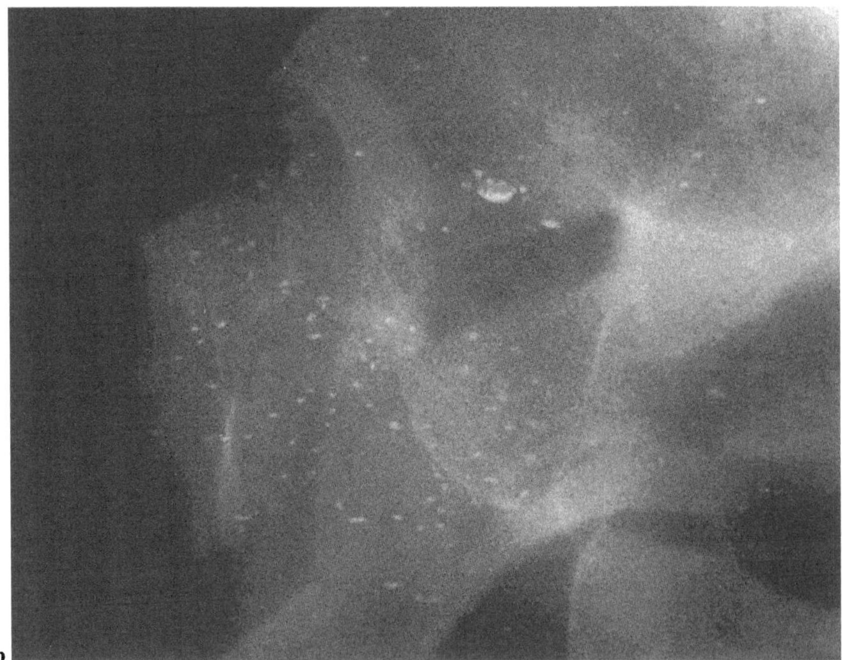

Fig. 7.19. Extensive microcalcifications are present in both cases. *Case 1:* **a** craniocaudad view, **b** lateral view (2 ×); *Case 2:* **c** lateral view (4 ×).

One of these cases is benign. Which one?

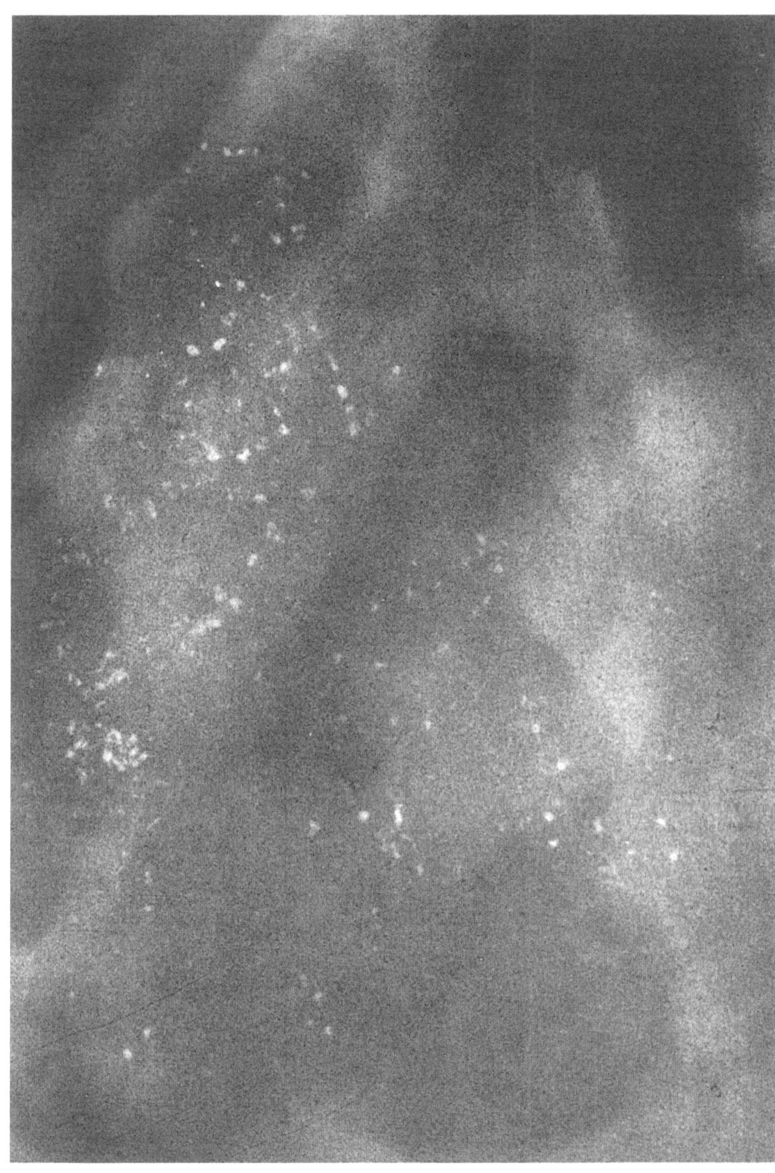

c

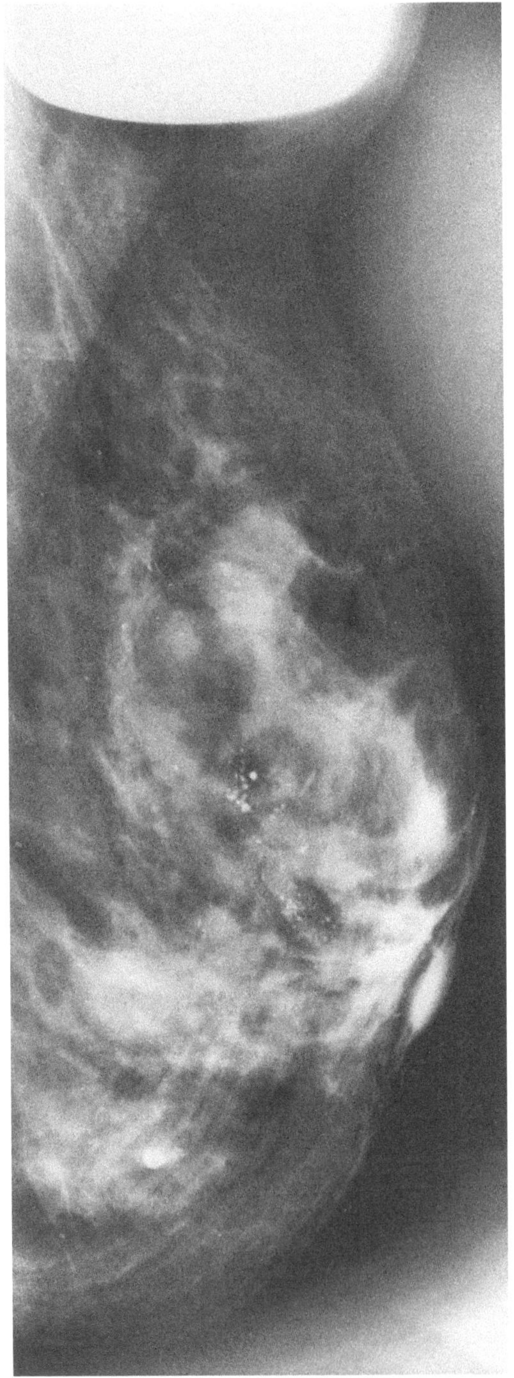

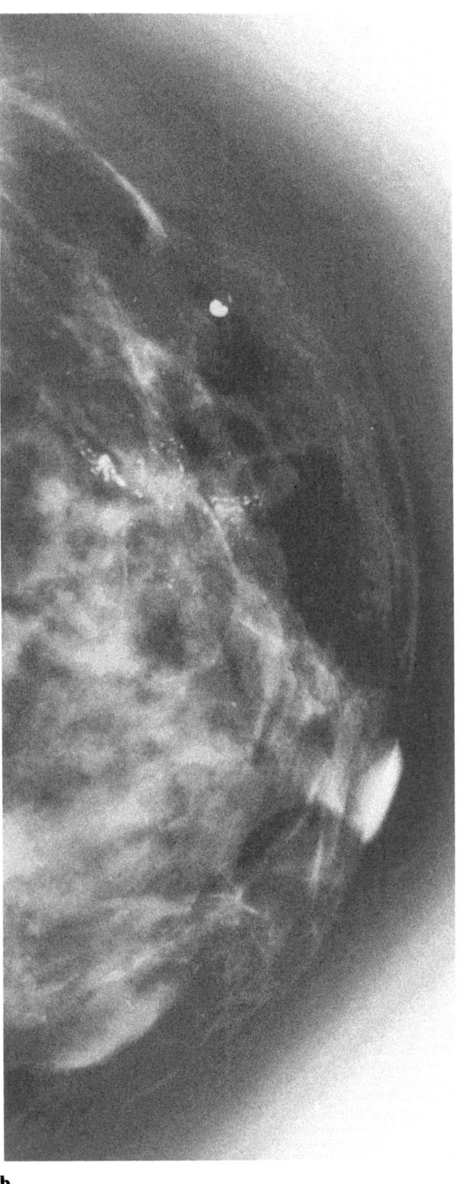

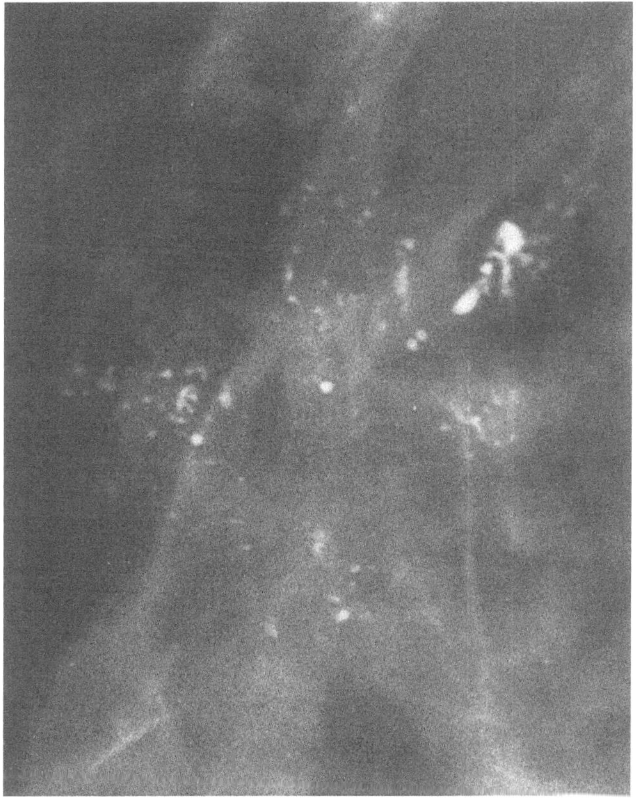

c

Fig. 7.20. Mammograms, original size. **a** Lateral view, **b** craniocaudad view, **c** detail of lateral view (4 ×). The case is referred to you for consultation. This 64-year-old woman has had a myocardial infarction, wears a pacemaker *(top)*, and is taking anticoagulant medication.

Do you think this is a carcinoma? Under the circumstances would you recommend biopsy or follow-up, since the microcalcification cluster might be benign?

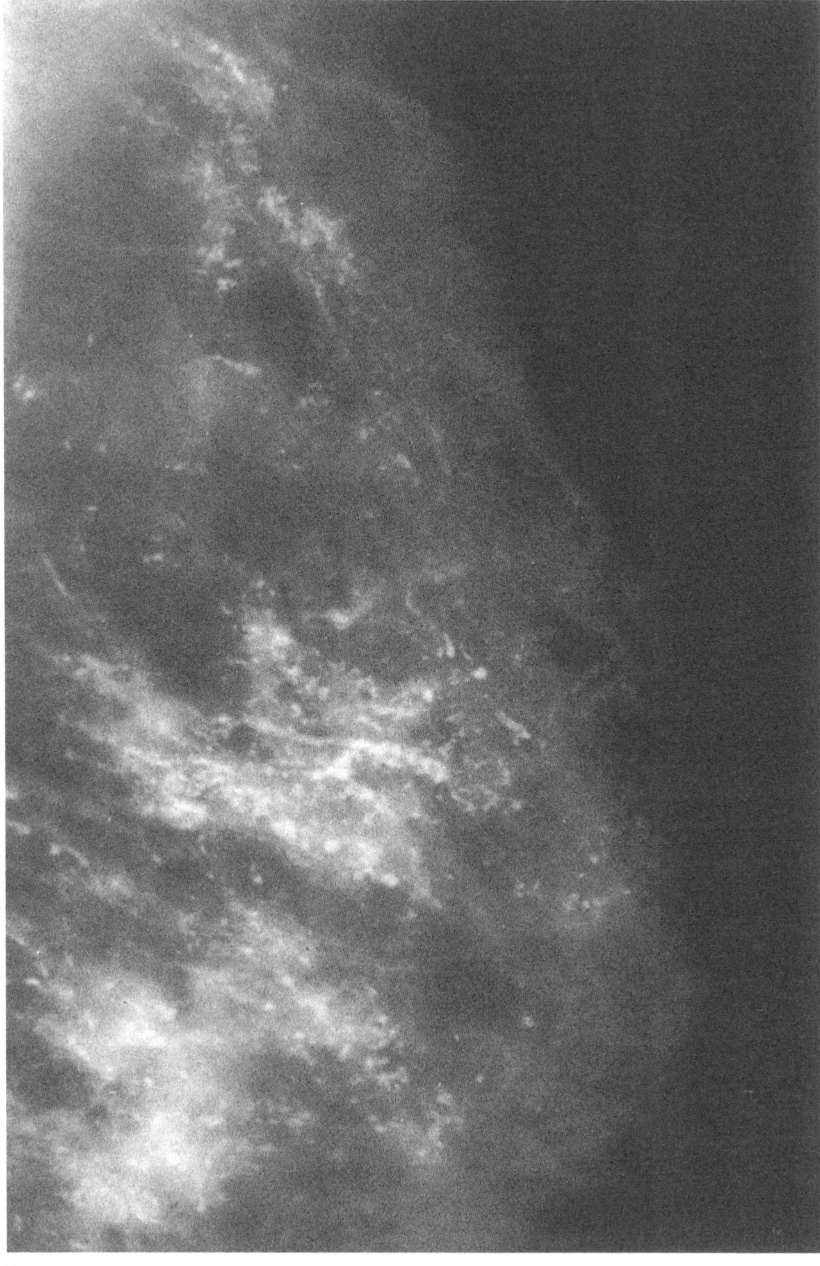

a

Fig. 7.21. Please list *all* the possible differential diagnoses for case **a** (slightly magnified) and for case **b** (3 ×).

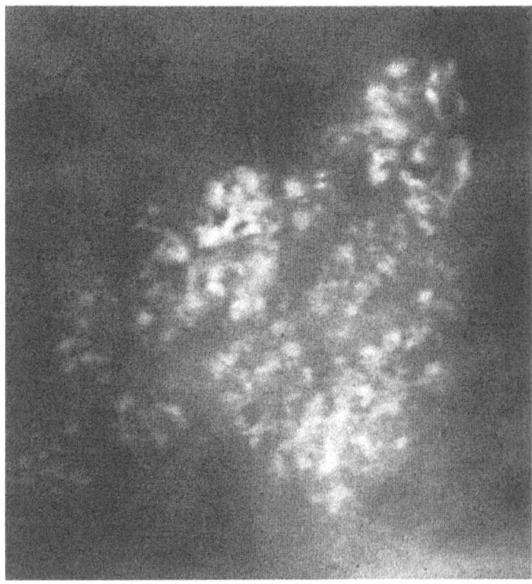

b

Answers

Fig. 7.2. Biopsy is indicated for *Case 1* because of minimal polymorphism of the microcalcifications on the craniocaudad view. Histology: ductal carcinoma.
Case 2: Liponecrotic microcysts.
Case 3: The previous biopsy was needlessly done for calcified sebaceous glands. A repeat biopsy is unnecessary.

Fig. 7.3. Biopsy is indicated for *Case 3:* classic intraductal carcinoma with infiltration, but without a palpable mass.
Case 1: Water-soluble contrast material on the skin.
Case 2: Diffuse, microcystic (blunt duct) adenosis. Note the "septa" between the cysts (diplococcuslike pattern).

Fig. 7.4. Biopsy is justified for *Case 2:* rectangular cluster of predominantly punctate microcalcifications with *minimal polymorphism*. Histology: predominantly papillary-cribriform, partly comedocarcinoma.
Case 1: Milk of calcium cysts with "teacup signs."
Case 3: Sclerosing adenosis, *ovoid* cluster of polymorphous microcalcifications.
Case 4: Fibroadenoma.

Fig.7.5. You should recommend biopsy for the following cases:

Case 1: Roughly triangular cluster of a few (6) microcalcifications with minimal polymorphism, suggestive of an *intraductal* lesion. Histology: carcinoma 4 mm in size.

Case 3: Triangular cluster of mostly punctate microcalcifications with two linear and one y-shaped calcification. Histology: comedocarcinoma 8 mm in size.

Case 4: Flat, possibly triangular or diamond-shaped cluster of barely perceptible microcalcifications with minimal polymorphism (see illustration). The apparent absence of the calcifications 6 months previously and the history of contralateral mastectomy should raise a suspicion of a second carcinoma. Histology: ductal carcinoma 2 cm (!) in size.

Case 5: The number of the slightly polymorphous, relatively large microcalcifications has increased in a 4-year period. The cluster shape (**f**) is roughly triangular. An intraductal process is suspected. Histology: hyalinized and calcified fibroadenoma.

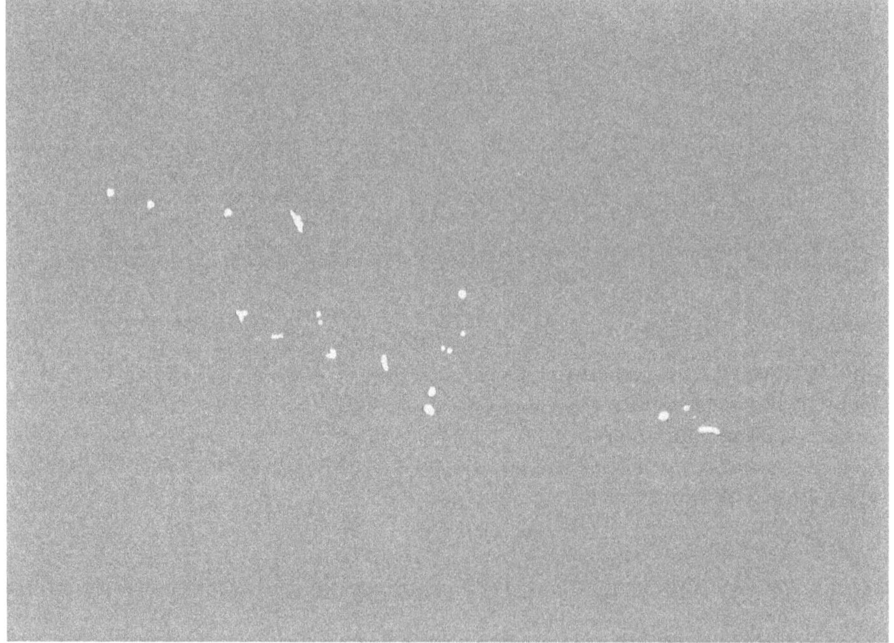

Biopsy is unnecessary in *Cases 2* and *6:*

Case 2: Artifact. (Referral; origin of artifact unknown).

Case 6: Ovoid cluster, 5 mm in size, of *monomorphously* punctate, occasionally facetted microcalcifications with septa. Microcystic (blunt duct) adenosis.

Fig. 7.6. Biopsy should be recommended for all cases except *Case 3,* which involves a rounded cluster of calcified sebaceous glands that cannot be entirely "projected out of" the breast, but whose nature is disclosed by the characteristic shape of the microcalcifications.

Case 1: The possibly triangular or diamond shape and the polymorphism of the faint microcalcifications signify an intraductal process, most likely a comedocarcinoma. Histology: comedomastitis.

Case 2: left Triangular cluster with posterior notch. Marked polymorphism. *Right* Smaller, similar cluster that is barely perceptible (see illustration). Histology: comedocarcinoma.

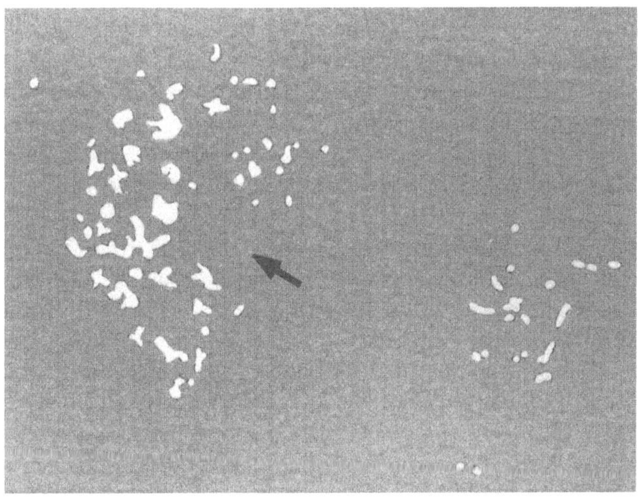

Case 4: The cluster shape changes with the plane of the projection. It is propeller-shaped on the craniocaudad view (**e**) and triangular on the lateral view (**f**). Polymorphism. Histology: comedocarcinoma.

Fig. 7.7. The correct answer: reexamine in 6 weeks. If the microcalcifications (butterfly-shaped cluster with minimal polymorphism) are still within the breast, a repeat biopsy must be recommended, as it was in this instance. The second biopsy uncovered the small, clinically occult carcinoma (predominantly cribriform, partly comedo) and confirmed the radiologic diagnosis. The type A and B lobular neoplasia was only a satellite lesion.

Fig. 7.8. The original histologic diagnosis is proper, and there is no need to call the surgeon. The picture is classic for sclerosing adenosis: dense, ovoid (kidney-shaped?) cluster of polymorphous microcalcifications. Areas of lobular neoplasia are sometimes found in association with sclerosing adenosis!

Fig. 7.9. The second answer is correct. The patient had an obvious comedocarcinoma 2 years previously. The first biopsy was done as an outpatient procedure in a gynecology office. At repeat biopsy, performed in a hospital, histologic proof of the carcinoma was finally obtained.

Fig. 7.10. The second answer is correct. The small, rounded cluster of microcalcifications showing minimal polymorphism represents sclerosing adenosis. Follow-up is appropriate.

Fig. 7.11. Biopsy is indicated for **a** and **c**. In **a** we see a very small number of calcifications that are definitely intraductal and taper toward the nipple. Similar calcifications, also definitely intraductal, are present in **c**. Both cases involved diffuse ductal carcinomas with varying degrees of calcification. The suspicious feature in **b** is an artery with circumscribed calcification.

Fig. 7.12. *Case 1:* Clustered milk of calcium cysts. The microcalcifications on the craniocaudal view (**a**) are rounded and faint, and those on the lateral view (**b**) are denser and streaklike (teacup sign). Biopsy is unnecessary.
Case 2: Partly clustered, partly scattered calcifications of microcystic (blunt duct) adenosis, showing the "septa" characteristic of this lesion. Biopsy is unnecessary.
Case 3: The supervisor is correct; this is a comedocarcinoma. But in the first two cases, please convey your opinion to your supervisor as tactfully as you can!

Fig. 7.13 a. The abnormality is visible only on the lateral mammogram, and so your colleague cannot tell whether it is located laterally, centrally, or medially. Regardless of the nature of the abnormality, "enucleation" would not be possible in the absence of a palpable mass.
b On closer inspection it is clear that the "abnormality" is a fingerprint!

Fig. 7.14. *Case 1:* Large punctate v-shaped calcifications occurring within an ovoid shadow are typical of *fibroadenoma,* i.e., intracanalicular in origin.
Case 2: If the cluster is visible only on the lateral view, it may represent an artifact or a group of milk of calcium cysts (since milk of calcium may be harder to see in the craniocaudad projection). Fluid levels (teacup signs) are seen only in *milk of calcium cysts,* i.e., lobular in origin.

Fig. 7.15. The cluster in *case 1* displays the classic pattern of comedocarcinoma: a triangular cluster with lateral processes, posterior notching, and polymorphism, showing a predominance of linear and branched calcification forms.
The cluster in *case 2* was identified histologically as a predominantly papillary-cribriform carcinoma with few comedo elements, accounting for the minimal polymorphism. The microcalcifications are predominantly punctate, and the cluster shape is triangular.
Case 3: This lesion is benign (hyalinized fibroadenoma), despite the marked increase in the number of calcifications (biopsy would not be inappropriate!).

Fig. 7.16. *Cluster 1* Multiple foci of microcystic (blunt duct) adenosis accompanied by two milk of calcium cysts with fluid levels. All the microcalcifications are therefore of lobular origin.
Cluster 2 Minimal polymorphism with predominantly punctate microcalcifications. The cluster shape is difficult to assess. A biopsy was recommended because of the uncertain nature of the findings. Histology: papillary carcinoma.

Fig.7.17. Triangular cluster of polymorphous microcalcifications. Biopsy is indicated.
Histology: sclerosing adenosis. Very small foci of sclerosing adenosis demonstrate the limitations of the method when they present a triangular or indefinite configuration, in which case they are indistinguishable from a very small carcinoma.

Fig.7.18. Extensive comedocarcinoma and, near the chest wall, a calcified fibroadenoma.

Fig.7.19. *Case 1:* Milk of calcium cysts, benign. The craniocaudad view (**a**) shows only punctate microcalcifications, while fluid levels are seen on the lateral view (**b**). *Case 2:* Comedocarcinoma. Large, triangular cluster of polymorphous microcalcifications containing islandlike zones that are devoid of microcalcifications.

Fig.7.20. Stellate cluster of polymorphous microcalcifications suggestive of ductal carcinoma. If the patient, with her cardiac condition, is at all able to tolerate biopsy, histologic confirmation is advised. Histology: comedocarcinoma.

Fig.7.21. If you listed any possible diagnosis other than carcinoma, please reread this book!

8 Clinically Occult, Mammographically Suspicious Microcalcification Clusters: Pre-, Intra-, and Postoperative Measures

Before the era of mammography, a breast malignancy was considered to be occult only if local or distant metastases had developed, but a primary tumor could not be palpated in the breast. In the modern view, a breast carcinoma is clinically occult if it cannot be detected by ordinary clinical means – regardless of whether the lesion is still at the preclinical stage (occult early carcinoma) or has already produced metastasis or nipple eczema as in Paget's disease (occult late carcinoma). With the increasing use of screening mammography for asymptomatic women, the problem of the localization of clinically occult suspicious findings arises more and more frequently. (HOMER 1982; LETTON and MASON 1980). A carcinoma may be clinically occult if:
– it is *too small* to be palpated
– it is *relatively too small* because of the large breast size or because it is located deep within the breast
– its *consistency* is similar to that of surrounding tissues, i.e., the healthy tissue is just as firm or firmer than the neoplastic tissue.

Microcalcifications characteristic of carcinoma are the classic example of an occult breast malignancy. This chapter covers problems relating to the localization of clinically occult, mammographically suspicious microcalcification clusters.

The entire procedure (localization and processing of the material) is normally carried out in three stages:
1) Preoperative localization
2) Intraoperative specimen radiography
3) Postoperative processing of the material for histologic examination.
These may be supplemented by:
a) Radiographic examination of the paraffin block
b) Postoperative mammograms.

8.1 Preoperative Localization

Geometric Localization

Preferably this should be done on the day before the biopsy, with the surgeon and patient in attendance. The location of the microcalcification cluster is determined on the craniocaudad and lateral mammograms using a coordinate system consisting of a horizontal axis (ordinate) and a vertical axis (abscissa) centered on the nipple (Fig. 8.1 a, b).

The coordinate system is transposed onto the patient's breast, and the skin site over the abnormality is marked (Fig. 8.1 d). The distance of the microcalcification cluster from the skin is indicated on both planes (Fig. 8.1 f). A sketch indicating the

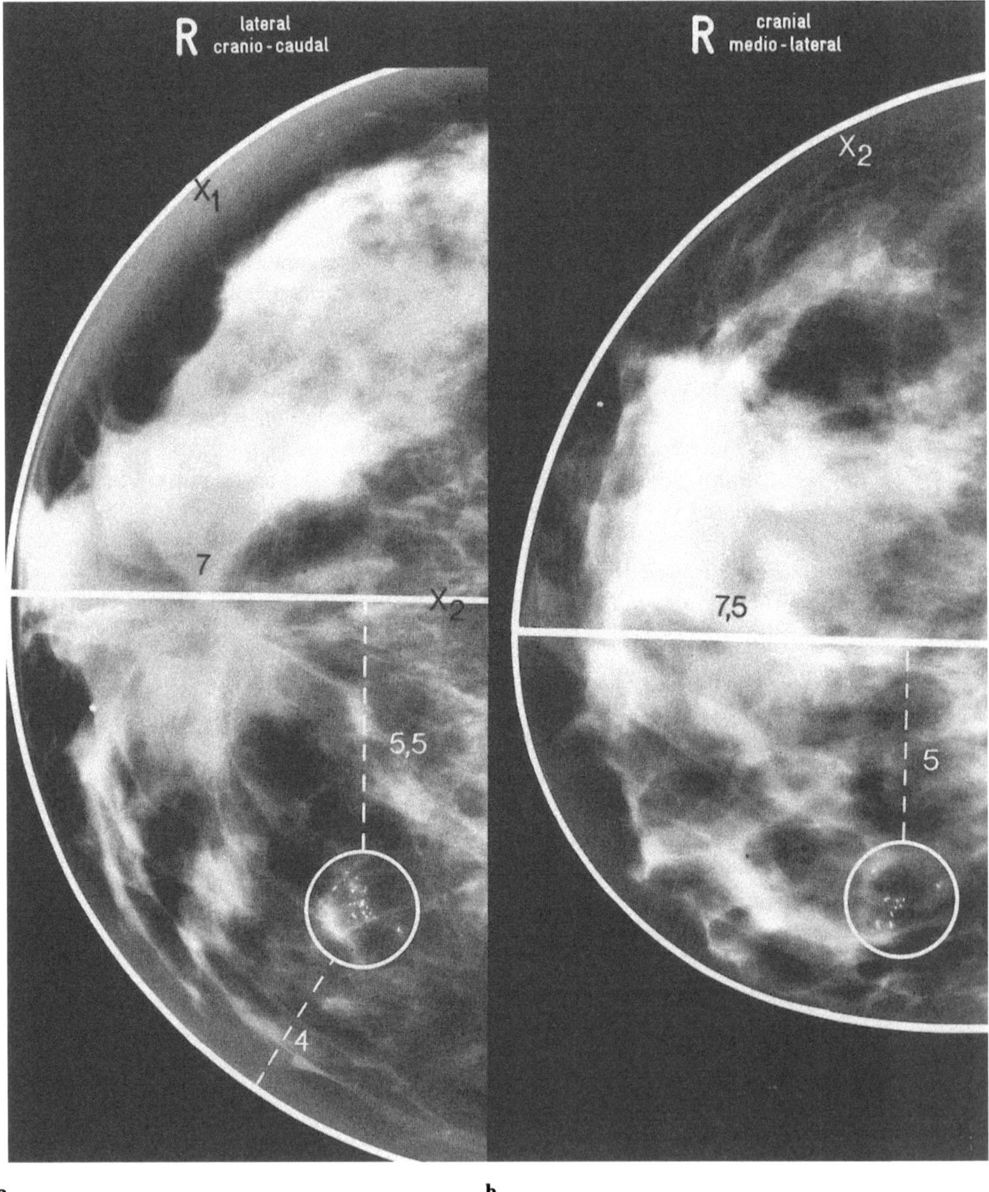

a

b

Fig. 8.1. a Craniocaudad mammogram. **b** Lateral mammogram. X_1, horizontal nipple line; X_2, vertical nipple line. The triangular cluster of polymorphous microcalcifications (**c** 3.5 ×) is in the lower medial quadrant, 7–7.5 cm behind the nipple, about 5–5.5 cm below and medial to the breast axis (X_1 or X_2), 4 cm from the skin surface. There is no palpable tumor. **d** The data are transposed onto the patient's breast. **e** Specimen radiograph: the microcalcification cluster is at the edge of the specimen between the numbers *0* and *1 (arrow)*. **f** The cluster is excised in a block. **g** Magnified view of the block (3.5 ×). Histology: noninfiltrating comedocarcinoma

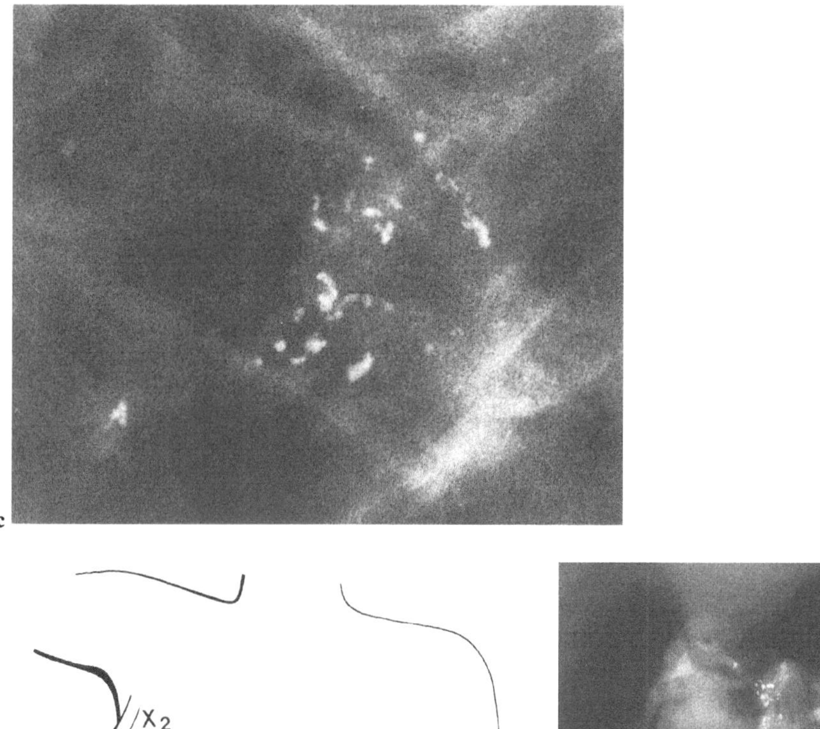

location is then made as a reminder for the surgeon. With this localization technique, it is extremely important that the affected breast and the affected quadrant be clearly marked. Care is taken to verify that the film was labeled correctly so that there will be no mistakes when the biopsy is performed. Geometric localization can be done with the patient standing and the breast resting on the film-holder table, as when the mammogram was taken, or the patient may be placed on her back or side, as she will for surgery.

The suspicious area can be localized even in the absence of the surgeon and patient by preparing a localization diagram. This is done by projecting the lateral and craniocaudad mammograms onto a diagram of the breast. In this way the suspicious area can be assigned to a particular quadrant. Again, the depth of the lesion should be indicated (Fig. 8.2). This technique, recommended by BERGER et al. (1966), does not require special management, but is somewhat uncertain. Geometric preoperative localization as described above is the simplest solution. Its disadvan-

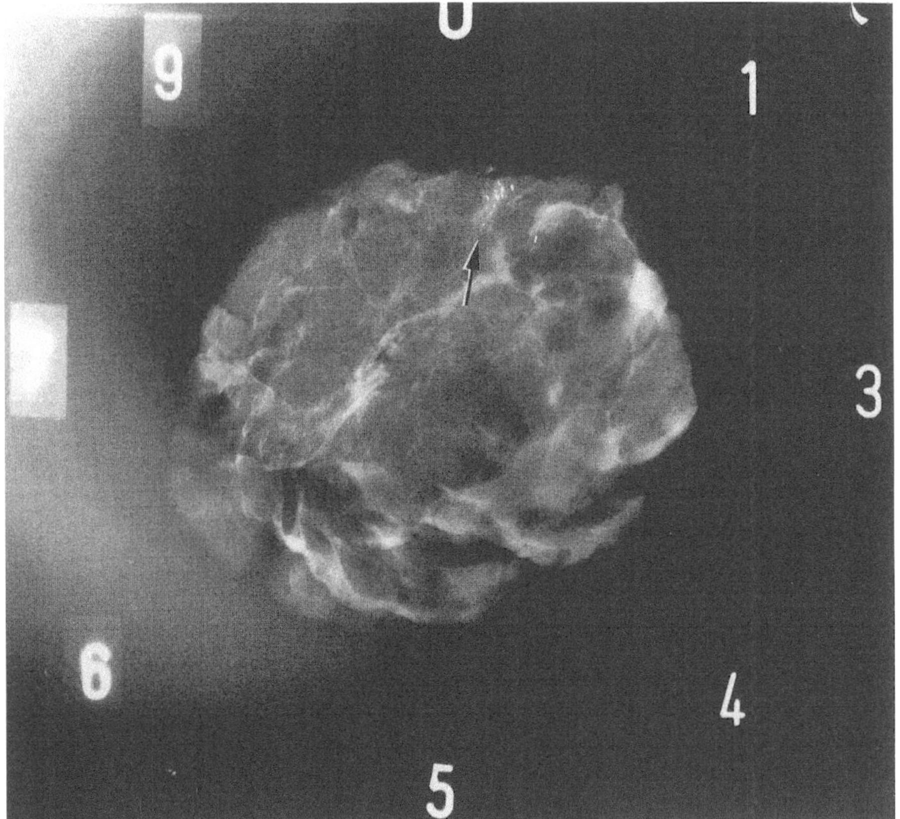

e

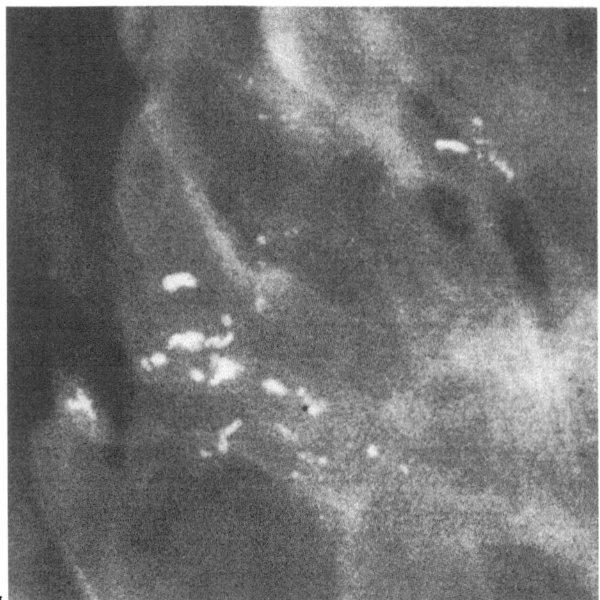

g

Fig.8.1e, g. Legend on p 234

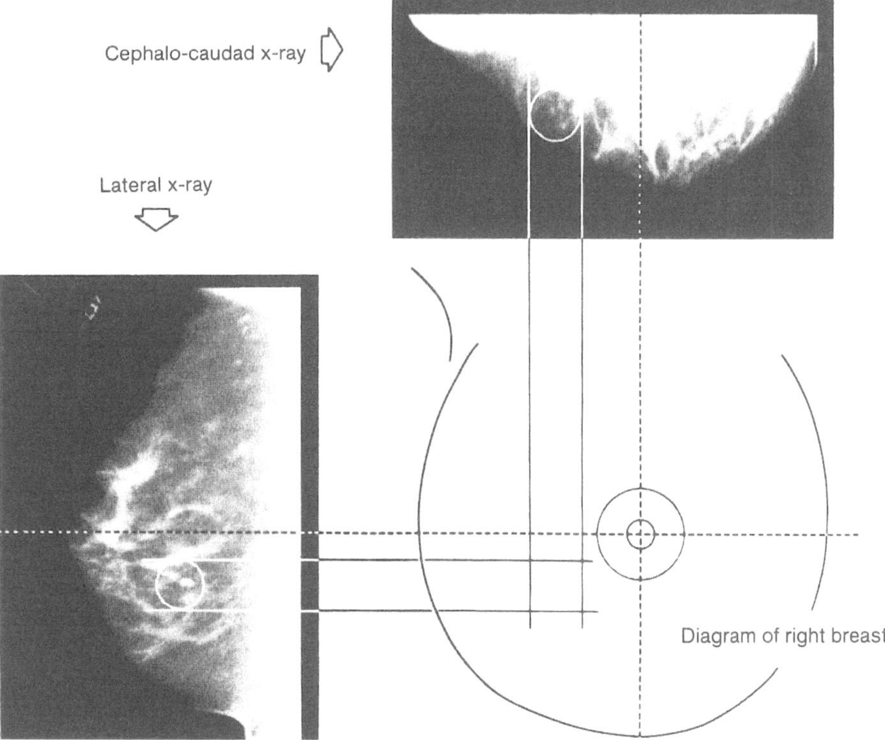

Fig. 8.2. Localization diagram of BERGER et al. (1966)

tage is its relative imprecision which can lead to greater surgical trauma, especially with deeply situated lesions.

Geometric Localization with a Needle, Hookwire, Contrast Medium, or Metal Ball

These techniques begin with geometric localization as described above. Shortly before the biopsy is performed, a needle (DODD et al. 1966; THREATT et al. 1974; LIBSHITZ et al. 1976) or a cannula of suitable gauge is inserted into the breast under local anesthesia, and either a flexible metal wire with a hooked end (Homer 1985) or a small shot (BARTH et al. 1977) is threaded through to the biopsy site.

Alternatively, the site may be marked by injecting a mixture of water-soluble contrast medium (or iodizedoil, e.g., Lipiodol, as recommended by RAININKO et al. 1976) and a visible dye (e.g., patent blue).

After the area has been marked by a suitable method, mammograms must be taken to check the accuracy of the localization. If the localization is imprecise, a second small shot may be inserted or a different dye (e.g., indocyanine green) injected. With HOMER's curved-end wire, made of a tough pseudoelastic alloy, repositioning is simple and easily accomplished. The disadvantage of dye localization is that the dye diffuses rapidly, staining the entire quadrant blue or green if the biopsy is not performed within about 30 min. The injection of carbomedicinal suspension is

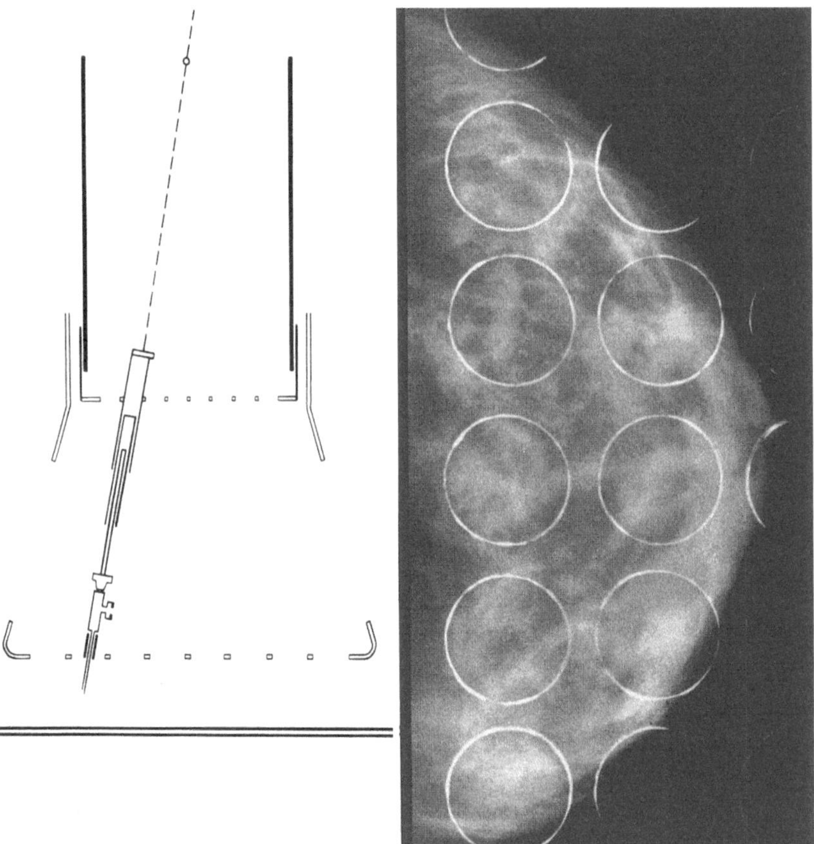

Fig. 8.3. Special apparatus with a perforated guide plate. The drawing shows the telescopic guide of the localization needle, in which a negative pressure is produced with a syringe. The needle is introduced through the appropriate hole of the perforated compression cone (Professor K. BRE- ZINA, Vienna)

longer lasting and thus obviates immediate transfer of the patient to the surgical suite.

Localization with Specialized Apparatus

The accurate localization of an occult microcalcification cluster is made more diffi- cult by the fact that compression of the breast displaces its internal structures. This problem is overcome by avoiding a change in breast position from mammography to biopsy. Means must be available for accurately determining the site of insertion of the needle, and the direction of the needle must follow that of the X-ray beam by which the abnormality was imaged. Also, the depth of needle insertion must be pre- cisely determined. BREZINA (1975a, b) and KRAMAN and FESER (1975) have designed special devices for the localization of occult breast lesions. These consist of a special film table, a telescopic needle guide, and a multiperforated compression

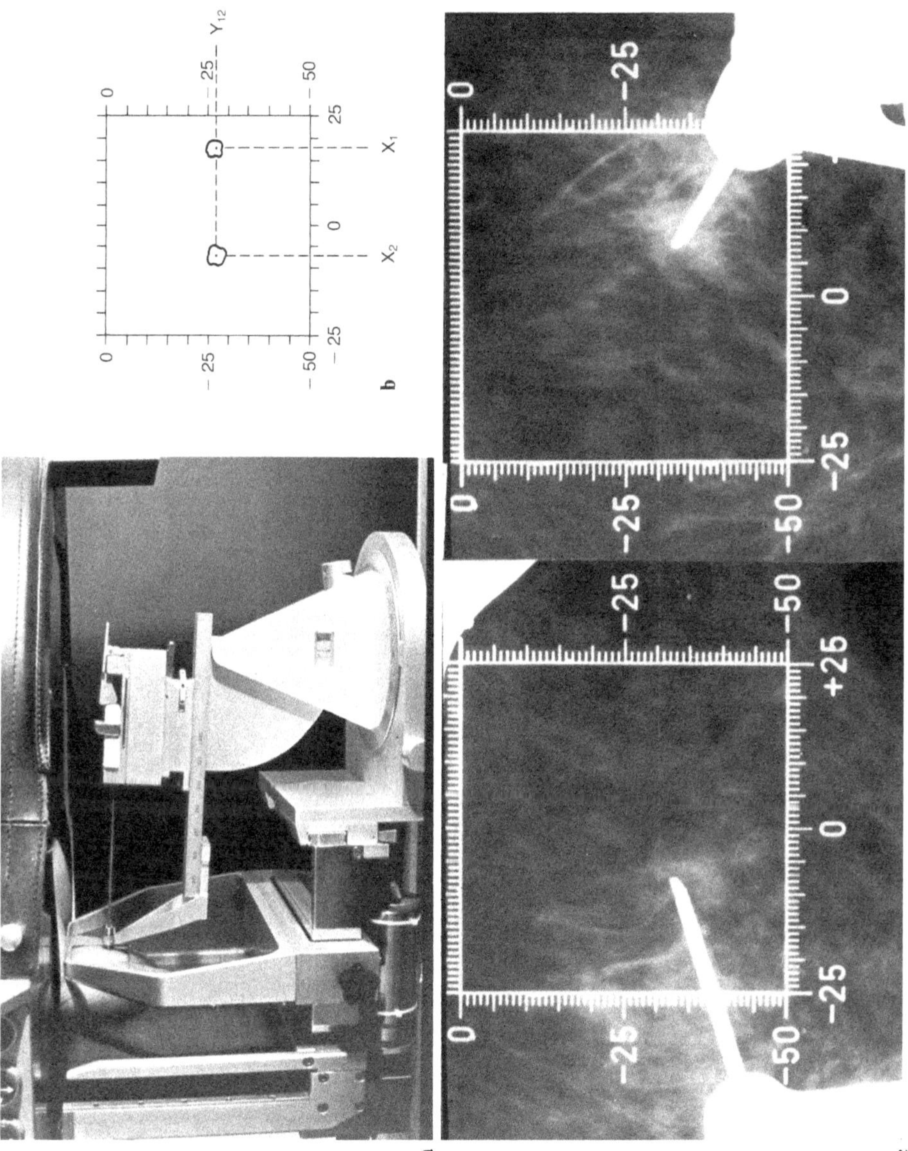

Fig. 8.4. a Stereotaxic instrument of NORDENSTRÖM for percutaneous needle biopsy of the breast. **b** The drawing shows the principle of the localization of an impalpable mammographic abnormality: one film 15° to the left (x_1) and one 15° to the right of the central beam (x_2) creates a parallax displacement of the abnormality. Localization is determined by measuring x_1, x_2, and y. **c** Check mammograms confirm the correct placement of the needle

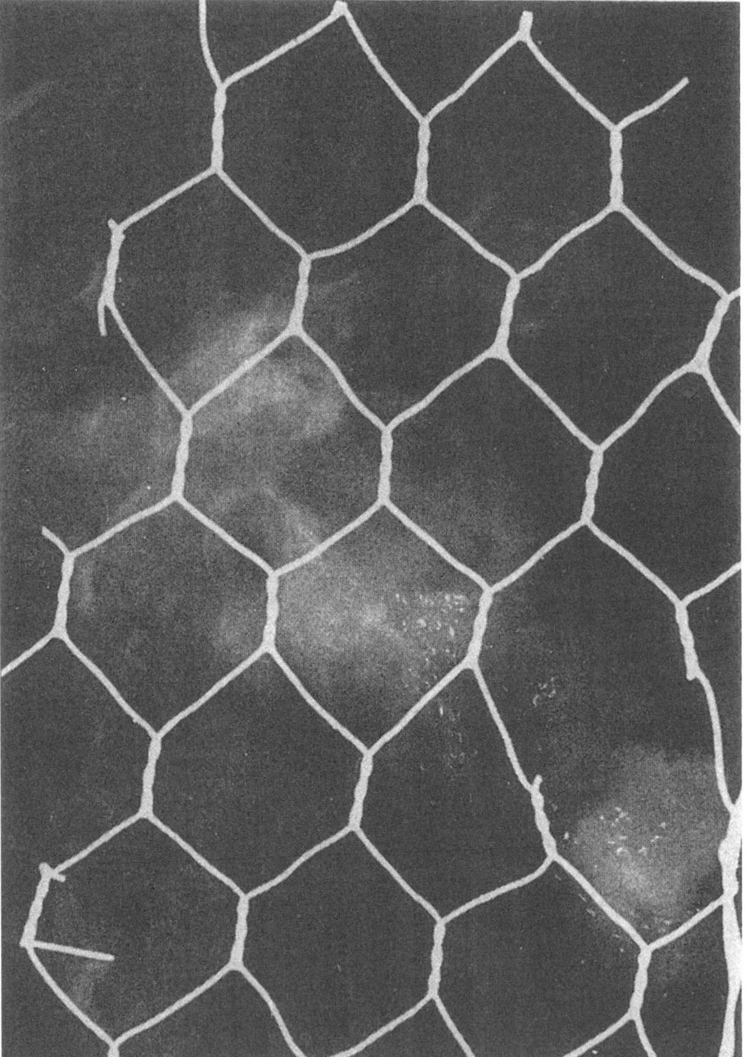

Fig. 8.5. The first specimen radiograph, published in 1951 by LEBORGNE. He used a wire mesh screen as a means of localizing the microcalcifications

device made of Plexiglas or sterilizable grid material (Fig. 8.3). A spot film is taken of the suspicious area, then the needle guide is mounted in place, and the needle is inserted while the breast remains compressed.

The stereotaxic instrument designed by NORDENSTRÖM (1977) is a self-contained system that has its own X-ray tube (BOLMGREN et al. 1977). Biopsy material is taken with a percutaneous screw needle and *histologically* (not cytologically) examined (Fig. 8.4a, b). The advantage of this technique is that excisional biopsy is necessary only with a positive result. The disadvantage is that the technique gives no

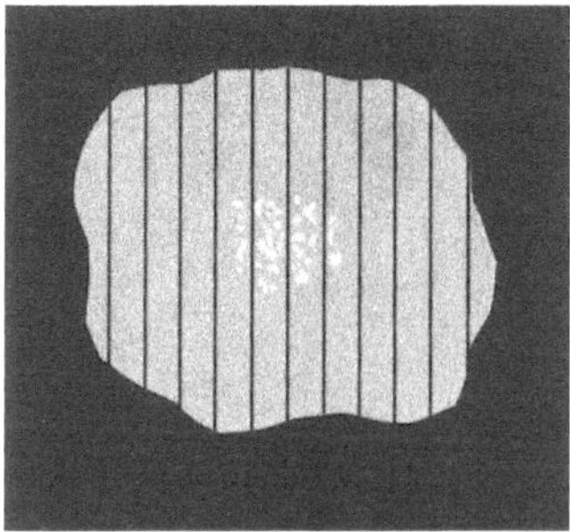

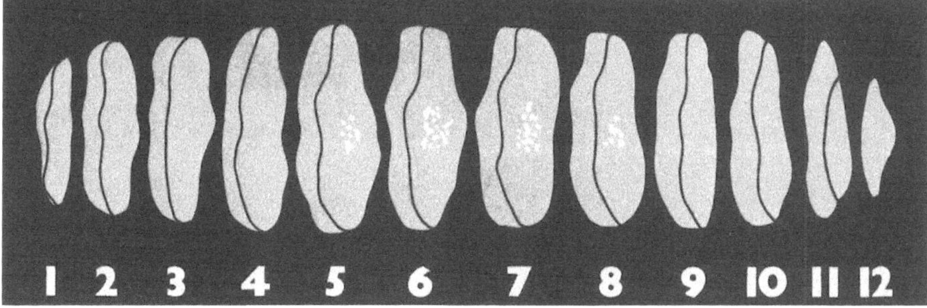

Fig. 8.6. The excised tissue is cut into slices, and radiographs are taken of the individual slices, which are labeled with lead numbers

information on the true extent of the lesion. Also, it produces some degree of iatrogenic trauma, and hematomas can form as in other percutaneous and excisional biopsies. DIXON (1983) recommends computed tomography for the preoperative localization of suspicious microcalcifications that are close to the chest wall.

8.2 Intraoperative Specimen Radiography

Decades ago, LEBORGNE (1951) addressed this problem as follows: "Only radiologic examination of the surgical specimen can enable us to localize the tiny microcalcifications for histologic examination and to find a small carcinoma that otherwise would be overlooked." He used a wire mesh screen as a way of localizing suspicious calcifications in the biopsy specimen (Fig. 8.5).

Where there is suspicion of occult mammary carcinoma, biopsy should be performed only in a hospital where facilities are available for intraoperative specimen radiography. A mammographic unit is indispensable. WILLGEROTH et al. (1978) designed a fluoroscopic device for the localization of microcalcifications in the operating room. Before the surgical wound is closed, a soft-tissue radiograph should be taken of the excised tissue to determine whether or not the radiographically suspicious area has been removed. If the microcalcification cluster is not visible on the specimen radiograph, then wider excision is necessary. Another film is then taken of the new specimen. Even with accurate localization, a small carcinoma sometimes may be found only after multiple specimens have been excised.

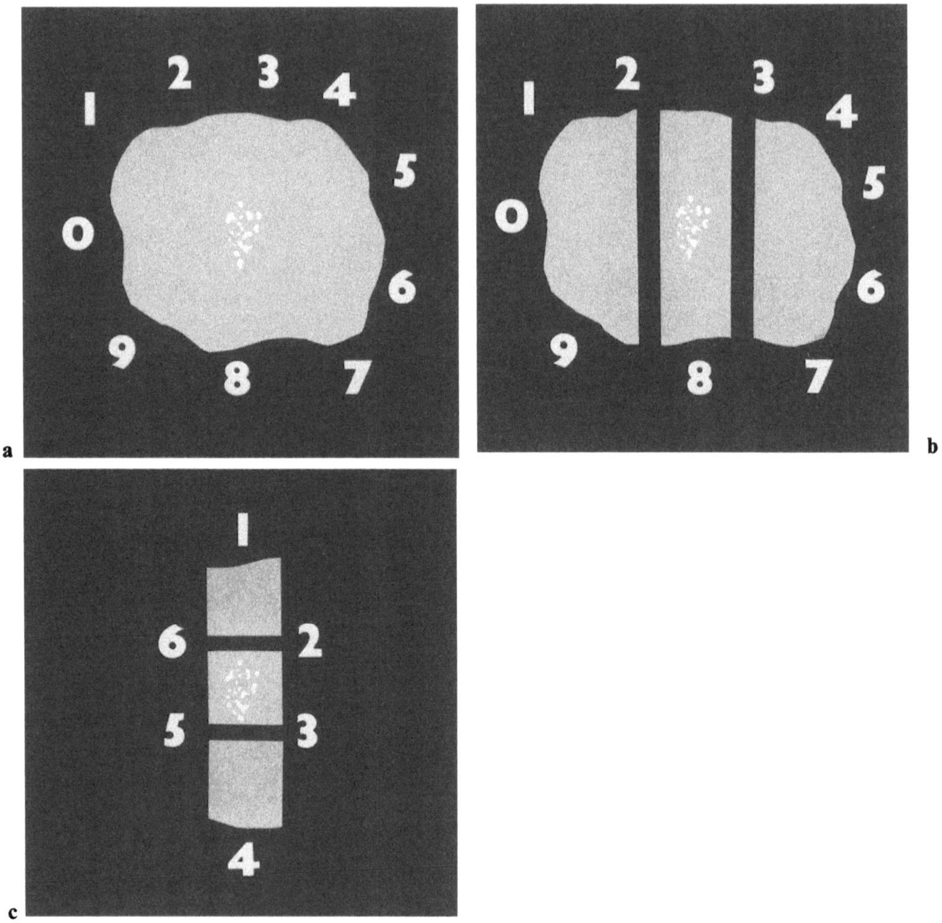

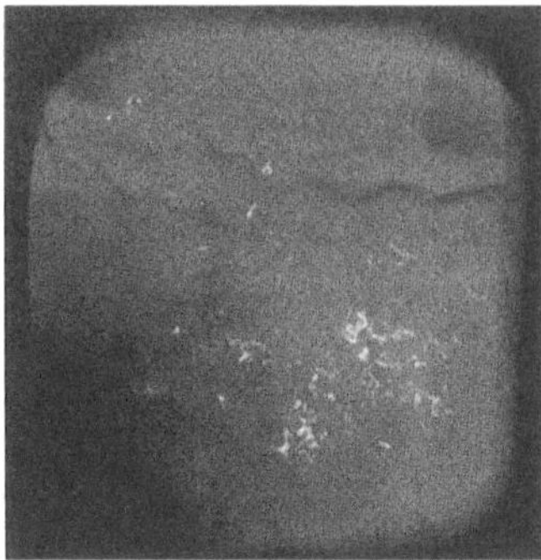

Fig. 8.7 a–c. Procedure for isolating a microcalcification cluster in several steps. **a** Lead numbers are placed around the specimen; the microcalcification cluster is centered between numbers *2, 3,* and *8.* **b** The areas of the specimen that do not contain microcalcifications are cut away, and the whole specimen is radiographed again. **c** The tissue containing the calcifications is cut to the size of a paraffin block. The block and the remaining tissue are sent separately for histologic evaluation

Fig. 8.8. Radiograph of a paraffin block with microcalcifications in a comedocarcinoma

8.3 Postoperative Study

Processing of the Specimen for Histologic Study

Postoperative processing of the specimen is important, because an intraductal carcinoma that has not yet infiltrated surrounding tissues may be occult for the pathologist.

A frozen-section examination is not advised, as the volume of material is usually so small that there may not be enough left for paraffin embedding if histologic findings are indefinite. In any case the result of the frozen-section examination is only tentative because, as ROSEN and SNYDER (1977) point out, a carcinoma may still be found in paraffin-embedded sections even if the frozen section is negative. The specimen can be processed in slices, and, after radiography, the suspicious slices containing microcalcifications can be sent to the pathologist for examination (Fig. 8.6). One can also "surround" the suspicious area, successively reducing its size under radiographic control until finally the block containing the microcalcifications is in effect "dissected free" for paraffin embedding (Fig. 8.7 a–c, Fig. 8.1 e–g). The individual slices should be marked with lead numbers. This also applies to the technique mentioned last; the specimen is encircled with lead numbers, and both the specimen and numbers are secured with tape before radiography. Not only the slices containing microcalcifications or the "isolated block" should be sent to the pathologist, but also the remaining tissue in a separate container.

Radiographic Examination of the Paraffin Block

If a ductal carcinoma is presumed from radiographs but is not found histologically, an explanation must be sought. In this case the paraffin block should be radiographed in two planes (HOLLAND 1984). Sections from the suspicious microcalcification cluster in the block will then permit a definite diagnosis to be made (Fig. 8.8).

Mammograms

Postoperative mammograms are recommended if the mammographic evidence of ductal carcinoma is still convincing despite a negative histologic result. They are particularly advised if the pathologist has found precancerous changes (e. g., proliferative lesion with atypia) or lobular neoplasia (which can occur in association with true carcinoma). It is best to obtain the mammograms about 6 weeks after the biopsy, by which time postoperative edema will have subsided.

The localization of occult mammary lesions and microcalcifications is a difficult challenge. It requires commitment on the part of the radiologist and close cooperation with the surgeon and pathologist.

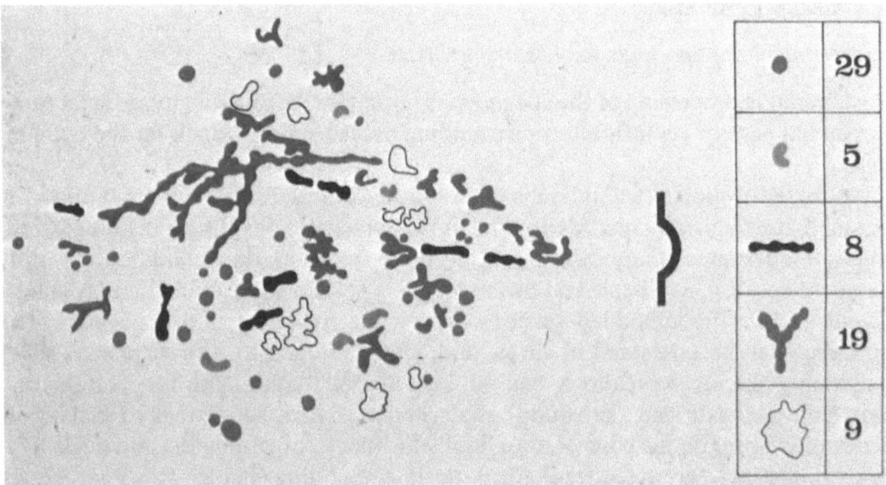

Fig. 4.77 b. Legend see also p. 110

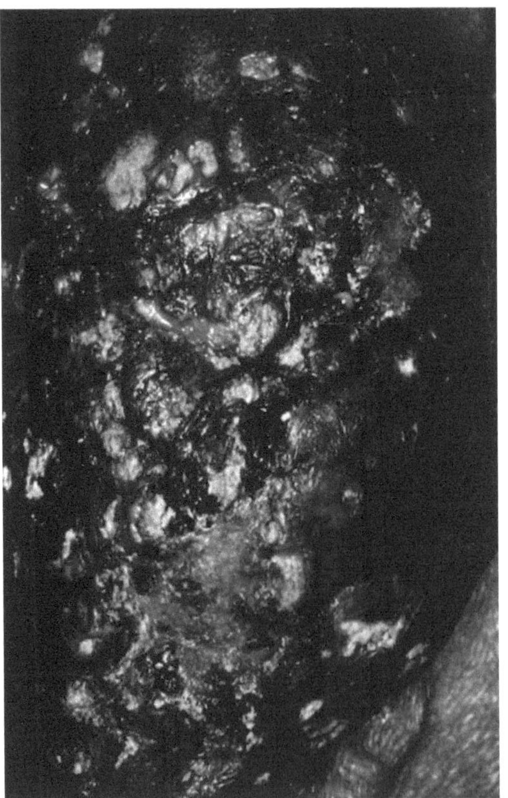

Fig. 6.31. c Photograph showing cutaneous necrosis with multiple ulcerations (see also p. 187)

References

Ahmed A (1975) Calcification in human breast carcinomas: ultrastructural observations. J Pathol 117: 247

Andersen JA (1977) Lobular carcinoma in situ of the breast. An approach to rational treatment. Cancer 39: 2597

Andersson I, Fex G, Petterson H (1977) Oil cyst of the breast following fat necrosis. Br J Radiol 50: 143

Azzopardi JG (1979) Problems in breast pathology. Saunders, Philadelphia

Bässler R (1978) Pathologie der Brustdrüse. Springer, Berlin Heidelberg New York (Spezielle pathologische Anatomie, vol 11)

Barth V (1977) Atlas der Brustdrüsenerkrankungen. Enke, Stuttgart

Barth V, Prechtel K (1982) Pathologie und Radiologie (Röntgendiagnostik und Thermographie) der Brustdrüse. In: Zuppinger A, Hellriegel W (eds) Mammatumoren. Springer, Berlin Heidelberg New York (Handbuch der medizinischen Radiologie, vol XIX/2)

Barth V, Behrends W, Haase W (1977) Methode zur präoperativen Lokalisation nicht palpabler suspekter Mikroverkalkungen im Brustdrüsenkörper (Kugelmarkierung). Radiologe 17: 219

Bassett LW, Gold RH, Cove HC (1978) Mammographic spectrum of traumatic fat necrosis: the fallibility of "pathognomonic" signs of carcinoma. AJR 130: 119

Basset LW, Gold RH, Mirra JM (1982) Nonneoplastic breast calcifications in lipid cysts: development after excision and primary irradiation. AJR 138: 335

Baum JK, Comstock CH, Joseph L (1980) Intramammary arterial calcifications associated with diabetes. Radiology 136: 61

Benjamin JL, Guy CL (1977) Calcification of implant capsules following augmentation mammaplasty. Plast Reconstr Surg 59: 432

Berger SM, Curcio BM, Gershon-Cohen J, Isard HJ (1966) Mammographic localization of unsuspected breast cancer. AJR 96: 1046

Bernstein JR (1977) Nonsuppurative nodular panniculitis (Weber-Christian disease). An unusual cause of mammary calcifications. JAMA 138: 1942

Bjurstam NG (1978) Radiogarphy of the female breast and axilla. Acta Radiol (Stockh) [Suppl 357]

Bloodgood JC (1923) The clinical picture of dilated ducts beneath the nipple frequently to be palpated as a doughy worm-like mass, the varicocele tumor of the breast. Surg Gynecol Obstet 36: 486

Bloodgood JC (1934) Comedocarcinoma (or comedoadenoma) of the female breast. Am J Cancer 22: 842

Bohmert H, Baumeister RG (1975) Die subkutane Mastektomie. Indikation und Technik. Fortschr Med 93: 697

Bolmgren J, Jacobson B, Nordenström B (1977) Stereotaxic instrument for needle biopsy of the breast. AJR 129: 121–125

Bouropoulov V, Anastassiades OT, Kontogeorgos G, Rachmanides M, Gogas I (1984) Microcalcifications in breast carcinomas. A histological and histochemical study. Pathol Res Pract 179: 51

Brandt G, Bässler R (1969) Pathomorphogenese experimenteller Verkalkungen in der weiblichen Brustdrüse. Ein Beitrag zur Calciphylaxie. Virchows Arch [A] 348: 139

Brandt G, Bässler R (1972) Die Wirkung der experimentellen Hyperkalzämie durch Dihydro Fachysterin auf Drüsenfunktion und Verkalkungsmuster der Mamma. Licht-, elektronenmikroskopische und chemischanalytische Untersuchungen. Virchows Arch [A] 365: 155

Brezina K (1975 a) Röntgenologisch gezielte Mammabiopsie. ROEFO 122: 330

Brezina K (1975 b) Ergebnisse der Mammographie mit gezielter Nadelbiopsie. Wien Klin Wochenschr 87: 666

Broks PDC (1976) Ausgedehnte subkutane Kalzifizierung der Mamma. ROEFO 125: 566

Brown RC, Zuehlke RL, Ehrhardt JC, Jochimsen PR (1981) Tattoos simulating calcifications on xeroradiographs of the breast. Radiology 138: 583

Bryant J (1981) Male breast cancer: a case of apocrine carcinoma with psammoma bodies. Hum Pathol 12: 751

Citoler P (1978) Microcalcifications of the breast. In: Grundmann E, Beck L (eds) Early diagnosis of breast cancer. Fischer, Stuttgart, p 113

Citoler P, Zippel HH (1975) Das Carcinoma in situ der Mamma. Ver Dtsch Ges Pathol 59: 549

Colbassini HJ J, Feller WF, Cigtay OS, Chun B (1982) Mammographic and pathologic correlation of microcalcification in disease of the breast. Surg. Gynecol Obstet 155: 689

Cornil V (1908) Les tumeurs du sein. Baillière, Paris

Dixon GD (1983) Preoperative computed-tomographic localization of breast calcifications. Radiology 146: 836

Dodd GD, Fry K, Delany W (1966) Preoperative localization of occult carcinoma of the breast. In: Management of the patient with cancer. Saunders, Philadelphia

Egan RL (1964) Mammography. Thomas, Springfield

Egan RL (1969) Fundamentals of mammographic diagnoses of benign and malignant diseases. Oncology 23: 126

Egan RL, Sweeney MB, Sewell CW (1980) Intramammary calcifications without an associated mass in benign and malignant diseases. Radiology 137: 1

Egger H, Müller S (1977) Das Fibroadenom der Mamma. Kann der Kliniker auf die Exzision verzichten? Dtsch Med Wochenschr 102: 1495

Farrow JH (1968) Clinical considerations and treatment of in situ lobular breast cancer. AJR 102: 652

Finsterbusch R, Gross F (1934) Kalkablagerungen in den Milch- und Ausführungsgängen beider Brustdrüsen. Röntgenpraxis 6: 172

Fisher ER, Fisher B (1977) Lobular carcinoma of the breast: an overview. Ann Surg 185: 377

Foote FW, Stewart FW (1941) Lobular carcinoma in situ. A rare form of mammary cancer. Am J Pathol 17: 49

Foote FW, Stewart FW (1945) Comparative studies of cancerous versus noncancerous breasts. Ann Surg 121: 6

France CJ, O'Connell JP (1970) Osseous metaplasia in the human mammary gland. Arch Surg 100: 238

Frantz VK, Pickren JW, Melcher GW, Auchincloss H (1951) Incidence of chronic cystic disease in so-called "normal breasts". A study based on 225 post mortem examinations. Cancer 4: 762

Friedrich M (1983) Folien-Raster-Kombinationen in der Mammographie. Lymphologie 7: 92

Friedrich M (1984) Schlitzblendentechnik für die Mammographie. ROEFO 141: 574

Friedrich M, Weskamp P (1976a) Bildgütefaktoren bei der Filmmammographie. I. Mitteilung. ROEFO 125: 259

Friedrich M, Weskamp P (1976b) Bildgütefaktoren bei der Filmmammographie. II. Mitteilung. ROEFO 125: 461

Friedrich M, Weskamp P (1984a) Komplexe Bewertung filmmammographischer Abbildungssysteme. Teil 1: Methodische Grundlagen. ROEFO 140: 585

Friedrich M, Weskamp P (1984b) Komplexe Bewertung filmmammographischer Abbildungssysteme. Teil 2: Vergleich von 18 Systemen mittels Signal-Rausch-Matrix. ROEFO 140: 707

Frischbier JH, Lohbeck HV (1977) Frühdiagnostik des Mammakarzinoms. Thieme, Stuttgart

Gajewski H (1973) Aufnahmetechnische Grundlagen der Mammographie. In: Hoeffken W, Lanyi M Röntgenuntersuchung der Brust. Thieme, Stuttgart

Galkin BM, Feig SA, Patchefsky AS, Rue JW, Gamblin WJ, Gomez DG, Marchant LM (1977) Ultrastructure and microanalysis of "benign" and "malignant" breast calcifications. Radiology 124: 245

Galkin BM, Frasca P, Feig SA, Holderness KE (1982) Non-calcified breast particles. A possible new marker of breast cancer. Invest Radiol 17: 119

Galkin BM, Feig SA, Frasca P, Muir HD, Soriano RZ (1983) Photomicrograph if breast calcifications: correlation with histologic diagnosis. Radiographics 3/3: 450

Gershon-Cohen J (1961) Breast roentgenology. Historical review. AJR 86: 879-883

Gershon-Cohen J (1970) Atlas of mammography. Springer, Berlin Heidelberg New York

Gershon-Cohen J, Ingleby H, Hermel MB (1955) Occult carcinoma of breast. Arch Surg 70: 385

Gershon-Cohen J, Ingleby H, Hermel MB (1956) Calcification in secretory disease of the breast. AJR 76: 132

Gershon-Cohen J, Berger SM, Curcio BM (1966) Breast cancer with micro-calcifications: diagnostic difficulties. Radiology 87: 613

Goldwyn RM (1977) Subcutaneous mastectomy (editorial). N Engl J Med 297: 503

Gregl A (1979) Farbatlas der Galaktographie, klinische radiologische Symptomatik und Therapie der sezernierenden Brust. Schattauer, Stuttgart

Gros Ch (1963) Les maladies du sein. Masson, Paris

Haagensen CD (1962) Lobular carcinoma of the breast. Clin Obstet Gynecol 5: 1093

Haagensen CD (1971) Diseases of the breast, 2nd edn. Saunders, Philadelphia

Haagensen CD, Laue N, Lattes R, Bodian C (1978) Lobular neoplasia (so-called lobular carcinoma in situ) of the breast. Cancer 42: 737

Hamperl H (1939) Über die Myothelien (Myo-epithelialen Elemente) der Brustdrüse. Virchows Arch [Pathol Anat] 305: 171

Hamperl H (1968) Zur Frage der pathologisch-anatomischen Grundlagen der Mammographie. Geburtshilfe Frauenheilkd 28: 901

Hassler O (1969) Microradiographic investigations of calcifications of the female breast. Cancer 23: 1103

Hermanutz D, Müller R (1970) Mammakarzinom und verkalkte Fettgewebstransplantate nach beidseitiger Mammavergrößerungsplastik. ROEFO 113: 530

Hoeffken W, Lanyi M (1973) Röntgenuntersuchung der Brust. Thieme, Stuttgart

Hofmann WD, Bosbach FW (1970) Die fibrosierende Adenose der weiblichen Brustdrüse. Klinik, Pathologie und Ergebnisse von Nachuntersuchungen nach Knotenexstirpation. Geburtshilfe Frauenheilkd 30: 526

Holland R (1984) New aspects and pitfalls in the diagnosis of breast cancer. Med Dissertation, Katholische Universität Nijmegen, Niederlande

Homer MJ (1981) Nonpalpable mammographic abnormalities: timing the follow-up studies. AJR 136: 923

Homer MJ (1982) Localisation of nonpalpable breast lesions: state of the art. Int J Breast Mammary Pathol Senologica 1: 215

Homer MJ (1985) Nonpalpable breast lesions: localisation using a curved-end retractable wire. Radiology 157: 259

Hüppe JR, Schneider HJ (1977) Zur Frage des richtigen Mammographiefilms. Radiologe 17: 195

Hutter RVP, Foote FW (1969) Lobular carcinoma in situ, long term follow-up. Cancer 24: 1081

Ingleby H, Gershon-Cohen J (1960) Comparative anatomy, pathology and roentgenology of the breast. University of Pennsylvania Press, Philadelphia

Ingelby H, Hermel MB (1956) Calcification in secretory disease of the breast. AJR 76: 132

Inoue Y, Ohya G, Maruyama M, Omoto R (1978) Die röntgenologischen Veränderungen nach Mammaplastik. ROEFO 129: 353

Jennings RJ, Fewell TR (1979) Filter-photon energy control and patient exposure. In: Logan WW, Muntz EP (eds) Reduced dose mammography. Masson, New York

Kiaer W (1954) Relation of fibroadenomatosis to cancer of the breast. Munksgaard, Copenhagen

Kindermann G, Rummel W (1973) Das Adenom der Mamille: eine Übersicht über Klinik und Morphologie. Geburtshilfe Frauenheilkd 33: 724

Koide T, Katayama H (1979) Calcification in augmentation mammoplasty. Radiology 130:337

Kraman B, Feser J (1975) Eine neue Methode zur Lokalisierung nicht tastbarer Laesionen der weiblichen Brust. ROEFO 123: 369

Lammers W, Kuhn H (1979) Verbesserte Bildqualität in der Mammographie durch Streustrahlenraster. Electromedica 1: 2

Lanyi M (1977a) Differentialdiagnose der Mikroverkalkungen. Die verkalkte mastopathische Mikrocyste. Radiologe 17: 217

Lanyi M (1977b) Differentialdiagnose der Mikroverkalkungen. Röntgenbildanalyse von 60 intraductalen Karzinomen, das "Dreiecksprinzip". Radiologe 17: 213

Lanyi M (1982a) Formanalyse von 153 Mikroverkalkungsgruppen maligner Genese. Das „Dreieckprinzip". ROEFO 136: 77

Lanyi M (1982b) Formanalyse von 136 Mikroverkalkungsgruppen benigner Genese. ROEFO 136: 182

Lanyi M (1983) Formanalyse von 5641 Mikroverkalkungen bei 100 Milchgangskarzinomen: die Polymorphie. ROEFO 139: 240

Lanyi M, Citoler P (1981) Differentialdiagnostik der Mikroverkalkungen: die kleinzystische (blunt duct) Adenose. ROEFO 134: 225

Lanyi M, Neufang KFR (1984) Möglichkeiten und Grenzen der Differentialdiagnostik gruppierter intramammärer Mikroverkalkungen. ROEFO 141: 4

Lauth G, Eulenburg R, Zwiens G, Duda V (1983) Erste klinische Erfahrungen mit der Rastermammographie. Röntgenblätter 36: 281

Leborgne R (1951) Diagnosis of tumors of the breast by simple röntgenography, calcifications in carcinomas. AJR 65: 1

Leborgne RA (1967) Esteatonecrosis quistica calcificata de la mama. Torax 16: 172

Le Gal M, Durand JC, Laurent M, Pellier D (1976) Condute à tenir devant une mammographie révelatrice de microcalcifications groupeés, sans tumeur palpable. Nouv Presse Med 5: 1

Le Gal M, Chavanne G, Pellier D (1984) Valeur diagnostique des microcalcifications groupées déconvertes par mammographies (A propos de 227 cas avec vérification histologique et sans tumeur du sein palpable). Bull. Cancer (Paris) 71/1: 57

Lendvai-Virágh K, Lendvai T, Rückner R (1983) Praktische Erfahrungen mit der Rastermammographie in der alltäglichen Praxis. Röntgenblätter 36: 289

Leonhardt T (1968) A case of Weber-Christian disease with roentgenographically demonstrable mammary calcifications. Am J Med 44: 140

Letton AH, Mason EM (1980) The treatment of nonpalpable carcinoma of the breast. Cancer 46: 980

Levitan LH, Witten DM, Harrison EG Jr (1964) Calcifications in breast disease mammographicpathologic correlation. 92/1: 29

Lewison EF (1964) Lobular carcinoma in situ of the breast. The feminine mystique. Milit Med 129: 115

Lewison EF, Finney GG Jr (1968) Lobular carcinoma in situ of the breast. Surg Gynecol 126: 1280

Libshitz HI, Feig SA, Fetouh S (1976) Needle localisation of nonpalpable breast lesions. Radiology 121: 557

Libshitz HI, Montague ED, Paulus DD (1977) Calcifications and the therapeutically irradiated breast. AJR 128: 1021

MacErlean DP, Nathan BE (1972) Calcification in sclerosing adenosis simulating malignant breast calcification. Br J Radiol 45: 944

Marinescu I, Damian A (1984) Primary hyperparathyroidism associated with galactophorous ducts calcification. Endokrinologie 22: 211

McDougal BA, Lukert BP (1977) Resolution of breast pain and calcification with renal transplantation. Arch Intern Med 137: 375

Menges V, Wellauer J, Engeler V, Stadelmann R (1973) Korrelation zahlenmäßig erfaßter Mikroverkalkungen auf dem Mammogramm und dadurch diagnostizierter Karzinome und Mastopathietypen. Radiologe 13/11

Menges V, Frank P, Prager P (1976) Zahlenmäßige Zunahme von Mikroverkalkungen, ein wichtiges röntgendiagnostisches Kriterium für das okkulte Mammakarzinom. ROEFO 124: 372–378

Mika N, Reiss KH (1968) Optimierung der Röntgenbelichtungstechnik mit Hilfe der Halbleiterspektometrie. Röntgenpraxis 21: 164

Millis RR, Davis R, Stacey AJ, Phil M (1976) The detection and significance of calcifications in the breast: a radiologic pathology study. Br J Radiol 49: 12

Moskowitz M (1979) Screening is not diagnosis. Radiology 133: 265

Muir R (1941) The evolution of carcinoma of the mamma. J Pathol Bacteriol 52: 155

Muir BB, Laub J, Anderson TJ, Kirkpatrick AE (1983) Microcalcification and its relationship to cancer of the breast: experience in a screening clinic. Clin Radiol 34: 193

Nordenström B (1977) Stereotactic screw needle biopsy of nonpalpable breast lesions: breast carcinoma. The radiologist's expanded role. Wiley Medical, New York

Nordenström B, Zajicek J (1977) Stereotaxic needle biopsy and preoperative indication of non-palpable mammary lesions. Acta Cytol (Baltimore) 21: 350–351

Ozello L (1970) Epithelial-stromal junction of normal and dysplastic mammary glands. Cancer 25: 586

Paterok EM, Egger H, Willgeroth F (1983) Mehr als 1500 radiologisch indizierte Mammabiopsien. Geburtshilfe Frauenheilkd 43: 721

Péntek Z, Balogh J, Bakó B, Élias S (1975) Mikrokalzifikation im männlichen Mammakarzinom. ROEFO 123/1: 90

Pilgram W, Lendvai-Viràgh K, Lendvai T, Michel R (1980) Die Behandlung maligner und präkanzeröser Prozesse der Mamma durch subkutane Mastektomie mit gleichzeitiger Augmentation. Geburtshilfe Frauenheilkd 40: 1009

Raininko R, Linna MI, Räsänen O (1976) Preoperative localization of non-palpable breast tumors. Acta Chir Scand 142: 575

Redfern AB, Ryan JJ, Su CT (1977) Calcification of the fibrous capsule about mammary implants. Plast Reconstr Surg 59: 249

Reinhardt K (1974) Verkalkung eines Fettgewebstransplantates in der Mamma. Röntgenblätter 27: 418

Rocek V, Sery Z, Sera D, Kamenicek O (1968) Verkalkungen beim männlichen Mammakarzinom ROEFO 109: 679

Rosen IW, Nadel HI (1966) Roentgenographic demonstration of calcification in carcinoma of the male breast. Radiology 86: 38

Rosen PP (1984) Lobular carcinoma in situ and intraductal carcinoma of the breast. In: McDivitt RW, Oberman HA, Ozello L, Kaufmann N (eds) The breast. International Academy of Pathology monograph. Williams and Wilkins, Baltimore

Rosen PP, Snyder RE (1977) Nonpalpable breast lesions detected by mammography and confirmed by specimen radiography – recent experience. Breast 3: 13

Rosen PP, Liebermann PH, Braun DW, Kosloff C, Adair F (1978) Lobular carcinoma in situ of the breast. Detailed analysis of 99 patients with average follow-up of 24 years. Am J Surg Pathol 2: 225

Rummel W, Kindermann G, Egger H, Weishaar J (1976) Mikrokalk in der Mammographie. Geburtshilfe Frauenheilkd 36/12: 1053

Sachs L (1978) Angewandte Statistik. Springer, Berlin Heidelberg New York

Salomon A (1913) Beiträge zur Pathologie und Klinik der Mammakarzinome. Arch Klin Chir 103: 573

Sandison AT (1958) A study of surgically removed specimens of breast, with special reference to sclerosing adenosis. J Clin Pathol 11: 101

Sang Y Han, Witten DM (1977) Diffuse calcification of the breast in chronic renal failure. AJR 129: 341

Schmitt EL, Threatt BA (1984) Relationship of mammographic intraarterial calcifications and diabetes. South Med 77: 988

Schöner E, Gutgesell H (1981) Osteochondrosarkom der Mamma. ROEFO 135: 714

Schwartz GF, Feig SA, Rosenberg AL, Patchefsky AS, Schwartz AB (1984) Staging and treatment of clinically occult breast cancer. Cancer 53: 1379

Sickles EA (1982) Mammographic detectability of breast microcalcifications. AJR 139: 913

Sickles EA (1986) Breast calcifications: mammographic evaluation. Radiology 160: 289

Sickles EA, Abele JS (1981) Milk of calcium within benign breast cysts. A characteristic mammographic finding not to be confused with carcinoma. Radiology 141: 655

Sigfússon BF, Andersson I, Ljungberg O (1982) Percutaneous injection of contrast medium into breast lesions for radiographic exclusion of malignancy. Br J Radiol 55: 26

Sigfússon BF, Andersson I, Aspegren K, Janzon L, Linell F, Ljungberg O (1983) Clustered breast calcifications. Acta Radiol [Diagn] (Stockh) 24: 273

Snyder RE (1966) Mammography and lobular carcinoma in situ. Surg Gynecol 122: 255

Stegner HE, Pape C (1972) Beitrag zur Feinstruktur der sog. Mikrokalzifikation in Mammatumoren. Lbl Allg Path Anat 115: 106

Tabár L, Márton Z, Kádas I (1972) Verkalkungen im männlichen Brustkrebs. ROEFO 117: 360

Tabár L, Dean PB (1983) Teaching atlas of mammography. Thieme, Stuttgart

Thiels C, Dumke K (1977) Mammaverkalkung nach Paraffininjektion. ROEFO 126: 173

Threatt B, Appelmann H, Dow R (1974) Percutaneous needle localisation of clustered mammary microcalcifications prior to biopsy. Am J Roentg 121: 839

Torell JA, Knight JP, Marcus PB (1984) Intraluminal calcium hydroxyapatite crystals in breast carcinoma: an ultrastructural study. Ultrastruct Pathol 6: 9

Urban JA, Adair FE (1949) Sclerosing adenosis. Cancer 2: 625
Wahlers B, Plum R, Fischedick O (1977) Die perkutane Darstellung von Milchgängen in gutartigen Mammatumoren. Fortschr. Röntgenstr 126: 345
Wegener HO (1977) Nachweis und Erkennbarkeit von Mikrokalzifikationen im Xeromammogramm. ROEFO 126/4: 350–360
Willgeroth F, Rummel W, Saebel M, Kuhn H, Ascherl E (1978) Intraoperativer Nachweis von Mikroverkalkungen der Brust mit einem Durchleuchtungsgerät. Geburtshilfe Frauenheilkd 38: 636
Willemin A (1972) Les images mammographiques. Karger, Basel
Zippel HH, Citoler P, Kievernagel G (1975) Verlaufsbeobachtungen bei Patientinnen mit lobulärer Neoplasie in der Mamma. Arch Gynaekol 219: 150

Subject Index

Numbers in *italics* indicate the page on which the keyword is covered in most detail.

C. Annonier, Paris

Female Breast Examination

A Theoretical and Practical Guide to Breast Diagnosis

Translated from the French by R. Chambers

1986. 155 figures, 6 tables. XIII, 228 pages.
ISBN 3-540-16302-6

Progress in diagnostic procedures and in the treatment of breast diseases has radically changed breast examination. In most cases, one procedure alone is no longer sufficient; rather, a comprehensive diagnostic strategy which combines different techniques is required.

This book clearly describes, compares, and evaluates different diagnostic methods. The actual capabilities and limitations of each technique are examined. The need for a combination of diagnostic procedures at various stages – in the decision-making process, actual examination, and final analysis – is demonstrated.

Springer-Verlag
Berlin Heidelberg New York
London Paris Tokyo

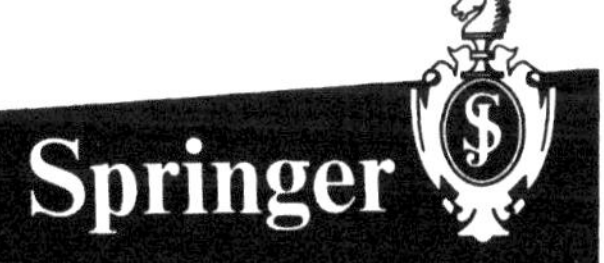